Springer
Tokyo
Berlin
Heidelberg
New York
Barcelona
Hong Kong
London
Milan
Paris
Singapore

N. Hayashi (Ed.)

Brain Hypothermia
Pathology, Pharmacology, and Treatment of Severe Brain Injury

With 88 Figures

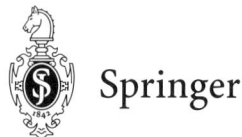 Springer

NARIYUKI HAYASHI, M.D., Ph.D.
Professor
Department of Emergency and Critical Care Medicine
Nihon University School of Medicine
30-1 Oyaguchi Kami-machi, Itabashi-ku
Tokyo 173-8610, Japan

ISBN 4-431-70277-6 Springer-Verlag Tokyo Berlin Heidelberg New York

Library of Congress Cataloging-in-Publication Data

Brain hypothermia : pathology, pharmacology, and treatment of severe brain injury / N. Hayashi (ed.).
  p. ; cm.
  Includes bibliographical references and index.
  ISBN 4431702776 (alk. paper)
  1. Brain damage—Treatment. 2. Cold—Therapeutic use. I. Hayashi, Nariyuki.
  [DNLM: 1. Brain Injuries. 2. Hypothermia. WL 354 B8127 2000]
  RC387.5 .B717 2000
  616.8′047—dc21
                                                                00-041320

Typesetting: Best-set Typesetter Ltd., Hong Kong
Printing and binding: Hirakawa, Japan
SPIN: 10752293

Preface

Rapid progress in new technologies and their application to diagnosis and monitoring of brain tissue temperature and metabolism have led to major advances in understanding the pathophysiology of brain damage and in therapy for critically brain-injured patients. In basic research, mild to moderate hypothermia promised to be very successful in neuroprotection against brain ischemia and trauma. However, clinical trials of hypothermia treatment have not produced the same results as those obtained in animal studies.

Recently, the mechanism of dynamic changes in brain tissue temperature has been discovered, and a new concept of brain hypothermia treatment for severely brain-injured patients has been developed. Dynamic change in brain tissue temperature is particularly relevant to the cerebral circulatory disturbances in stress-induced systemic catecholamine surge commonly encountered in patients with severe brain injuries. For a long time, however, we have been managing the injured brain using information from basic studies, obtained at 37°C. Therefore, we have been working under a number of misunderstandings regarding mechanism and technique in the management of severely brain-injured patients in ICU.

The new concept of brain hypothermia therapy clarified many targets of treatment which had not been discussed previously, such as brain thermal pooling, masking brain hypoxia associated with catecholamine surge, the metabolic shift from glucose to lipids which depends on the level of brain tissue temperature, and selective radical damage of dopamine in the central nervous system.

It was both appropriate and timely that the First Meeting of the Japanese Association of Brain Hypothermia and the International Symposium on Brain Hypothermia were scheduled for October 9–10, 1998, in Tokyo. At committee level, the Japanese Association of Brain Hypothermia also discussed starting an English journal of brain hypothermia. The symposium was intended to make known the newly discovered advantages of brain hypothermia treatment and to summarize what the issues are and what basic and clinical studies are necessary in the future. Brain hypothermia treatment is one of the possible methods for achieving a breakthrough in the survival of severely brain-injured patients.

I greatly appreciate the support of our colleagues from Japan and abroad who are interested in brain hypothermia treatment.

NARIYUKI HAYASHI, M.D., Ph.D.
First President of the Meeting of the Japanese Association of Brain Hypothermia
and the International Symposium on Brain Hypothermia

Contents

4. Clinical Studies of Brain Hypothermia

a. Mechanism

b. Diagnosis

c. Treatment

5. Panel Discussion

6. Summary

1. Brain Injury Mechanism

Enhanced Neuronal Damage in Severely Brain-Injured Patients by Hypothalamus, Pituitary, and Adrenal Axis Neurohormonal Changes

Nariyuki Hayashi

Summary. Brain edema, brain ischemia, and elevation of intracranial pressure have been considered major brain injury mechanisms. Therefore, factors that promote these pathophysiological changes, such as hypotension, hypoxia, free radicals, blood–brain barrier dysfunction, excitatory amino acid, and increased intracellular Ca^{++}, have been considered targets of treatment. This concept of brain injury mechanism has long been supported by many animal studies. Information from animal studies was obtained under conditions of anesthesia with body temperature controlled at 37°C. Therefore, harmful stress induced by pathophysiological changes from stimulation of the hypothalamus–pituitary axis have not been included. A new concept of brain injury mechanisms in severe brain-injured patients is presented in this chapter. When the brain is injured, progression of its pathophysiological state typically exhibits a certain time window. The initial stages of brain injury involve destruction of the brain tissue, localized brain ischemia, cytokine inflammation, and synaptic dysfunction with release of vascular agonists, catecholamines, dopamine, neurogenous agonists such as choline, excitatory amino acids, and K^+ ions. However, the prognosis of dying neurons in injured tissue is strictly influenced by two other extracerebral factors. One is the change in systemic circulation and metabolism associated with catecholamine surge, and the other is the inflammatory reaction associated with release of hypothalamus–pituitary axis hormones. The dying neurons need enough oxygen and an adequate metabolic substitute to make a neuronal recovery. Three types of brain hypoxia and energy crisis occur in the primarily injured neurons. One is rapid consumption of residual oxygen for maintaining intracellular homeostasis and neuroexcitation. Second, the catecholamine surge produces unstable cardiopulmonary dysfunction, hyperglycemia, and difficulty in washing out the elevated brain tissue temperature. The elevation of brain tissue temperature by brain thermopooling, hemoglobin dysfunction (difficulty in releasing oxygen from hemoglobin), reduced oxygen delivery, and intestinal blood shift produce neuronal hypoxia even with normal intracranial pressure, cerebral perfusion pressure, and PaO_2. This is specific neuronal hypoxia, masking brain hypoxia, has not been monitored previously. High temperature (above 38°C) and systolic blood pressure lower than 90–100 mmHg after reperfusion were the clinical conditions for producing brain thermopooling. This new pathophysiological change, brain thermopooling, masking brain hypoxia, progresses within 3–6 h after insult. Such specific pathophysiological conditions gen-

Department of Emergency and Critical Care Medicine, Nihon University School of Medicine, 30-1 Oyaguchi Kami-machi, Itabashi-ku, Tokyo 173-8610, Japan

erally precede cerebral edema and intracranial hypertension. After 6h, the third stage of brain hypoxia occurs with blood–brain barrier dysfunction and cytokine encephalitis associated with stimulation of the hypothalamus–pituitary axis, such as excess release of vasopressin and growth hormone. Hyperglycemia activates the release of vasopressin, blood–brain barrier dysfunction, and cytokine encephalitis by a feedback mechanism of macronutrient intake. Damage to the hypothalamus is important in understanding the brain injury mechanism. The hypothalamus is also important as the site for control of the mind—thinking, volition, emotion, love and anxiety—by means of the function of the dopamine A10 nervous system. After severe brain injury, dopamine leak from the dopamine nervous system permits selective radical damage to the dopamine A10 nervous system and facilitates development of a vegetative state or mental retardation. These entirely new brain injury mechanisms are triggered by a harmful stress response. The many neurons in primary injured brain tissue need restoration therapy before the start of neuroprotection therapy. Systemic neurohormonal pathophysiological changes are the most important initial target for neuronal restoration in injured brain tissue.

Key words. Brain thermopooling, Brain hypoxia, Hyperglycemia, Blood–brain barrier

Introduction

It is difficult for primary brain-injured tissue to survive; therefore, secondary brain injury such as brain edema, brain ischemia, and reduced cerebral perfusion pressure (CPP) caused by elevation of intracranial pressure (ICP) has been considered as a target of treatment. The promoting factors of these pathophysiological changes—free radicals, blood–brain barrier (BBB) dysfunction, excitatory amino acids, and increased intracellular Ca^{++}—also have been considered as the target of treatment. This concept of brain injury mechanism has been supported by many animal studies [1,23,29,33,35].

However, recent clinical studies elucidate three clinical issues about the previous concept of brain injury mechanism concerning the management of severe brain injury. First, many clinical experiences have been reported about the recovery of primary injured tissue using CT scan and MRI studies in brain trauma [21,22]. The recovery of primary brain injury without clinical deficits could be explained such as "all neurons in the primary injured brain tissue do not die immediately, but are going to die." Therefore, primary brain injury is also an initial target of treatment for neuronal restoration in the acute stage.

The second issue is the incidence of the very difficult mechanism of neuronal recovery in injured tissue by systemic pathophysiological changes [6,16–18]. These brain injury mechanisms associated with excess neurohormone release, such as catecholamine surge, vasopressin, and growth hormone, have been found to strongly affect the reversibility and prognosis of injured neurons [7,21,22]. These new brain injury mechanisms are difficult to determine precisely by anesthetized experimental animal studies because these neurohormonal excess reactions are retarded. Anesthesia conceals the severity of these stresses and thus makes these new brain injury mechanisms unclear in animal studies.

The third issue is brain thermopooling associated with unstable cardiopulmonary dysfunction that is caused by stress-induced catecholamine surge [16,17,20]. Elevations of brain tissue temperature, 40° to 44°C, are recorded in severely brain-injured patients with trauma and subarachnoid hemorrhage (SAH) or after resuscitation of cardiopulmonary arrest (CPA) [18]. However, all experimental data using animal studies were obtained at 37°C of controlled body temperature (brain temperature about 37°–37.5°C).

These new concepts of brain injury mechanisms are not demonstrated by experimental animal studies. The mechanism of brain injury which is observed in animal studies is not similar to clinical cases, especially in severely brain-injured patients. These new brain injury mechanisms are also not covered by previous neuroprotective treatment such as management of brain edema, ICP elevation, brain ischemia, and free radical reactions.

In this chapter, a new brain injury mechanism that was determined by clinical studies is presented, with discussion about the initial target of treatment of severe brain injury.

Clinical Studies

Extracerebral mechanisms unfavorable to severe brain injury were studied with 313 severe head injury patients.

Vasoactive Neurohormonal Release at Time of Admission in Coma Patients

To analyze the effect of vasoactive neurohormonal release into the systemic circulation, cerebral glucose metabolism, the changes of cardiopulmonary functions that directly influence the development of secondary brain injury, and serum vasoactive catecholamines (epinephrine, norepinephrine, and dopamine) and vasopressin were studied. Serum catecholamines were measured by high performance liquid chromatography using ECD-300 with Eicomopak CA-50D3, 3.1 mmf × 150 mm (EICOM, Tokyo, Japan). Vasopressin was measured by RIA using a γ-counter (ARC-950; ALOKA, Tokyo, Japan). These vasoactive hormones will be expected to change by influence of treatment, medications, severity of injury, and time after trauma. All head trauma patients (ten cases) had a Glasgow Coma Scale (GCS) less than 9 and were admitted at our emergency and critical care medical center between 14 and 48 min after trauma. Blood samples were obtained before the start of treatment.

Elevation of Brain Tissue Temperature by Brain Thermopooling

Monitoring of brain tissue temperature (BTT) of herniated terminal head trauma patients (10 cases) was recorded at 40°–44°C of BTT in all patients. After recording hyperthermia in severe brain injury, we have been interested in the mechanism of pathophysiological changes of BTT and interactions between changes of BTT, core temperature, tympanic membrane temperature, and jugular venous blood temperature. The mechanism of elevation of BTT after severe brain injury was studied in 45 cases. BTT was directly monitored by Mon-a-therm Luer Lock Temperature Sensor (MARINCLOT JAPAN, Tokyo, Japan). The tympanic membrane temperature, jugular venous temperature, and core temperature were recorded by continuously using a Sher-1-Temp series 400 compatible probe (JAPAN SHAW WOOD, Tokyo, Japan), an H-catheter for monitoring of jugular venous blood temperature and oxygen saturation (ABBOTT LABORATORIES, North Chicago, IL, USA), and a Swan–Ganz catheter (ABBOTT), respectively, at the same time.

Hemoglobin Function Evaluated by Changes of Hemoglobin Enzyme: 2,3-Diphosphoglycerate

Hemoglobin dysfunction measured by reduced 2,3-diphosphoglycerate (DPG) produces a difficult release of oxygen from hemoglobin and causes unsuccessful neuronal oxygenation even when enough oxygen is inhaled [9,32]. The abnormal reduction of hemoglobin enzyme, DPG, could be caused by severe hyperglycemia and acidosis.

From this basic research information, we wondered about the incidence of hemoglobin dysfunction after severe brain injury. We have monitored the two types of DPG, red blood cell DPG (RBC-DPG) and hemoglobin-binding DPG (Hb-DPG), in arterial blood through a femoral artery catheter and in jugular venous blood through a jugular venous H-catheter (Abbott), respectively. All these changes (17 cases) in the acute stage were measured using a double-beam photospectroanalyzer 220 (Hitachi, Tokyo, Japan).

Hyperglycemia and Prognosis

Hyperglycemia has been understood as a negative factor to activate anaerobic metabolism and increase lactate in injured brain tissue [30,35]. Our preliminary studies about the effect of hyperglycemia on hemoglobin dysfunction, BBB dysfunction, and cytokine encephalitis suggested that hyperglycemia has a deeper meaning for promoting secondary brain injury and also for preventing neuronal restoration in injured brain tissue. To analyze the critical level of hyperglycemia for clinical deterioration, the level of hyperglycemia expected to fall in coma was studied in children (12 cases), adults (124 cases), and older patients (74 cases), respectively.

Activation of Hypothalamus–Pituitary Axis Neurohormonal Functions

Recent clinical studies about severe brain injury suggested that harmful stress activates the release of growth hormone (GH) that is associated with poor prognosis [7]. The mechanism of neurohormonal brain injury is still unclear. The hypothalamus is the major center for adapting to harmful stress such as severe brain injury, subarachnoid hemorrhage (SAH), and ischemic cerebral apoplexy by two mechanisms: one is catecholamine surge, and the other is activation of the neurohormonal immune system through the hypothalamus–pituitary axis function [3,5,8,14,27,36]. The author hypothesized that inadequate activation of hypothalamus function by excess release of vasopressin, GH, pyrogen (IL-1 and IL-6), and adrenocorticotropic hormone (ACTH) related to the catecholamine surge might influence neuronal recovery. Hyperglycemia and increased brain tissue glucose also activate these negative factors by the feedback mechanism of hypothalamus neural control of macronutrient intake.

To analyze the secondary mechanism of brain injury by activation of the hypothalamus–pituitary axis, sequential changes of vasopressin, growth hormone, cerebrospinal fluid (CSF), and blood cytokines IL-1 and IL-6, and BBB dysfunction evaluated by changes of CSF/serum albumin [24,25] were measured during 1 week after trauma. The interaction between changes of vasopressin, activation of cytokines, and BBB dysfunction was also studied in severe brain injury.

Effect of Hyperglycemia and Brain Tissue Glucose on the Release of Vasopressin

Hyperglycemia or increased brain tissue glucose theoretically activates the feedback mechanism of neural and metabolic control of macronutrient intake of the hypothalamus [2,28,36]. At this time, excess release of vasopressin and insulin also could be emphasized. The severe hyperglycemia associated with harmful stress is one of the major negative factors that activates anaerobic metabolism, especially in severe brain injury. However, the effects of hyperglycemia and increased brain tissue glucose on the release of vasopressin and damage of BBB function in severe brain injury are not understood. Vasopressin is one of the modulators of BBB function and vasoconstriction. From these new concepts of brain injury mechanism, the author studied the interaction between changes of serum hyperglycemia, increased brain tissue glucose and vasopressin release, changes of BBB function, increase of CSF IL-6, and increased brain tissue glutamate in severely brain-injured patients using CMA Microdialysis AB System (CMA/MICRODIALYSIS, Solna, Sweden) and the Neurochem Coulochem Electrode Array System (MC MEDICAL, Tokyo, Japan).

Results

Vasoactive Neurohormonal Release at Time of Admission in Coma Patients

All head injuries studied were severe, evaluated as GCS 6, five cases, GCS 5, three cases, GCS 4, two cases, and GCS 3, two cases. Time before admission to the hospital was variable, from 14 to 48 min. Serum vasoactive hormones of all patients were recorded at a very high level (Fig. 1). The level of epinephrine was 45 to 3990 pg/ml, which is 3 to 266 times higher than normal values; the level of norepinephrine was 88 to 6000 pg/ml, which is 4.4 to 300 times higher than normal values; the level of dopamine was 25 to 510 pg/ml, 1.3 to 25.5 times higher than normal values; and the level of vasopressin was 10 to 550 pg/ml, about 14 times higher than control values.

The most interesting information was that the increased catecholamine surge was well correlated with the severity of hyperglycemia, and the specific time of each change was recorded

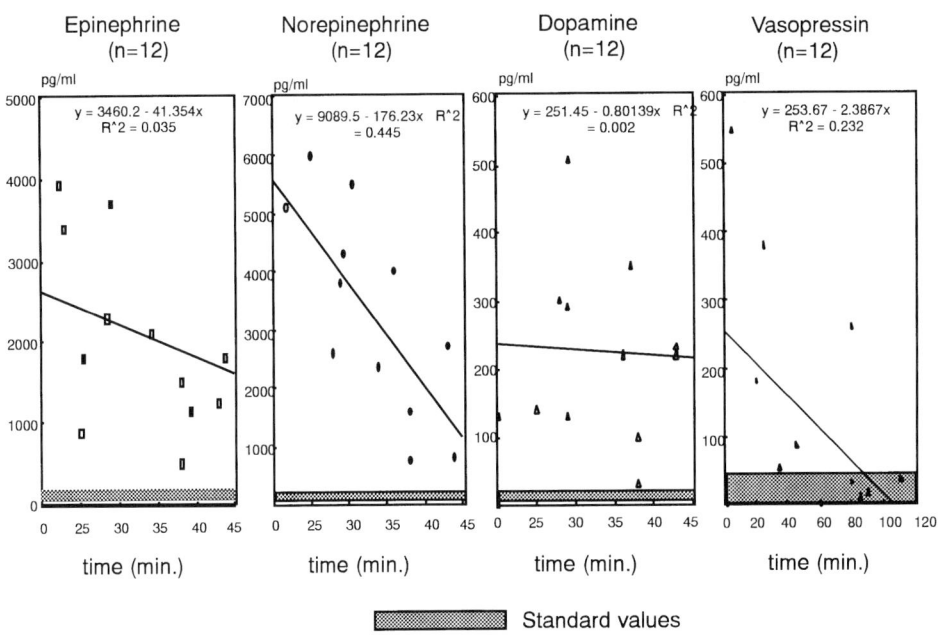

FIG. 1. Sequential changes of catecholamines and vasopressin after severe brain damage

for each vasoactive hormones (see Fig. 1). Epinephrine increased within 3 h, norepinephrine increased within 1 h, dopamine increased after more than 3 h, and vasopressin was increased within 2 h. All these data suggested that the neurohormonal protective system for the systemic circulation was limited to within 1 to 3 h and that the possibility of the hazard of excess release of vasoactive neurohormones develops after 3 h.

Brain Thermopooling

The normal value of BTT is 0.2° to 0.6°C higher than core temperature (blood temperature). A positive correlation was observed between changes of BTT and tympanic membrane temperature (TMT) and jugular venous blood temperature (JvBT). BTT change was more highly correlated to the changes of JvBT than of TMT (Fig. 2). The BTT changed dynamically in the acute stage of severe brain injury. The four major factors, core temperature, blood pressure or CPP, and cerebral blood flow (CBF), were influenced by the dynamic changes of BTT.

The major clinical issue is unstable cardiopulmonary dysfunction, which is caused by excess catecholamine surge after harmful brain injury. In most cases, it is very difficult to manage lowered systemic blood pressure at time of hospital admission in the acute stage. In most cases of GCS less than 6, that is, severely brain-injured patients, systolic blood pressure could be controlled between 90 and 100 mmHg; however, it is very difficult to maintain systolic blood pressure above 100 mmHg without adequate fluid resuscitation. This uncontrollable lower blood pressure triggers the occurrence of brain thermopooling because of the difficulty in washing out the elevated brain tissue temperature. Promoting factors of elevation of BTT are a body temperature of more than 38°C, after reperfusion, systolic blood pressure below 90 to 100 mmHg, and reduced CBF.

Figure 3 shows a typical case of brain thermopooling (BTT elevated to 42°C) after severe brain injury without elevation of ICP. The patient, a 56-year-old man, immediately went into

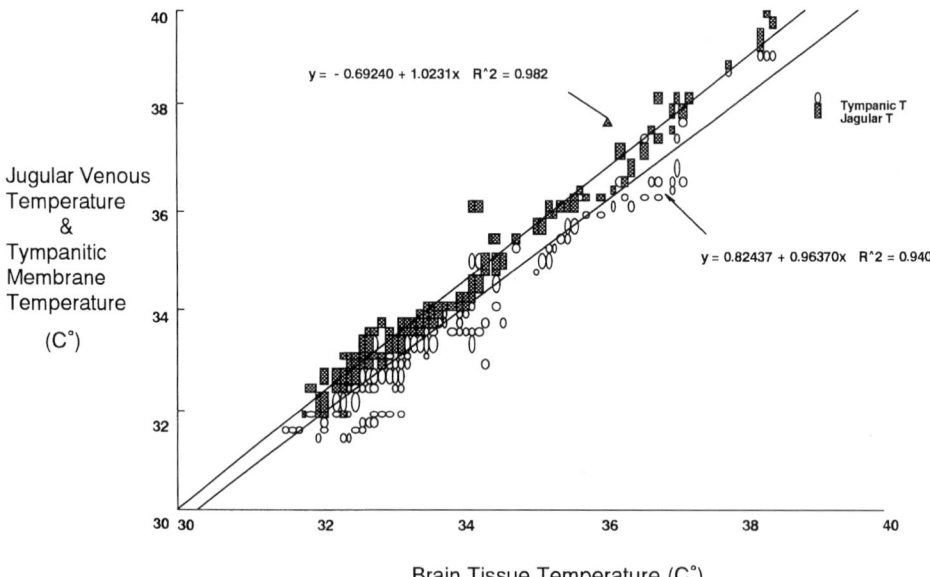

FIG. 2. Relationship between changes of brain tissue temperature, jugular venous temperature, and tympanic membrane temperature

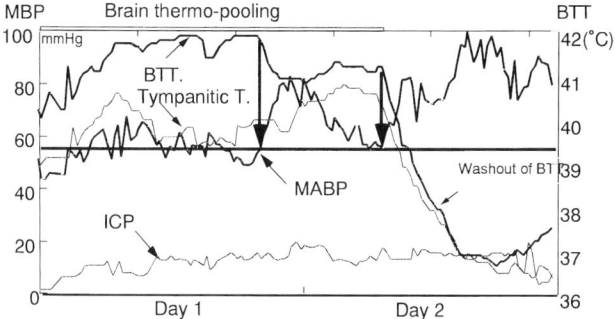

FIG. 3. Brain thermopooling (elevation of brain tissue temperature, BTT) is produced by mean arterial blood pressure (MABP) lower than 55-mmHg. BTT was dramatically reduced after MABP increased to above 55 mmHg. The brain thermopooling phenomenon is not associated with elevation of intracranial pressure (ICP). Brain thermopooling was produced by conditions such as body temperature higher than 38°C and systolic blood pressure lower than 90–100 mmHg after reperfusion

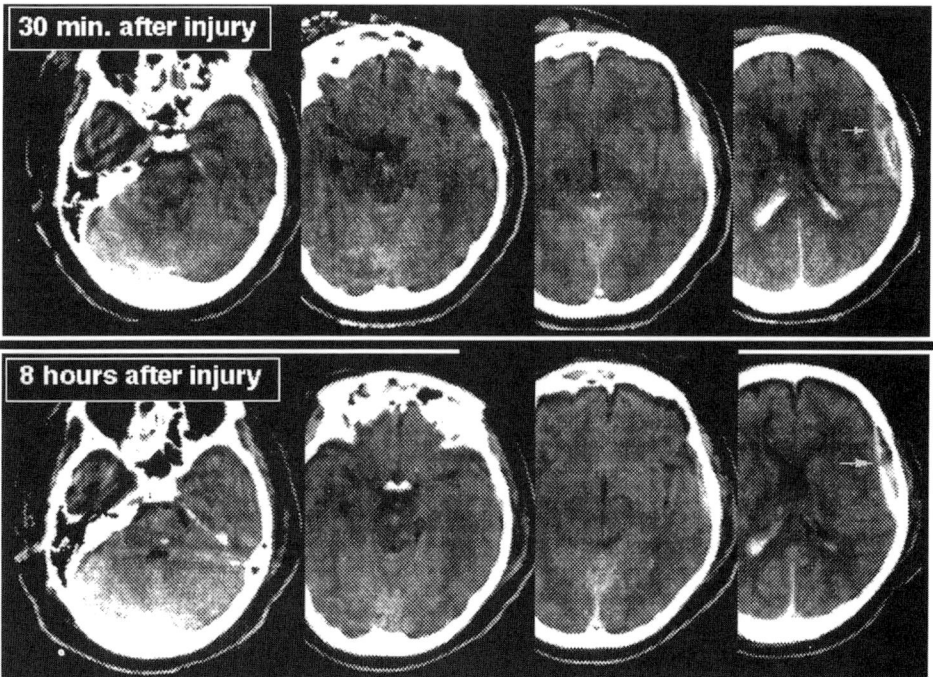

FIG. 4. CT scan of case of brain thermopooling

shock with pulmonary contusion, diffuse brain injury, and a small epidural hematoma (Fig. 4). ICP was controlled below 20 mmHg (Fig. 3). There was no relationship between change of ICP elevation and clinical prognosis. At time of admission, we immediately started fluid resuscitation with dopamine. Systolic blood pressure temporarily recovered to 110 to 120 mmHg, and he was hospitalized. However, we faced the difficult control of hypotension caused by lower cardiac output during 6 h; mean arterial blood pressure (MABP) lower than 55 mmHg

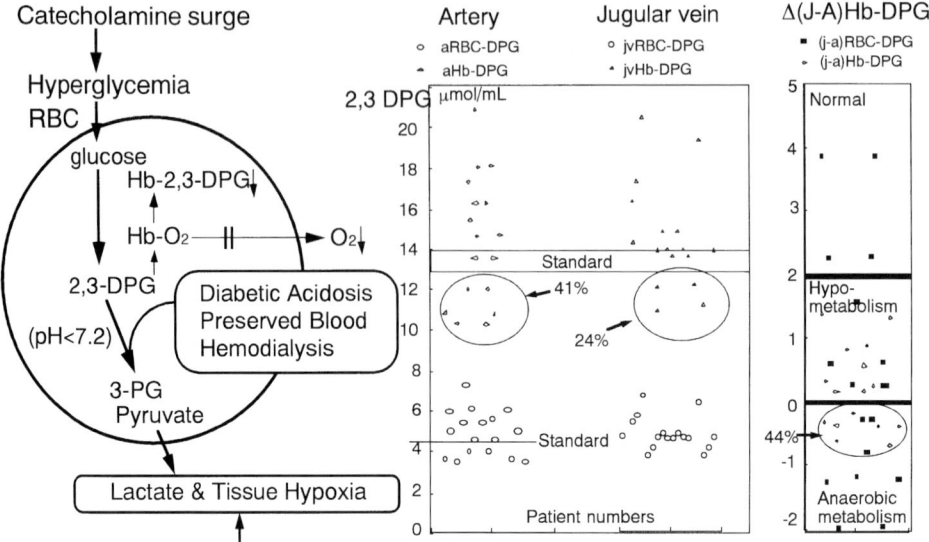

FIG. 5. Disturbance of O_2 release from hemoglobin was 24%, and anaerobic metabolism was recorded at 44% even with normal PaO_2 in the acute stage of severe brain injury

produced typical brain thermopooling for 24 h. In this patient, the critical level of MABP to wash out the elevated BTT was 55 mmHg. As a result of this new finding of the secondary brain injury mechanism, we have started management of BTT and brain hypothermia treatment because the previous neuroprotective treatment was not expected to have any effect on the elevated BTT at 42°C.

Reduction of 2,3-Diphosphoglycerate (DPG) in the Severely Brain-Injured Patient

The normal values of total blood DPG, RBC-DPG, and Hb-DPG were 1.6 to 2.6 mmol/ml, 4.8 to 5.3 mmol/ml, and 13 to 14 mmol/ml, respectively. Hemoglobin function in arterial blood was reduced in 6 of 17 cases (41%). However, lower jugular venous blood Hb-DPG, actual hemoglobin dysfunction in release of oxygen in the brain tissue, was recorded in 4 of 17 cases (24%), even with normal PaO_2 (Fig. 5). In all these patients, serum pH was recorded at lower than 7.2, associated with severe hyperglycemia, higher than 220 mg/dl, and severe acidosis.

The difference of jugular venous blood Hb-DPG and arterial Hb-DPG suggests the level of oxygenation for the brain tissue. In this study, hemoglobin dysfunction was recorded in 6 of 17 cases (41%), dysfunction of hemoglobin enzyme in 4 of 17 (24%), and anaerobic metabolism was recorded in 6 of 16 cases (44%) (see Fig. 5).

The High Incidence of Coma with Severe Hyperglycemia

The severity of hyperglycemia in 218 severely brain-injured patients (GCS < 8) was studied. In 184 of 218 cases (84%), hyperglycemia was very severe, more than 180 mg/dl. As to clinical deterioration, coma was closely related to the severity of hyperglycemia. Moderate hyperglycemia, 160 to 179 mg/dl, was only found in a few cases of coma, 6 of 218 (3%) adults. These

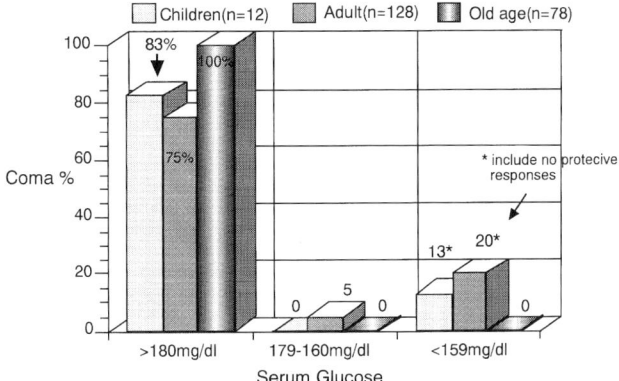

Fig. 6. Effect of hyperglycemia on induction of coma of children, adults, and older persons after severe brain injury

patients with moderate hyperglycemia did not have severe brain injury; it was limited to those of GCS 8. No recording of moderate hyperglycemia among children and older patients was statistically analyzed. No response of hyperglycemia was observed in 2 of 12 cases (13%) in children and 26 of 128 cases (20%) among adults. In this group, two different types of clinical deterioration were observed: one is a patient not so severely injured, of GCS 8, and the other occurs in patients suddenly seriously damaged. Most cases of serious injury were patients who underwent a sudden shock.

Severity of hyperglycemia associated with clinical deterioration was strongly correlated to the older group (100%) and next to younger patients (83%) (Fig. 6). Monitoring of hyperglycemia was very useful to evaluate the severity of harmful stress.

Activation of the Hypothalamus–Pituitary Axis

The hypothalamus–pituitary axis hormones are stimulated by excess release of catecholamines [27]. In recent studies on the changes of BBB function by vasopressin and poor prognosis with elevated serum GH, the sequential changes of hypothalamus–pituitary axis function, release of vasopressin, growth hormone (GH), adrenocorticotropic hormone (ACTH), the CSF cytokines IL-1 and IL-6, serum IL-1 and IL-6, and blood–brain barrier function were studied. Attention was focused on the interaction among these factors, especially the role of vasopressin that is an indirect parameter of hypothalamus function.

After severe brain injury (GCS 3–6), serum vasopressin immediately increased to 200 to 600 pg/ml over 2 h, which is 130 to 400 times higher than the standard value, and then continued at high levels of 10 to 20 pg/ml for 5 to 6 days (Figs. 1, 7). The peak release of vasopressin was observed at the last day. This release pattern of vasoactive and osmotic regulator hypothalamus hormone was very similar to the changes of CSF IL-1 and IL-6 cytokines and the severity of BBB dysfunction (Fig. 7).

The change in BBB dysfunction was also a very similar pattern to the changes of serum ACTH. However, the statistical analysis of correlation between changes of BBB dysfunction, ACTH, and vasopressin suggested that vasopressin was much related to the BBB dysfunction and increase of CSF IL-1 and IL-6 cytokines (Fig. 8).

Direct relationships between changes of serum GH and vasopressin were not observed. The first day was peak time to release of vasopressin; however, GH release revealed two peak times,

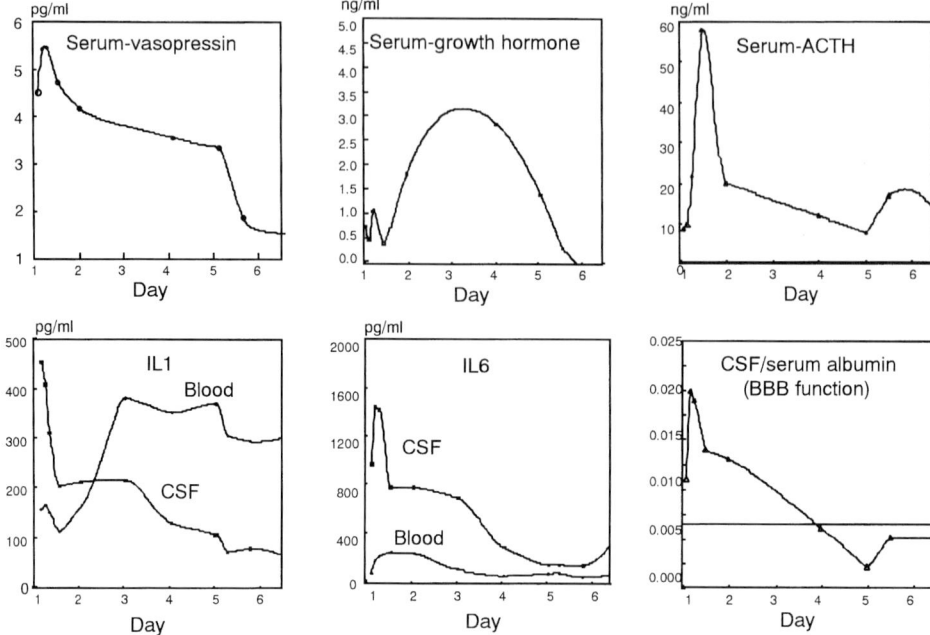

FIG. 7. Changes in neurohormonal inflammatory cytokines and BBB function in brain-injured patients after brain hypothermia treatment

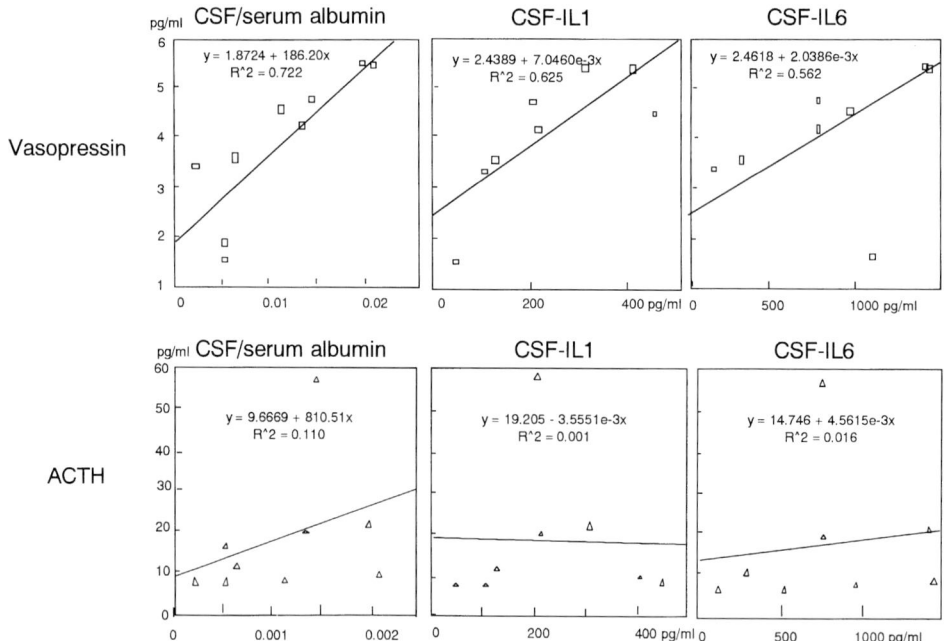

FIG. 8. Relationships between changes of BBB function (CSF/serum albumin ratio), CSF proinflammatory cytokines, and neurohormonal release after traumatic brain injury

a relatively small amount in the first day and large amounts 3 to 4 days after severe brain injury. Elevation of serum IL-1 preceded the second large release of GH (Fig. 8).

High Correlation of Brain Tissue Glucose to the Release of Serum Vasopressin

Macronutrient intake is regulated by the feedback mechanism of vasopressin through the stimulation of hypothalamus neuropeptide Y receptors [2,27]. Immunoanatomical studies revealed the presence of neuropeptide Y not only in the hypothalamus [5], but also on the vascular walls of brain, lung, and heart [12]. The neuropeptide Y in brain tissue and vascular walls acts as a receptor of norepinephrine and glucose [2,14,27]. Therefore, neuropeptide Y receptors might be regulating systemic circulation and brain metabolism. We wondered whether the catecholamine surge-induced hyperglycemia could be stimulated very strongly by the hypothalamus neuropeptide Y system. The hypothalamus neuropeptide Y is also the appetite center and stimulates by means of hyperglycemia or increased brain tissue glucose.

We have studied the correlative changes of vasopressin release, serum glucose, and interstitial brain tissue glucose using a microdialysis monitor. As a result, both brain tissue glucose and serum glucose were found to be related to the changes of BBB dysfunction associated with release of vasopressin. The interstitial brain tissue glucose was more highly correlated to the release of vasopressin, BBB dysfunction, and cytokine reactions than serum hyperglycemia (Fig. 9). However, no relationship with release of vasopressin and brain tissue glutamate was recorded.

Discussion

Previous Brain Injury Mechanism

The initial stage of brain injury involves destruction of brain tissues and vasculature and release of vasoactive substances such as endogenous opiates [29], catecholamines [1], serotonin [1,25], asparate [1], excitatory amino acids, and K ions [1]. These changes immediately develop in cerebral ischemia, which accompanies synaptic paralysis and cardiopulmonary dysfunction. In animal studies, initial release of the excitatory amino acid, glutamate, which is modulated by constitutive NO radicals, has been noted to increase intracellular Ca^{++} ion in injured brain tissue [35]. The release of glutamate, increasing intracellular Ca^{++} ion, and constitutive free radical attack causes severe damage by intracellular homeostasis and membrane dysfunction [30,35]. The pathophysiological changes in injured brain tissue [35], protection mechanism [4,26,31], the relationships between secondary brain injury and systemic circulation, and prognosis are summarized in Fig. 10.

Cerebral ischemia and neuroexcitatory synaptic injury are considered as major pathophysiological changes in the initial stage of severe brain injury. In injured brain tissue, tissue destruction, vascular engorgement, brain edema, and cytokine inflammation have been considered as pathophysiological changes followed by elevation of ICP [30,35]. Before the elevation of ICP and progression of brain edema, functional changes of vascular permeability start between 2 and 15 h. Before the progression of widespread brain edema, selective specific neuronal damage of basal ganglia has been reported [15]. In animal studies, the neuroexcitatory amino acid glutamate is nominated as a major factor to promote synaptic injury in cerebral ischemia [23,30,35].

After the passage of 24 h, brain edema and intracranial hypertension begin to progress, which accompany increased inducible second free radical reactions [34,35]. At this stage,

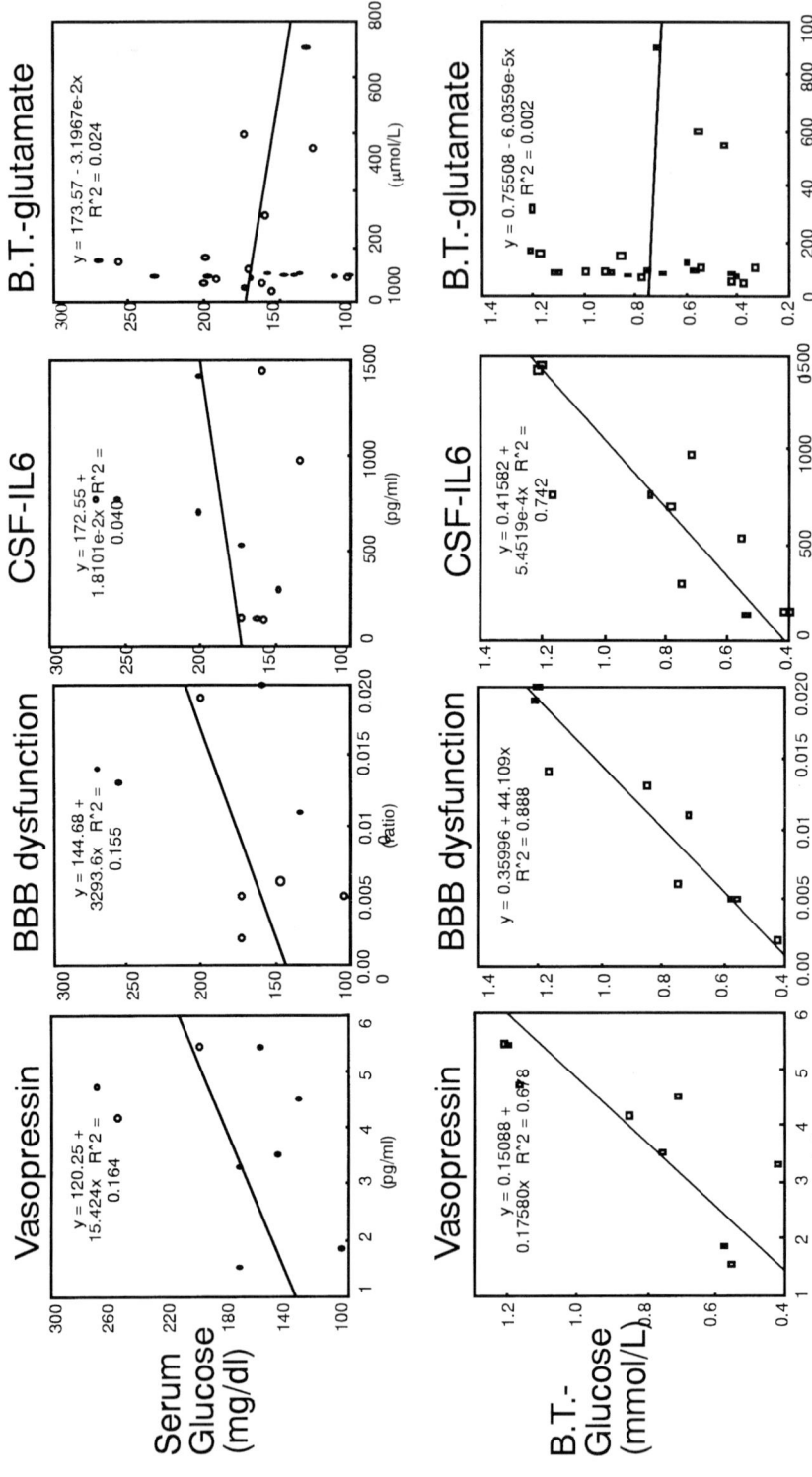

FIG. 9. Effects of hyperglycemia and cerebral glucose metabolism on vasopressin-associated BBB dysfunction and cytokine inflammation. *B.T.*, brain tissue; *BBB*, brain blood barrier; *CSF*, cerebrospinal fluid

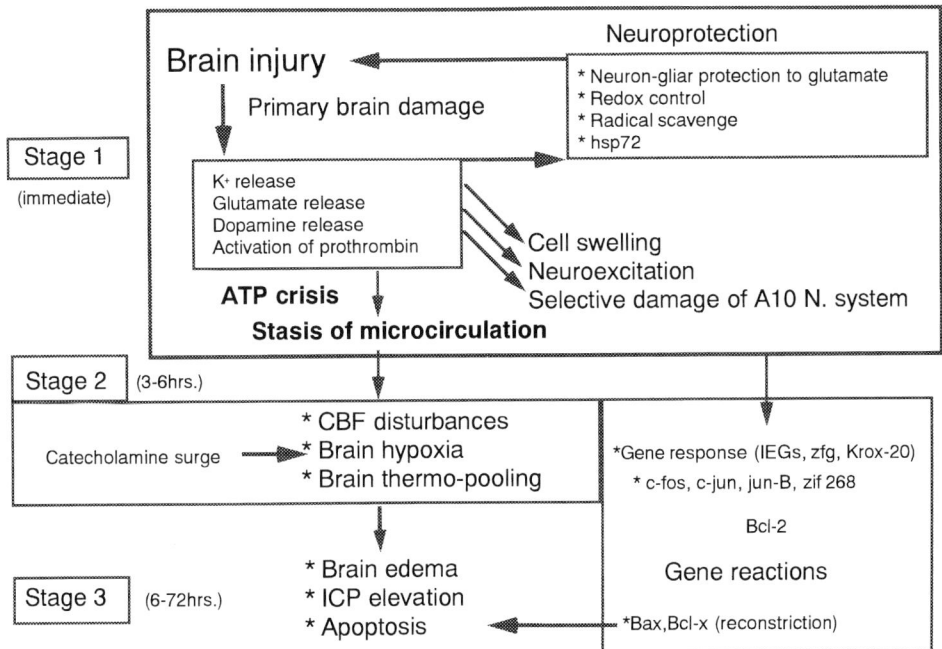

FIG. 10. Time window schema of pathophysiological changes in injured brain tissue and systemic reactions

intravascular release of thromboplastin, activation of intravascular coagulability, and consumption of thromboplastin fibrinolysis agents with changes of microcirculation of vascular permeability occur. The vascular engorgement, disturbances in microcirculation, ICP elevation, and inducible free radical reactions produce a malignant ischemic circle and cause progression of brain edema and intracranial hypertension.

The responses of systemic immunoprotective cells, the neutrophils and macrophages, to the stress of the trauma produce cytokines and inducible NO and superoxide anion radicals [35]. The release of cytokines causes changes of intravascular coagulation, producing adhesion molecules on the intima of vascular walls and damage of vascular function. Systemic attack by delayed inducible free radicals from activation of neutrophils and macrophages causes more extensive damage by these changes and produces increased vascular permeability, leakage of immunological protective γ-globulin into the extracellular space, osmotic extracellular edema by low protein, and results in the complication of hyperdynamic severe infections. The clinical issue is introducing the concept of this brain injury mechanism based on experimental animal studies [35].

Why Are Brain Edema, Brain Ischemia, ICP Elevation, and Reduced CPP Not Sufficient to Explain the Brain Injury Mechanism in Severely Injured Patients?

Brain edema, ICP elevation, brain ischemia, and decreased CPP have been considered as major targets of treatment at the acute stage. This concept of brain injury mechanism has been supported for a long time by many animal studies. However, in animal studies, neurohormonal pathophysiological changes caused specifically by the harmful stress of severe brain injury are not seen under anesthesia. In clinical studies, brain hypoxia caused by hemoglobin dysfunction and elevated BTT, brain thermopooling [22], hyperglycemia-associated BBB dysfunction, and cytokine encephalitis-associated BBB dysfunction are elucidated.

Catecholamine Surge-Induced Masking Brain Hypoxia Disturbs Neuronal Restoration in Injured Brain Tissue

When the brain is severely injured, brain hypoxia occurs in the primarily injured tissue, accompanied by abrupt cell swelling with K^+ ion release causing Na^+ channels to open, synaptic paralysis leading to respiratory arrest, and low cerebral perfusion elicited by cardiac dysfunction with a 50- to 200-fold increased catecholamine surge (see Fig. 1). The severe catecholamine surge produces masking brain hypoxia, which is not recorded by previous monitors by brain thermopooling, circulation shift into the intestinal organs, lower oxygen delivery and hemoglobin dysfunction. Excess release of catecholamines produces two metabolic disturbances, such as severely increased cyclic AMP and hyperglycemia with consumption of ATP and glycogen in major organs, heart, and liver (Fig. 11). Increased cyclic AMP immediately produces vascular contraction and cardiac ischemia due to coronary spasm and contraction myocytolysis. The ST elevation on electrocardiogram (ECG) and the difficulty of maintaining systolic blood pressure for wash out of elevated BTT are recorded within 3 h after severe brain injury.

In the case of lower systolic blood pressure, less than 90 to 100 mmHg, after reperfusion, inability to wash out BTT occurs and BTT rises to 40°–44°C with neuronal hypoxia in the injured tissue [17,18,20]. This new pathophysiological condition starts as cerebral oxygen metabolism advances regardless of cerebral ischemia between 2 and 15 h after insult. Such specific pathophysiological conditions generally precede brain tissue hypoxia with lavish perfusion [18].

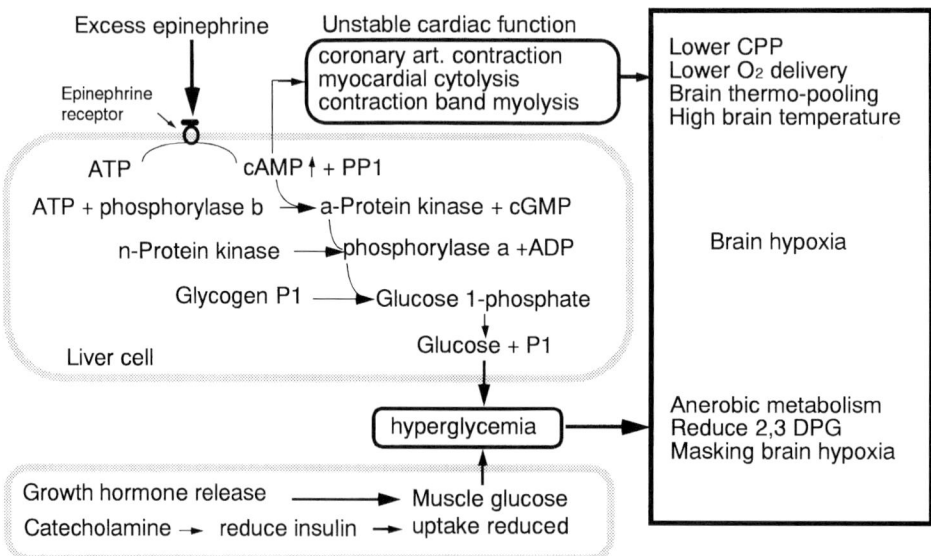

Fig. 11. Cardiopulmonary and metabolic changes following excess autonomic nerve and neuroendocrinological reactions after severe brain injury

From about 3 h after brain injury, dopamine-dominant systemic circulation occurs (see Fig. 1). Dopamine increases cardiac output (CO); however, it causes selective vasodilatation of intestinal vasculature and renal blood vessels. This specific dopamine-dominant catecholamine imbalance makes possible a blood shift into the intestine rather than brain even with normal CPP and normal oxygen delivery. Clinically, this phenomenon is recorded by elevated rectal temperature rather than BTT and TMT [18]. In normal conditions, BTT is always higher than rectal or bladder temperature. It is very difficult for brain-injured patients to survive when the BTT/rectal temperature ratio (or TMT/rectal temperature ratio) becomes less than 0.96 [18].

The meaning of severe hyperglycemia after severe brain injury is summarized as consumption of ATP and glycogen in heart and liver, activation of anaerobic metabolism in the brain tissue, difficulty in release of oxygen from hemoglobin because of reduced DPG, BBB dysfunction with vasopressin release, and production of proinflamary cytokines. In this study, 41% of patients with GCS less than 6 recorded hemoglobin dysfunction as shown by lower arterial blood Hb-DPG. In 24% of patients with GCS less than 6, oxygen was not released from hemoglobin in the brain even with normal PaO_2 as shown by lower jugular venous Hb-DPG (in Fig. 5). This result means that oxygen inhalation is not useful under the condition of reduced hemoglobin enzyme, DPG. Our preliminary studies suggested that severe ketoacidosis and pH < 7.2 promote progressive metabolization of DPG to the lactate. This harmful stress-induced hyperglycemia with reduced DPG must be considered as one cause of masking brain hypoxia in initial management.

From this study of stress-induced catecholamine surge, we must understand that normal control of ICP, CPP, and PaO_2 are not always correct as care management for the survival of injured neurons. The control of BTT at 34°–32°C could only prevent excess release of catecholamine surge and allow easy care of masking brain hypoxia.

The main purpose of brain hypothermia treatment is to halt or retard these pathophysiological changes by precise lowering of BTT and to make available sufficient oxygen and metabolic substrates. Previous procedures to control ICP and prevent brain edema are inadequate for handling masking brain hypoxia and brain thermopooling-related pathophysiological changes.

Elevation of BTT by Brain Thermopooling Must be Prevented for Neuronal Restoration and Secondary Brain Damage

Brain temperature is influenced by cerebral blood flow (CBF); however, its precise regulatory mechanism has not yet been clarified. We have found that change in BTT is determined by four factors, the first three being (1) body temperature (core temperature), (2) cerebral perfusion pressure, which carries the core temperature into the brain tissue, and (3) brain metabolism (as shown in Fig. 12) [20,22]. Therefore, BTT is highest, 37.0° ± 0.29°C, then core temperature, 36.3° ± 0.23°C, tympanic membrane temperature, 36.7° ± 0.27°C, and bladder temperature, 36.6° ± 0.25°C, under physiological conditions. BTT is controlled by (4) the final factor, CBF. BTT is maintained consistently very close to the body core temperature. Excess accumulation of BTT is prevented by the CBF washout mechanism [22] (see Fig. 3). In other words, CBF works as a biphasic function to regulate BTT: one function is as a carrier of thermal energy into the brain and the other is a washout mechanism to prevent excess elevation of thermal energy in the brain tissue [20,22] (see Fig. 12).

In complete cerebral ischemia, BTT decreases because transporting of core temperature is limited. However, incomplete brain ischemia will elevate local BTT. Causes of brain ther-

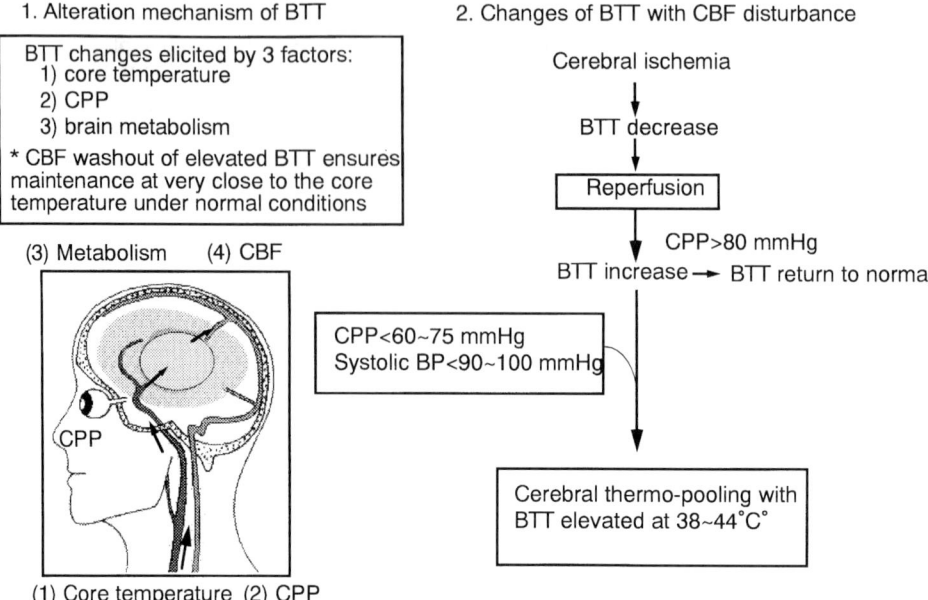

1. Alteration mechanism of BTT   2. Changes of BTT with CBF disturbance

BTT changes elicited by 3 factors:
1) core temperature
2) CPP
3) brain metabolism
* CBF washout of elevated BTT ensures maintenance at very close to the core temperature under normal conditions

Cerebral ischemia

BTT decrease

Reperfusion

CPP>80 mmHg
BTT increase → BTT return to normal

CPP<60~75 mmHg
Systolic BP<90~100 mmHg

(3) Metabolism   (4) CBF

CPP

(1) Core temperature (2) CPP

Cerebral thermo-pooling with BTT elevated at 38~44°C°

FIG. 12. Schema of brain tissue temperature (BTT) alteration mechanism under physiological conditions and during cerebral ischemia

mopooling have been found to be fever above 38°C, after reperfusion, systolic blood pressure lower than 90–100 mmHg in adults, and CPP below 60–75 mmHg.

The Meaning of Harmful Stress-Associated Hyperglycemia in the Acute Stage

To protect cardiopulmonary function and neuronal function against harmful brain injury, the hypothalamus–pituitary–adrenal glands release norepinephrine, epinephrine, and dopamine. This catecholamine surge can maintain CBF and coronary circulation and protect the brain and heart when the release of catecholamines is appropriate. However, in severe brain injury cases, catecholamines 50 to 200 times higher than normal produce cardiopulmonary dysfunction and a energy crisis in the liver and heart (see Fig. 11).

To cause hyperglycemia, the catecholamine surge promotes the metabolic change of adenosine triphosphate (ATP) to cyclic AMP. Cyclic AMP is metabolized in liver and heart, and then cAMP shifts to glucose by consuming organ ATP and glycogen. Therefore, serum hyperglycemia could be evaluated as an indirect parameter of the severity of catecholamine surge (Fig. 11). Hyperglycemia after harmful stress is an unavoidable metabolic change in severely brain-injured patients. On the other hand, no response of hyperglycemia after severe brain injury means harmful stress is light, even with unconsciousness or no physical protective response time by a rapid serious brain injury.

Prolonged severe hyperglycemia (serum glucose higher than 220 mg/dl) suggests not only the presence of hypothalamus–adrenal gland-stimulating pathophysiological changes but also the consumption of ATP in liver and heart. The ATP crisis, however, of hyperglycemia in liver and heart causes an unstable cardiopulmonary circulation, lower CPP, blood shift into the intestine, and changes in the reactivity to antishock drugs.

Hyperglycemia, especially at more than 180 mg/dl, is closely related to deterioration of consciousness into coma (Fig. 6). The background of this harmful stress-associated hyperglycemia can be summarized not only by systemic circulatory metabolic changes but also by direct secondary brain damage from the occurrence of anaerobic brain metabolism, unsuccessful neuronal oxygenation with hemoglobin dysfunction, and progress of BBB dysfunction by activating vasopressin release through the feedback mechanism of macronutrient intake reactions.

Response of the Hypothalamus–Pituitary Axis

The release of neurotransmitters, such as excitatory amino acids, glutamate, and AMPA, promotes secondary brain damage by delayed neuronal death [1,11,33]. By the same mechanism, in cases of severe brain injury, vasopressin is released from the hypothalamus by stimulation of mechanical injury, hyperglycemia [27], and inflammatory cytokines [3,25]. Therefore, the pattern of vasopressin release is variable depending on the severity and causes of brain injury.

In severe brain trauma, two patterns of vasopressin release were recorded in this study (see Figs. 1, 7). Initial peaks 130 to 400 times higher than the usual level of serum vasopressin were recorded within 2h after brain injury. The initial response of vasopressin release could be explained by feedback control of hyperglycemia through norepinephrine (1-h catecholamine surge) stimulation of the hypothalamus neuropeptide Y system [2,14,27,28]. The hypothalamus neuropeptide Y receptor also contributes to regulating the release of vasopressin, insulin, and corticotropin by macronutrient intake [2,27]. In this study, the role of brain tissue glucose in release of vasopressin was demonstrated. Hyperglycemia is one factor that causes brain tissue glucose increase. In severely brain-injured patients, sometimes it is very difficult to control serum glucose at 120 to 140mg/dl precisely for a long time. Therefore, after 2h, a continued high level of serum vasopressin, 20 to 10pg/ml for 5 to 6 days, was recorded with increased brain tissue glucose (see Fig. 7). This caused hyperglycemia 2h later and also could produce a metabolic imbalance between the glucose supply and its consumption in brain tissue, resulting in increased brain tissue lactate. The prolonged release of vasopressin without precise control of serum glucose between 120 and 140mg/dl was not controlled. This management is especially important during brain hypothermia treatment.

Vasopressin is an antidiuretic hormone; therefore, the prolonged release of vasopressin could be understood as a protection response for hyperglycemia-induced hyperosmolarity. However, excess release of vasopressin activates inflammatory cytokines, as shown by increased CSF IL-1, and damages BBB function (see Figs. 7, 8). Management of brain hypothermia could be prevention of the initial release of vasopressin. However, the second stage of prolonged vasopressin release is not prevented by brain hypothermia without control of hyperglycemia. This uncontrolled release of vasopressin by the hypothermia mechanism is one of the major pitfalls of brain hypothermia. The precise mechanism of the pitfalls of brain hypothermia treatment is described in the chapter by Hayashi et al. (this volume).

In experimental studies on the function of vasopressin, vascular constriction in lung and coronary artery [12] and a poor prognosis of severe brain injury were observed. Immunoanatomical studies have demonstrated the presence of neuropeptide Y like a mesh on the surface of cerebral vessels [2,12]. However, the precise mechanism of the vascular reaction in the cerebral vessels is not understood. In this clinical study, the association of vasopressin with BBB function and changes of inflammatory cytokines was recorded (see Figs. 8, 9).

In recent clinical studies, increased serum GH and poor prognosis were reported [7]. The high level of GH release stimulates the increase of serum IFN-γ [3], which activates proinflamatory cytokines such as IL-1, IL-6, and tumor necrotizing factors [8]. The proinflammatory cytokines stimulate the release of GH [3]. This phenomenon is also observed in Fig. 7.

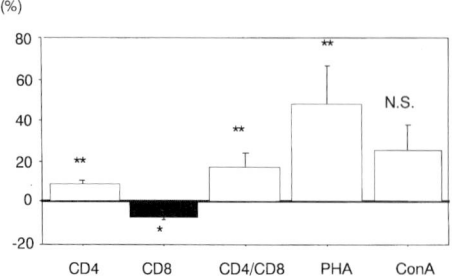

FIG. 13. Percent changes in T-cell markers after administration of growth hormone ($n = 7$)

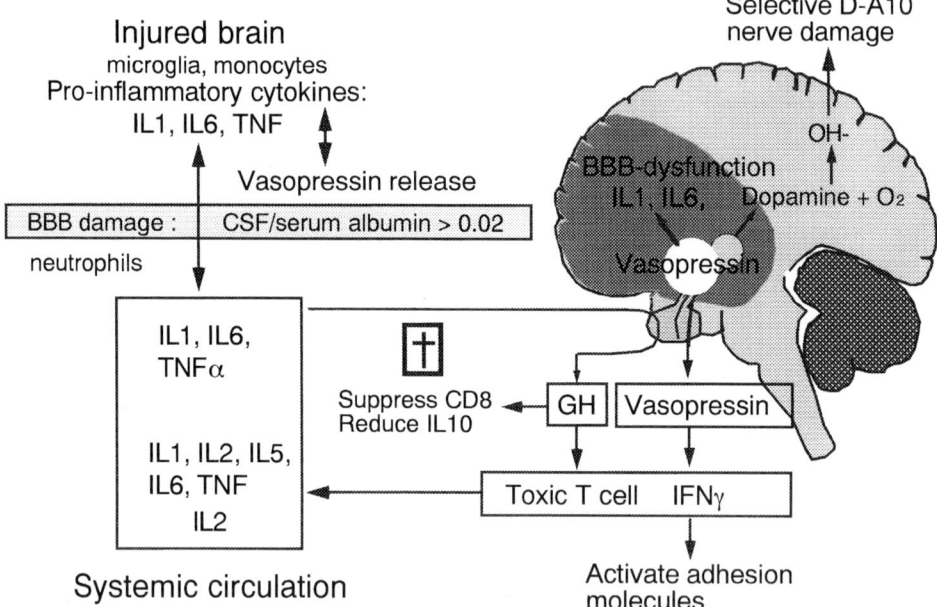

FIG. 14. Neurohormonal-inflammatory brain damage after severe brain injury

The peak time of GH release is 3 to 4 days after trauma. In many cases who did not survive, we have recorded progressive increase of IL-6 and suppression of IL-10. Our preliminary studies concerning replacement therapy of GH to patients in immune crisis suggested that GH activates CD4 and cellular immune function but suppresses CD8 with reduced antiinflammatory cytokine IL-10 [18,20] (Fig. 13). Therefore, in the acute stage of brain-injured patients, excessive release of GH promotes cytokine encephalitis in injured brain tissue and reduces the possibility of recovery of injured neurons by suppression of the antiinflammatory cytokine IL-10 (Fig. 14).

In cases of severe BBB dysfunction with a recorded CSF/serum albumin ratio greater than 0.02, increased serum cytokines by GH and pulmonary infections easily penetrate the BBB. This dangerous BBB dysfunction-associated cytokine encephalitis is most often seen 3 to 4 days after severe brain injury. The relationships between changes of hypothalamus–pituitary axis neurohormonal dysfunction and BBB dysfunction must be considered as to their effect on increasing serum glutamate when planning enteral and parenteral nutrition.

New Concept of Brain Injury Mechanism

When the brain is injured, its pathophysiological state typically progresses, showing a certain time window. The initial stages of brain injury involve destruction of the brain tissues, localized brain ischemia, cytokine inflammation, and synaptic dysfunction with release of vascular agonists (endogenous opiates) [29] catecholamines, dopamine, neurogenous agonists such as choline [1,11], excitatory amino acids, and K^+ ion [1,11]. However, the prognosis of dying neurons in injured tissue is strictly influenced by two extracerebral factors: one is the changes in the systemic circulation and metabolism associated with catecholamine surge, and the other is inflammatory reactions associated with the release of hypothalamus–pituitary axis hormones (Fig. 15).

The dying neurons require sufficient oxygen and adequate metabolic substrate if they are to recover successfully. Three different types of brain hypoxia and energy crisis occur in the primarily injured neurons. In injured brain tissue, the injured neurons initially release potassium ions with changes of membrane depolarization [35]. The injured neurons expend oxygen to maintain the intracellular status. Neuroexcitation by excitatory amino acid release also consumes residual oxygen in injured neurons [11]. As a mechanism of adaptation of localized injured tissue, glial regulation mechanisms for release of neuronal transmitters and intracellular proton storm have been reported [31]. For these reasons, residual oxygen is rapidly consumed.

As a second mechanism of brain hypoxia, poor neuronal oxygen supply with systemic circulatory–metabolic imbalance is the most important target of initial treatment, as shown by this clinical study. The harmful stress-induced catecholamine surge produces unstable cardiopulmonary dysfunction and hyperglycemia. The unstable cardiopulmonary function produces brain thermopooling with insufficient CBF. Excess release of catecholamines also produces brain hypoxia by hemoglobin dysfunction, reduced oxygen delivery, and intestinal blood shift caused by the dopamine-dominant circulation. This type of brain hypoxia sometime shows normal ICP, normal CPP, and normal PaO_2 (Fig. 16). The previous neuroprotec-

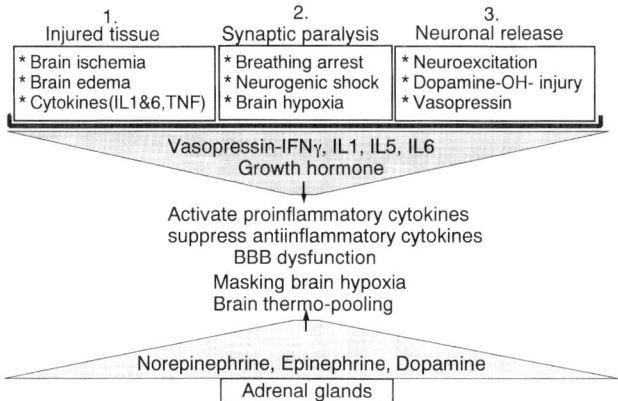

Fig. 15. Interactions between changes of intracerebral brain damage and systemic neurohormonal circulatory metabolic changes after severe brain injury

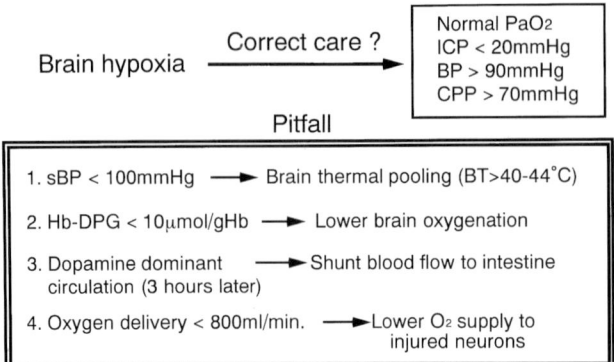

FIG. 16. The pitfalls in management of brain hypoxia

tion management methods, such as control of ICP, CPP, oxygen inhalation, and brain edema, cannot provide recovery from these types of brain hypoxia.

In ICU management and brain hypothermia treatment, neuronal hypoxia in injured brain tissue even with normal ICP, CPP and PaO_2 must be carefully handled. We call this specific neuronal hypoxia masking brain hypoxia, which is not monitored by previous methods. In critical cases with severe catecholamine surge, the coronary spasm and contraction band myolysis associated with the epinephrine and norepinephrine surge allows easy misdiagnosis the acute myocardiac infarctions. We recorded 40°–44°C of BTT after reperfusion of severe brain injury and cardiac arrest brain ischemia in the acute stage. A high fever (more than 38°C) and systolic blood pressure lower than 90–100 mmHg after reperfusion are clinical conditions producing brain thermopooling. This new pathophysiological condition progresses relative to the advance of cerebral oxygen metabolism regardless of cerebral ischemia between 3 and 6h after insult. Such specific pathophysiological conditions generally precede cerebral edema and heavy perfusion.

The third type of brain hypoxia is caused by the secondary brain damage mechanism of brain edema, ICP elevation, and brain ischemia, as described previously. After the passage of 6h, the third stage of brain hypoxia progresses with brain edema and ICP elevation accompanying activation of the hypothalamus–pituitary axis, BBB dysfunction, and cytokine encephalitis. The management of masking brain hypoxia, hyperglycemia, reduced serum albumin, and control of BTT at 32°–34°C is a useful basis for treatment of these three types of brain hypoxia. Regarding delayed neuronal injury, animal studies have demonstrated that with release of glutamate, that is, excitatory amino acid, delayed neuronal cell death occurs with increased intracellular Ca levels accompanying excessive neuronal excitation (see Fig. 10).

The presence of brain damage of the hypothalamus is important in understanding the brain injury mechanism and also in designing ICU management. In this study, the hypothalamus–pituitary neurohormonal axis brain injury mechanism was presented. However, the hypothalamus is also the important location for control of mind, thinking, volition, emotion, love, and anxiety by means of the function of the dopamine A10 nervous system [21,22]. After severe brain injury, dopamine leak from the dopamine nervous system permits selective radical damage of the dopamine A10 nervous system and facilitates development of vegetation or mental retardation [10,11,13,21,22]. This issue and the management method of mental retardation will be presented at later.

Conclusion

As a brain injury mechanism, not only the pathophysiological changes in injured brain tissue but also the systemic circulatory metabolic changes associated with neurohormonal pathophysiological responses have been elucidated. Masking brain hypoxia, even with normal ICP, CPP, and PaO_2, brain thermopooling, hyperglycemia-related BBB dysfunction, and hypothalamus–pituitary axis-related cytokine encephalitis are summarized as a new brain injury mechanism. This entirely new brain injury mechanism is triggered by a harmful stress response. Therefore, studies in anesthetized animals cannot easily demonstrate this clinical systemic brain injury mechanism. The many neurons in primary injured brain tissue need restoration therapy before the start of neuroprotection therapy. Systemic neurohormonal pathophysiological changes provide a good target for neuronal restoration in injured brain tissue.

References

1. Baker AJ, Zornow MH, Scheller MS, Yaksh TL, Skilling SR, Smullin DH, Larson AA, Kuczenski R (1991) Changes in extracellular concentrations of glutamate, asparate, glycine, dopamine, serotonin, and dopamine metabolites after transient global ischemia in the rat. J Neurochem 57:1370–1379
2. Beck B (2000) Quantitative and macronutrient-related regulation of hypothalamic neuropeptide Y, galanin and neurotensin. In: Berthoud HR, Seeley RJ (eds) Neural and metabolic control of macronutrient intake. CRC Press, Boca Raton, pp 455–464
3. Billiau A, Vankelecom H (1992) Interferon-γ: general biological properties and effects on the neuro-endocrine axis. In: Bartfai T, Ottoson D (eds) Neuro-immunology of fever. Pergamon Press, Oxford, pp 65–77
4. Boise LH, Gottschalk AR, Quintans J, et al (1995) Bcl-2 and Bcl-2-related proteins in apotosis regulation. Curr Top Microbiol Immunol 200:107–121
5. Chronwall BM, Di Maggio DA, Massari VJ, Pickel VN, Ruggiero DA, O'Donohue TL (1985) The anatomy of neuropeptide Y-containing neurons in rat brain. Neuroscience 15:1159
6. Clifton G, Robertson C, Kyper K, Tayloe AA, Dhenkne RD, Grossman R (1983) Cardiovascular response to severe head injury. J Neurosurg 59:447–457
7. Corte FD, Mancini A, Valle D, Gallizzi F, Carducci P, Mignani V, De Marinis L (1998) Provocative hypothalamopituitary axis tests in severe head injury: correlations with severity and prognosis. Crit Care Med 26(8):1419–1426
8. Davila DR, Breif S, Simon J, et al (1987) Role of growth hormone in regulating T-dependent immune events in aged, nude, and transgenic rodents. J Neurosci Res 18:108–116
9. Dudariev VP, Lanovenko II (1999) Changes in the oxygen-binding properties of the blood in white rats under the influence of hypoxia and its pharmacological correction. Fiziol Zh 45(1–2):97–103
10. Globus MYT, Ginsberg MD, Haris SI, Busto R, Dietrich WD (1987) Role of dopamine in ischemic striatal injury. Neurology 37:1712–1719
11. Globus MYT, Busto R, Dietolich WD, Martinez E, Valdes I, Ginsberg MD (1998) Effect of ischemia on the in vivo release of striatal dopamine, glutamate, and γ-aminobutyric acid studied by intracerebral microdialysis. J Neurochem 51:1455–1464
12. Goadsby PJ, Edvinsson L (1997) Extrinsic innavation: transmitters, receptors, and functions — the sympathetic nerve system. In: Welch KMA, Caplan LR, Reis DJ, Siesjø Bo K, Weir B (eds) Primer on cerebrovascular diseases. Academic Press, San Diego, pp 60–63

13. Gualtieri CT, Chandler M, Coons TB (1989) Review. Amantadine: a new clinical profile for traumatic brain injury. Clin Neuropharmacol 12:258–270
14. Harfstrand A, Eneroth P, Abnati L, Fuxe K (1987) Further studies on the effects of central administration of neuropeptide Y on neuroendocrine function in the male rat: relationship to hypothalamic catecholamines. Regul Pept 17:167
15. Hayashi N, Hirayama T, Utagawa A, Ohata M (1993) Complete cerebral ischemia-induced circuit damage of the basal ganglia, substantia nigra and deep cerebellar nucleus in clinical cases. In: Tomita M, Mchedlishvili G, Rosenblum W, Heiss W-D, Fukuchi Y (eds) Microcirculatory stasis in the brain. Excerpta Medica, Amsterdam, pp 555–562
16. Hayashi N, Hirayama T, Utagawa A, Ohata M (1994) Systemic management of cerebral edema based on a new concept in severe head injury patients. Acta Neurochir (Suppl) 60: 541–543
17. Hayashi N, Hirayama T, Utagawa A (1994) The cerebral thermo-pooling and hypothermia treatment of critical head injury patients. In: Nagai H (ed) Intracranial pressure, vol IX. Springer, Tokyo, pp 589–599
18. Hayashi N (1995) Cerebral hypothermia treatment. In: Hayashi N (ed) Cerebral hypothermia treatment. Sogo Igaku, Tokyo, pp 1–105
19. Hayashi N (1996) Advance of cerebral hypothermia treatment. J Crit Med 8:295–300
20. Hayashi N, Kinoshita K, Shibuya T (1997) The prevention of cerebral thermo-pooling, damage of A10 nervous system, and free radical reactions by control of brain tissue temperature in severely brain injured patients. In: Teelken AW (ed) Neurochemistry. Plenum, New York, pp 97–103
21. Hayashi N (1997) Combination therapy of cerebral hypothermia, pharmacological activation of the dopamine system, and hormonal replacement in severely brain damaged patients. J Jpn Intensive Care Med 4:191–197
22. Hayashi N (1997) Prevention of vegetation after severe head trauma and stroke by combination therapy of cerebral hypothermia and activation of immune-dopaminergic nervous system. Proc Annu Meet Soc Treatment Coma 6:133–145
23. Kirino T (1982) Delayed neuronal death in the gerbil hippocampus following ischemia. Brain Res 239:57–69
24. Kossmann T, Hans V, Imhof HG, Stocker R, Grob P, Trentz O, Morgani-Kossmann MC (1995) Intrathecal and serum interleukin-6 and acute-phase response in patients with severe traumatic brain injuries. Shock 4:311–317
25. Kossmann T, Hans V, Lenzlinger PM, Csuka E, Stsahel PF, Trentz O, Morgani-Kossmann MC (1996) Analysis of immune mediator production following traumatic brain injury. In: Schlag G, Redel H, Traber D (eds) Shock, sepsis and organ failure. Springer, Berlin, Heidelberg, New York, pp 263–297
26. Krajewski S, Mai JK, Krajewaska M, et al (1995) Upregulation of bax proteins in neurons following cerebral ischemia. J Neurosci 15:6364–6376
27. Leibowiz SF, Sladek C, Spencer L, Temple D (1988) Neuropeptide Y, epinephrine and norepinephrine in the paraventricular nucleus: stimulation of feeding and the release of corticosterone, vasopressin and glucose. Brain Res Bull 21:905
28. Leibowitz SF (1999) Macronutrients and brain peptides: what they do and how they respond. In: Berthoud HR, Seeley RJ (eds) Neural and metabolic control of macronutrient intake. CRC Press, Boca Raton, pp 389–406
29. McIntosh TK, Hayes R, DeWitt D, Agura V, Faden AI (1987) Endogenous opioids may mediate secondary damage after experimental brain injury. Am J Physiol 258:E565–574
30. MacIntosh TK (1994) Neurological sequele of traumatic brain injury: therapeutic implications. Cerebrovasc Brain Metab Rev 6:109–162
31. Oppennheim RW, Houenou LJ, Johnson JE, et al (1995) Developing motor neurons rescued from programmed and axtonomy-induced cel death by GDNF. Nature 373:344–346
32. Pas'ko SA, Volosheniuk TG (1990) Disordered phosphorus metabolism and its correction in the acute period of severe craniocerebral trauma. Zh Vopr Neirokhir Im N N Burdenko 3:14–16
33. Sajia A, Hayes R, Lyeth B, Dixon E, Yamamoto T, Robinson S (1988) The effect of concussive head injury on the central cholinergic neurons. Brain Res 452:303–311

34. Silvka A, Coben G (1985) Hydroxyl radical attack on dopamine. J Biol Chem 260:15466–15472

35. Spuler A, Tan WKM, Meyer FB (1996) Molecular events in cerebral ischemia. In: Raffel C, Harsh GR (eds) The molecular basis of neurosurgical disease. Williams & Wilkins, Baltimore, pp 248–269

36. Stanley BG (1993) Neuropeptide Y in multiple hypothalamic sites controls eating behavior, endocrine, and autonomic system for body energy balance. In: Colmers WF, Wahlestedt C (eds) Biology of neuropeptide Y and related peptides. Humana Press, Totowa, NJ, p 457

2. Pathophysiology of Hypothermia

Molecular System Controlling Mammalian Hibernation with Circannual Rhythm

Noriaki Kondo*, Takashi Ohtsu, and Tsuneo Sekijima

Summary. Mammalian hibernation brings about remarkable physiological adaptation by which animals survive an extremely low body temperature lasting several days. Such adaptation has been suggested to be due to readjustment of cells and organs to a new physiological state. As hibernation occurs with circannual rhythm, this physiological readjustment has been suggested to be under the control of a circannual rhythm. Recently, a novel protein complex (HP), found in the blood of chipmunks, a mammalian hibernator, was defined as a unique factor regulated by gene expression associated with the endogenous circannual rhythm of hibernation. Biochemical studies of HP regulation revealed two hormones controlled through the hypothalamohypophyseal tract as candidate molecules involved in regulation of HP in the liver, suggesting that this system plays an important role in physiological adaptation for hibernation. Furthermore, circannual changes in HP level were found in the cerebrospinal fluid, and its content was up-regulated during hibernation, suggesting substantial involvement of HP in the control of hibernation in the brain. Thus, recent studies of HP have suggested a molecular mechanism of control of hibernation.

Key words. Mammalian hibernation, Circannual rhythm, Hibernation-specific protein, Gene expression, Hormone

Introduction

Mammalian hibernators have the ability to survive temporarily at low body temperatures close to 0°C during hibernation. Even in extreme hypothermia, the organisms maintain homeostasis and show resistance to low temperature and severe ischemia [4]. The marked depression of metabolism during hibernation has been reported to prolong longevity [12]. Thus, hibernators may possess a mechanism for preventing lethal damage during hibernation, suggesting that hibernation is a mechanism by which cells and organs are readjusted to a new physiological state.

Hibernation Control Project, Kanagawa Academy of Science and Technology, Mitsubishi Kasei Institute of Life Sciences, 11 Minamiooya, Machida, Tokyo 194-8511, Japan
* Present address: Hibernation Control Group, Mitsubishi Kasei Institute of Life Sciences, 11 Minamiooya, Machida, Tokyo 194-8511, Japan

Hibernation has been reported to occur circannually in ground squirrels kept under conditions of constant cold and darkness [14]. The behavioral and physiological changes in organisms such as body weight and blood hormone contents also showed a circannual rhythm linked to hibernation [18]. Electrophysiological studies of hearts of rodent hibernators revealed readjustment of the cellular calcium ion regulatory system during hibernation [2,6,11]. Such readjustment was circannually observed even under nonhibernating conditions [7], suggesting that the physiological regulation is endogenously induced at the cellular level without lowering body temperature. Based on these studies, a circannual hibernation rhythm has been suggested to control functions of cells and organs for maintenance of their life at low body temperatures. This control system has not been examined at the molecular level because of a lack of molecular probes controlled by an endogenous circannual rhythm.

Recently, we found a novel hibernation-specific protein (HP) in the blood of chipmunks, the contents of which were regulated by the differential expression of genes in association with hibernation [10,17]. This finding suggested that HP expression is under the control of a hibernation rhythm. In fact, although a few studies have been reported on differential gene expression during hibernation [1,16], no factors controlled by a circannual rhythm other than HP have been identified. These studies on the mechanism of regulation of HP have suggested that a molecular system controls hibernation. Our recent progress in this field is reviewed herein.

Animals

Male chipmunks (*Tamias sibiricus asiaticus*), caught in China within a few months after birth, were purchased from Tokyo Experimental Animal Co., Tokyo, Japan. Animals were usually kept under conditions of constant warmth (23°C) and a light/dark cycle (LD) (L/D = 12:12) with standard rat chow diet and water ad libitum. Most of the animals did not enter hibernation because of the high environmental temperature, although a few animals showed slight torpor. After more than 6 months under these conditions, some of the animals were transferred to a cold, dark room maintained at 5°C to perform hibernation experiments. Throughout our studies, animals were kept under these conditions.

HP Controlled by a Circannual Rhythm

Hibernation-specific protein (HP) has been found in the blood of chipmunks as a factor linked to hibernation [10]. HP was shown to be comprised of four novel proteins, three of which were structurally homologous and formed a complex (HP20C) with collagen-like domains in their NH_3-terminal regions. The other protein was a new member of the serpin superfamily (HP55) and associated with HP20C in the blood. The contents of HP in the blood changed with a clear circannual rhythm linked to hibernation in animals kept under conditions of constant darkness and cold (5°C) [9]. Before hibernation the HP level was markedly decreased. This reduced level of HP was maintained during hibernation and then returned to the normal level before termination of hibernation. During the hibernation season, animals showed a repeated constant torpid–arousal cycle where they periodically showed arousal for 10–20h after a state of continuous torpor for approximately 1 week. In this arousal state, the blood HP content remained reduced, indicating that rhythmic regulation of HP was not affected by periodical arousal.

A similar circannual rhythm of HP was observed even in animals kept under conditions of constant warmth (23°C) and LD (12L:12D) where hibernation was disturbed by a high environmental temperature [9]. When HP was reduced as observed in the hibernating state, animals began to hibernate immediately after exposure to cold, but animals died of cold when the body temperature was dropped without reducing HP. These studies clearly indicated that reduction of HP in the blood was not due to low body temperature but was controlled by an endogenous circannual rhythm of hibernation. Furthermore, it was assumed that the physiological readjustment of organisms controlled by a circannual rhythm enables them to lower their body temperatures without dysfunction of cells and organs. This assumption was supported by the previous finding that hearts were adapted to low body temperatures by the enhanced function of the calcium ion regulatory system [8]. Thus, a circannual rhythm controls physiological systems that protect organisms from the lethal damage caused by low body temperature. HP represents the first factor under control of a circannual rhythm, providing a new pathway for understanding the system responsible for control of hibernation.

Factors Regulating HP

The protein complex HP has been shown to be produced in the liver, and its production is regulated by gene expression associated with hibernation [17]. This finding suggested that the hibernation rhythm is transmitted to the liver probably through neural or humoral factors.

To screen for factors involved in regulation of HP production in the liver, primary cultures of hepatocytes from chipmunks were established. The level of production of HP in hepatocytes from hibernating animals was much lower than that in those from nonhibernating animals just after seeding, reflecting a reduction of HP during hibernation. With subsequent culture, the reduced production of HP was restored to a level similar to that observed in hepatocytes from nonhibernating animals. These observations indicated that HP production in the liver was inhibited during hibernation rather than activated during nonhibernation. These culture experiments suggested the existence of inhibitory factors. Therefore, the effects of various hormones and neurotransmitters on the production of HP in hepatocytes from nonhibernating animals were examined. The neurotransmitters tested (α- and β-adrenoceptor stimulants, Sigma Chemical Co., St. Louis, USA; histamine, Sigma; serotonin, Wako Pure Chemical Co., Osaka, Japan; acetylcholine, Daiichi Pharmaceutical Co., Tokyo, Japan) did not affect HP production, whereas of the 21 hormones tested thyroxine (Sigma) and testosterone (Sigma) induced a marked decrease and an increase in HP production, respectively [13]. Thyroxine inhibited HP production at concentrations above 10^{-11} M, and the up-regulation by testosterone was observed at 10^{-5} M (Fig. 1). As HP concentration in the blood has been shown to be markedly decreased during hibernation, thyroxine is a promising candidate for inducing biochemical changes similar to those that occur during hibernation. On the other hand, the increase in HP evoked by testosterone may contribute to the transition from the hibernating to the nonhibernating state.

The effects of these hormones on HP production were further examined in vivo (Fig. 2). Daily intraperitoneal administration of thyroxine ($25\,\mu g/100\,g$ body weight) decreased the HP (one half to one-fifth of that before treatment) 7 days after treatment, and the decreased level of HP was maintained during the period of administration. This inhibitory effect of thyroxine disappeared following cessation of administration. On the other hand, daily subcutaneous administration of testosterone ($1\,mg/100\,g$ body weight) gradually increased the HP in the blood, reaching a level three times that in the controls after 19 days of treatment. These results indicated that both hormones are effective in organisms as well as in cultured hepatocytes.

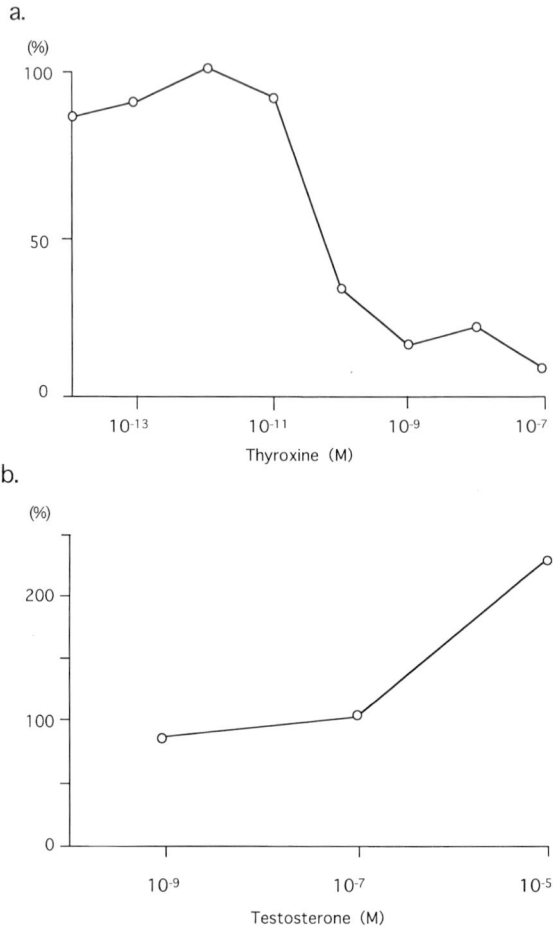

FIG. 1. Effects of thyroxine (**a**) and testosterone (**b**) on the production of the protein complex HP in cultured hepatocytes from nonhibernating animals. Both hormones were dissolved in dimethylsulfoxide and applied to culture media 6 days after seeding. HP contents in the culture media were measured 6 days after treatment. *Vertical* and *horizontal axes* show HP contents (% of control) and hormone concentrations (*M*), respectively

The involvement of hormones and glands in hibernation has been investigated in detail [5,18]. As thyroxine has important effects on metabolism and thermogenesis, many studies have been carried out in hibernators. Most of these studies suggested that thyroid activity is depressed during hibernation, although a few studies demonstrated that thyroid function continued during hibernation [3]. There have also been conflicting reports concerning the relation between gonadal activity and hibernation [5,18]. Thus, the effects of hormones on hibernation are obscure because of the influence of low body temperature and of differences in animal species, methodology, and experimental conditions. Our findings that thyroxine and testosterone induced changes in the HP level corresponding to those linked to the onset and

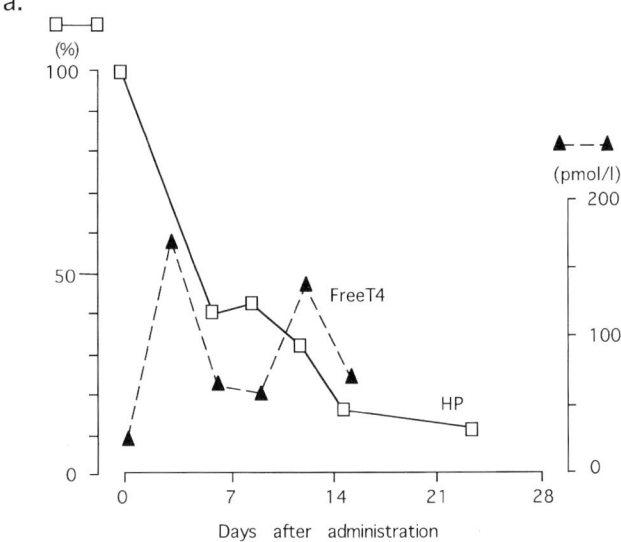

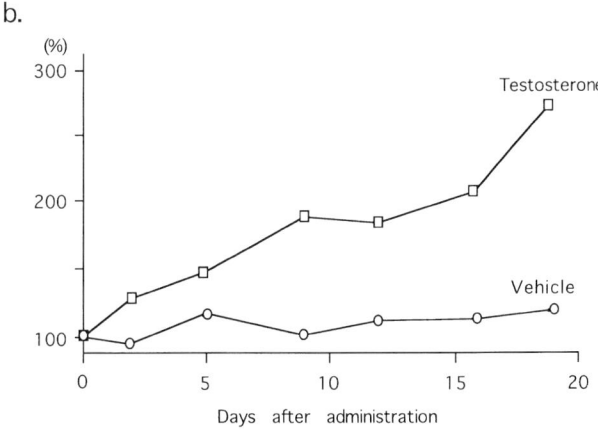

FIG. 2. Effects of thyroxine (**a**) and testosterone (**b**) on the blood HP contents in nonhibernating animals. Thyroxine was dissolved in 0.1 N NaOH and administered after neutralization with phosphate-buffered saline (25 μg/100 g body weight). Testosterone (1 mg/100 g body weight) was administered after dissolving in oil. These hormones were administrated every day. **a** HP (*solid line*) and free thyroxine (*broken line*) contents in the blood. *Vertical axes* show HP contents (% of before administration, *left*) and free thyroxine concentrations (pmol/l, *right*). **b** Testosterone (*squares*) and vehicle (*circles*) were administered, and HP contents in the blood were measured. The *horizontal axis* indicates time in days after administration of these hormones

termination of hibernation strongly suggested that these two hormones regulate a system responsible for hibernation and awakening by carrying hibernation signals to peripheral organs. These findings further suggested that hibernation is controlled through the hypothalamohypophyseal system, probably regulated by a higher center generating a circannual hibernation rhythm (a circannual clock), although less activation of this system during hibernation has been shown by morphological studies [18].

a.

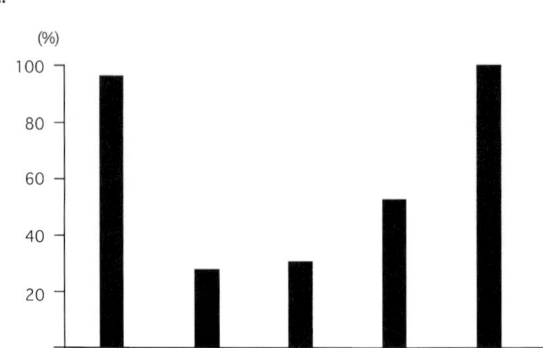

b.

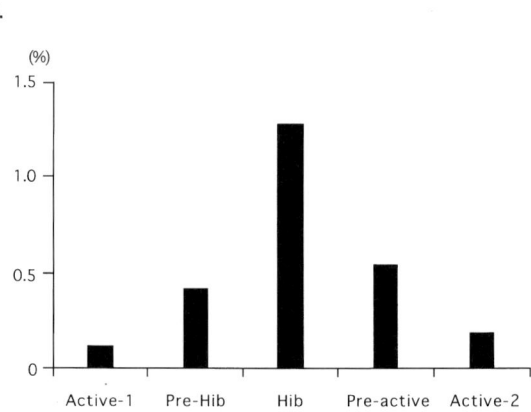

Fɪɢ. 3. HP contents in the blood (**a**) and cerebrospinal fluid (CSF) (**b**) in active, prehibernation (*Pre-Hib*), hibernation (*Hib*) and preactive (*Pre-active*) states. *Active-1*, 1 month before hibernation; Pre-Hib, 10 days before the onset of hibernation; *Hib*, 2 months after hibernation; *Pre-active*, 10 days before the termination of hibernation; *Active-2*, 2 months after the termination of hibernation. Values are expressed as means (*n* = 5). The *vertical axis* shows percent of HP content in the blood at Active-2

Possible Role of HP

Although HP has been identified as a unique molecule controlled by the hibernation rhythm, its physiological role in hibernation remains to be clarified. In a recent study, HP was detected in cerebrospinal fluid (CSF) collected from the lateral ventricle of chipmunks [15]. In the non-hibernating state, the concentration of HP in CSF was less than 1/1000 of that in the blood. HP in CSF began to increase prior to the onset of hibernation and remained high during hibernation and then decreased before its termination. These observations indicated that HP is up-regulated during hibernation only in the brain despite its down-regulation in the blood (Fig. 3). Similar circannual changes in HP in CSF were observed even in animals kept under conditions of constant warmth and a light-dark cycle where lowering of body temperature was disturbed. These results indicated that HP in CSF was regulated by a circannual rhythm similar to that in the blood, assuming that the HP contents in both CSF and the blood were controlled through a hibernation signal transduction system, probably the hypothalamohypophyseal tract.

Analysis of HP in CSF using gel permeation liquid chromatography and Western blotting revealed that HP, which exists as a complex of HP20C and HP55 in the blood [10], was structurally changed in CSF and existed as dissociated HP20C and HP55. This suggested that HP20C functions in the brain through dissociation from HP. As an increase in HP level in CSF was induced simultaneously with decreases in the blood HP level, and no HP gene expression was detected in the brain [17], HP appears to be actively transported across the blood–CSF barrier, probably via the choroid plexus. This suggested the existence of a mechanism by which HP, which has a high molecular weight (140 kDa), can pass through the blood–CSF barrier in association with a circannual hibernation rhythm, strongly indicating the requirement of HP for hibernation. Based on these results, it is reasonable to conclude that HP plays an important role in readjustment of cells and organs for physiological adaptation to hibernation probably through hormonal signal transduction.

Conclusions

Studies of HP expression controlled by a hibernation rhythm can facilitate elucidation of phenomena related to hibernation and hibernation control mechanism. A cirannual rhythm of HP was generated even under conditions of constant warmth where lowering of the body temperature was disturbed, and animals survived low body temperatures only during the period of reduced HP level (hibernation phase). These observations implied that the lowering of the body temperature during hibernation is merely one phenomenon of hibernation, and the greater significance of hibernation is to readjust physiological systems to allow survival of severely reduced body temperatures, which would generally be harmful resulting in cold and ischemic injury of cells and organs. From this point of view, hibernation is considered to be a mechanism by which cells and organs are protected from various injuries.

Recent molecular studies revealed that the HP level is down-regulated in the liver by differential gene expression under the control of humoral signals probably carried by thyroxine and testosterone. This suggests that these hormones, regulated through the hypothalamohypophyseal tract, protect cells and organs by controlling intrinsic cellular activities through differential gene expression. The two hormones presented here with catabolic and anabolic effects on cells, which are promising candidates for carriers of hibernation signals, are common to mammals including humans. Thus, we speculated that the hibernation rhythm may be functioning in humans without lowering the body temperature. The positive correlation between the brain HP content and hibernation emphasizes that HP functions in the brain for controlling hibernation. Understanding the hibernation control mechanism will provide factors and systems for protecting organisms from various harmful conditions and for establishing an artificial state similar to hibernation in nonhibernators.

References

1. Andrews MT, Squire TL, Bowen CM, Rollins MB (1998) Low-temperature carbon utilization is regulated by novel gene activity in the heart of a hibernating mammal. Proc Natl Acad Sci USA 95:8392–8397
2. Belke DD, Pehowich DJ, Wang LCH (1987) Seasonal variation in calcium uptake by cardiac sarcoplasmic reticulum in a hibernator, the richardson's ground squirrel. J Therm Biol 12:53–56

3. Demeneix BA, Henderson NE (1978) Thyroxine metabolism in active and torpid ground squirrels, *Spermophilus richardsoni*. Gen Comp Endocrinol 35:86–92
4. Frerichs KU, Hallenbeck JM (1998) Hibernation in ground squirrels induces state and species-specific tolerance to hypoxia and aglycemia: an in vivo study in hippocampal slices. J Cereb Blood Flow Metab 18:168–175
5. Hudson JW, Wang LCH (1979) Hibernation: endocrinologic aspects. Annu Rev Physiol 41:287–303
6. Kondo N (1986) Excitation-contraction coupling in myocardium of nonhibernating and hibernating chipmunks myocardium: effects of isoprenaline, a high calcium medium and ryanodine. Circ Res 59:221–228
7. Kondo N (1987) Identification of a pre-hibernating state in myocardium from nonhibernating chipmunks. Experientia 43:873–875
8. Kondo N (1997) Physiological and biochemical studies on hibernation control mechanism in mammalian hibernation. In: Hayaishi O, Inoue S (eds) Sleep and sleep disorders: from molecular to behavior. Academic, Tokyo, pp 129–143
9. Kondo N, Joh T (1996) Endogenous circannual rhythm of hibernation-specific proteins associated with hibernation in chipmunks. In: Geiser F, Hulbert AJ, Nicol SC (eds) Adaptation to the cold. University of New England Press, Armidale, pp 341–345
10. Kondo N, Kondo J (1992) Identification of novel blood proteins specific for mammalian hibernation. J Biol Chem 267:473–478
11. Kondo N, Shibata S (1984) Calcium source for excitation-contraction coupling in myocardium of nonhibernating and hibernating chipmunks. Science 225:641–643
12. Lyman CP, O'Brien RC, Greene GC, Papafrangos ED (1981) Hibernation and longevity in the turkish hamster *Mesocricetus brandti*. Science 212:668–670
13. Ohtsu T, Kondo N (1996) Effects of various hormones on the expression of hibernation-specific proteins in hepatocyte primary cultures from chipmunks. Jpn J Physiol 46(suppl):S117
14. Pengelley ET, Asmundson SJ (1974) Circannual rhythmicity in hibernating mammals. In: Pengelley ET (ed) Circannual clock: annual biological rhythms. Academic, San Francisco, pp 95–160
15. Sekijima T, Kondo N (1998) Transport of hibernation-specific proteins (HP) in the brain of chipmunks. Jpn J Physiol 48(suppl):S675
16. Srere HK, Wang LC, Martin SL (1992) Central role for differential gene expression in mammalian hibernation. Proc Natl Acad Sci USA 89:7119–7123
17. Takamatsu N, Ohba KI, Kondo J, Kondo N, Shiba T (1993) Hibernation-associated gene regulation of plasma proteins with a collagen-like domain in mammalian hibernators. Mol Cell Biol 13:1516–1521
18. Wang LCH (1982) Hibernation and the endocrines. In: Lyman CP, Willis JS, Malan A, Wang LCH (eds) Hibernation and torpor in mammals and birds. Academic, San Diego

3. Basic Research of Hypothermia Treatment

Therapeutic Hypothermia in Experimental Models of Traumatic Brain Injury

W. Dalton Dietrich

Introduction

The beneficial effects of mild-to-moderate hypothermia in experimental models of traumatic brain injury (TBI) have been demonstrated in many laboratories [4,11,21,40,45,67]. Using models of diffuse and focal injuries, brain cooling has been shown to both protect against neuronal damage and improve behavioral outcome. Recently, post-traumatic hypothermia has also been reported to protect against axonal damage [39,43]. In addition, the blood–brain barrier (BBB) consequences of TBI are also attenuated by moderate hypothermia [37,57]. Taken together, these investigations using different animal models and various morphological and functional endpoints emphasize how remarkably effective hypothermia can be in protecting the brain. Importantly, these experimental findings with therapeutic hypothermia have been supported by clinical data where hypothermic protection has been demonstrated in patients with severe brain injury [12,13,42].

In contrast to hypothermia, periods of delayed hyperthermia (>39°C) have been reported to worsen outcome in various animal models of brain injury [3,9,18,19]. Clinical data indicate that periods of core and brain hyperthermia occur in head-injured patients [33,35,59]. Therapeutic hypothermia may therefore improve outcome by attenuating the pathophysiological mechanisms associated with brain injury as well as by inhibiting transient elevations in brain temperature.

The purpose of this chapter is to review some of the experimental data regarding the importance of brain temperature in models of TBI. Specific mechanisms by which post-traumatic temperature alterations may affect the pathogenesis of brain injury and outcome will also be reviewed.

Histopathological Protection

Quantitative strategies have been developed to evaluate the effects of post-traumatic temperature on patterns of neuronal vulnerability in models of TBI. The effect of post-traumatic hypothermia on histopathological outcome was first evaluated in a model of parasagittal fluid-

Department of Neurological Surgery, Neurology and Cell Biology and Anatomy, University of Miami School of Medicine, P.O. Box 016960, Miami, FL 33101, USA

percussion (F-P) brain injury [21]. In that study, brain temperature was selectively decreased to 30°C starting 5 min after moderate trauma (1.7–2.2 atm) and maintained for a 3-h period. Three days later, contusion volume and the frequency of damaged cortical neurons were compared in hypothermic vs normothermic (37.5°C) rats. Post-traumatic hypothermia significantly decreased contusion volume and reduced the frequency of damaged cortical neurons. In a controlled cortical impact model in rats, mild hypothermia (32°–33°C) initiated 30 min before trauma and continued for 2 h significantly decreased contusion volume at 14 days [45]. In a model of diffuse traumatic brain injury coupled with hypoxia and hypotension, Yamamoto and colleagues [67] reported that moderate hypothermia (30°C) initiated 15 min after injury and maintained for 60 min provided almost complete protection against secondary insults.

Recently, the progressive nature of histopathological damage after TBI has been emphasized [5,56]. In one study, progressive atrophy was reported up to 1 yr after F-P brain injury [56]. Based on data from studies of cerebral ischemia [14,20], these new TBI findings raised the possibility that post-traumatic hypothermia provided temporary but not long-lasting protection. Thus, the long-term effects of post-traumatic hypothermia have recently been evaluated in a parasagittal F-P model [5]. Following normothermic TBI (2.0–2.3 atm), widespread atrophy of gray matter structures and enlargement of the lateral ventricle were reported at 2 months after trauma. Post-traumatic hypothermia (30°C/3 h) significantly attenuated the degree of cortical atrophy and inhibited the significant increase in ventricular enlargement. Thus, restricted periods of moderate hypothermia immediately after TBI appear to provide some degree of long-term histopathological protection.

Diffuse axonal injury (DAI) leads to disconnection of various brain regions, a condition that translates into much of the morbidity seen with head injury [1,2,28,47,49]. Moderate hypothermia has recently been reported to reduce axonal injury after experimental TBI [39,43]. Marion and White in 1996 first reported that post-traumatic hypothermia after cortical impact injury significantly decreased the frequency of immunoreactive-damaged axons [43]. Taken together, these histopathological and immunocytochemical studies clearly demonstrate that a brief duration of moderate hypothermia following TBI improves neuronal survival and protects against some types of axonal injury.

Behavioral Improvement with Post-traumatic Hypothermia

The histopathological assessment of the injured brain is considered to be an important endpoint for evaluating neuroprotective strategies; nevertheless, it is critical to determine whether histopathological protection correlates with improved behavioral performance. In 1991 Clifton and colleagues first reported that post-traumatic hypothermia (30° and 33°C) improved beam-balance and beam-walking tasks compared to normothermic rats (38°C) after midline F-P brain injury (2.10–2.25 atm) [11]. Subsequent studies using the F-P model demonstrated that post-traumatic hypothermia (30°C/3 h) improved both sensorimotor and cognitive behavioral deficits compared to normothermic rats [4,40]. Cognitive deficits including memory impairments are commonly observed in humans suffering brain injury. Thus, the ability to improve cognitive function after TBI by hypothermic strategies appears to be an exciting direction for treating the post-injured patient.

In clinical studies, post-traumatic hypothermia has also been reported to be beneficial [13,41,42,51,54]. Recently, Marion and colleagues demonstrated that post-traumatic hypothermia (32°–33°C/24 h) in patients with severe TBI and coma scores on admission of 5–7 hastened neurologic recovery and may have improved outcome [42]. These clinical findings are important because they indicate that preclinical data are relevant to the clinical condition of TBI.

Post-traumatic Hyperthermia

In contrast to hypothermia, post-traumatic hyperthermia (>39°C) has been shown to worsen outcome in experimental models of brain injury [9,18,19,25]. In one study, artificially elevating brain temperature to 39°C for a 3-h period, 24 h after moderate parasagittal F-P injury increased mortality compared to normothermic rats [25]. In that study, delayed hyperthermia also significantly increased contusion volume and increased the frequency of abnormal appearing myelinated axons. Many head-injured patients experience fever, and recent data indicate that bladder temperature and rectal temperature often underrepresent brain temperature after TBI, particularly when the patient is hypo- or hyperthermic [33,35]. Thus, delayed elevations in brain temperature may represent a clinically important secondary-injury mechanism. In the clinical setting, especially following severe brain trauma, fever should be aggressively treated.

Mechanisms of Hypothermic Protection

The pathophysiology of brain injury is complex, and many injury processes have been reported to be temperature-sensitive (for recent reviews see [14,24]). In addition to slowing oxygen consumption, post-traumatic hypothermia has been reported to blunt the rise in extracellular levels of excitatory amino acids after parasagittal F-P injury [30]. However, in a model of controlled cortical impact, hypothermia failed to attenuate the rise in extracellular asparate and glutamate, although contusion volume was significantly reduced by cooling [45]. Thus, variables including injury severity and where neurochemical samples are obtained in relation to contusion may significantly affect neurochemical results with therapeutic hypothermia. Post-traumatic hypothermia has also been reported to reduce the production of hydroxyl radicals compared to normothermic trauma [30]. Indeed, it has become clear that a reason why temperature is such an important factor in traumatic and ischemic outcome is because variations in temperature have dramatic effects on multiple pathophysiological mechanisms.

Blood-Brain Barrier Damage

Alterations in BBB dysfunction and cerebrovascular damage after TBI and other acute neurological states are believed to participate in neuronal damage [6,16,22,46,60]. Alterations in BBB permeability may contribute to the detrimental effects of TBI through excitotoxic processes, as well as by allowing abnormal passage of blood-borne exogenous neurotransmitters into the brain and influencing injury processes [48]. Experimental data have demonstrated that post-injury temperature modulations significantly influence vascular permeability. For example, while moderate hypothermia after transient global ischemia attenuates the degree of postischemic horseradish peroxidase (HRP) extravasation compared to normothermia, hyperthermia aggravates the permeability alterations [18]. In models of TBI, the detrimental consequences of TBI on BBB damage have also been reported to be reduced by post-traumatic hypothermia [37,57]. In addition, delayed post-traumatic hyperthermia induced 24 h after moderate F-P brain injury has been reported to increase HRP extravasation compared to normothermia [25]. Thus, post-traumatic temperature alterations may influence traumatic outcome by altering the vascular and permeability consequences of TBI.

Gene Expression and Apoptosis

Brain trauma has been reported to induce a variety of genes and proteins that would be expected to influence traumatic outcome [32,34,50,62]. Alterations in post-traumatic temperature may potentially affect the induction of various genes in the injured brain. For example, hypothermia was reported to attenuate the normal increase in interleukin-1beta RNA in traumatized rats [31]. In a model of transient global forebrain ischemia, Kamme and colleagues reported that hypothermia selectively increased the expression of specific genes [38]. In addition, the late induction of other genes occurred earlier under hypothermic conditions. Taken together, these results suggest that hypothermia may protect nervous tissues by attenuating the expression of genes associated with cell death and/or by enhancing the expression of neuroprotective or repair genes. Apoptosis has recently been implicated in the pathophysiology of traumatic brain injury [15,52]. Importantly, recent data indicate that hypothermia may also be neuroprotective by reducing neuronal apoptosis. In an experimental model of hypoxia-ischemia, moderate hypothermia reduced the fraction of apoptotic cells but not cells undergoing necrosis [27]. The consequences of therapeutic hypothermia on gene expression after TBI represents an exciting direction on trauma research.

Nitric Oxide

Recent data have implicated the importance of nitric oxide (NO) in the pathophysiology of TBI. Using a moderate F-P model, Wada and colleagues reported the immediate but transient increase in constitutive nitric oxide synthase (cNOS) activity within the histopathologically injured cortical region [64]. This increase in cNOS activity was followed by a sustained reduction in cNOS activity below control levels. In that study, post-treatment with L-arginine, the precursor of NO, reduced overall contusion volume. In another study, inducible NOS (iNOS) activity was shown to increase at 7 days after TBI [65]. Additionally, inhibition of iNOS activity by aminoguanidine treatment reduced the number of damaged cortical neurons. Recently, the effects of post-traumatic hypothermia on NOS activity have been reported [7]. Hypothermia (30°C) decreased the acute activation of cNOS, preserved cNOS activity at later post-traumatic periods, and prevented the delayed induction of iNOS compared to normothermic traumatized animals. Taken together, these studies indicate that therapeutic hypothermia may improve outcome after TBI by targeting the NO pathway.

Cerebral Blood Flow

The consequences of brain trauma on local cerebral blood flow (lCBF) have been documented in clinical studies and in several experimental models [17,23,26,29,36,58]. Perfusion deficits and cerebral ischemia are believed to represent important secondary injury mechanisms after TBI [44,68]. The hemodynamic consequences of moderate and severe F-P brain injury have recently been shown to differ. While moderate injury leads to reductions in lCBF of approximately 40% of control [23,29] severe trauma leads to reductions in lCBF that reach ischemic levels [26]. Most recently, the consequences of early post-traumatic brain hypothermia on lCBF have been reported after moderate F-P brain injury. In 1999, Zhao and colleagues reported that moderate hypothermia (30°C/3h) significantly lowered lCBF at 6 h after TBI compared to normothermic animals [69]. As a consequence, a state of mild metabolism-greater-than-blood-flow dissociation was demonstrated. Thus, post-traumatic brain hypothermia does not appear to improve outcome by increasing post-traumatic lCBF.

Inflammation

Inflammatory processes are believed to participate in the pathogenesis on TBI [10,53,63]. Strategies that target inflammation after cerebral ischemia have been reported to improve outcome. Of interest to the present discussion is the fact that therapeutic hypothermia has been reported to reduce the accumulation of polymorphonuclear leukocytes (PMNL) after focal cerebral ischemia [61]. Chatzipanteli and colleagues have recently demonstrated that therapeutic hypothermia after moderate F-P brain injury also reduces the degree of PMNL accumulation in damaged areas at 3 h and 3 days after TBI [8]. In that study, myeloperoxidase (MPO) activity was used as an indicator of PMNL accumulation. Additionally, post-traumatic brain hyperthermia (39°C/3 h) elevated MPO activity compared to normothermic values at both 3 h and 3 days after TBI. Taken together, these findings indicate that temperature-dependent alterations in PMNL accumulation after TBI may influence traumatic outcome.

Summary and Future Directions

Based on experimental data, mild-to-moderate hypothermia appears to be one of the most potent therapeutic approaches to treating brain trauma. Clearly the ability of temperature to target multiple pathophysiological processes may help explain why hypothermia works in multiple trauma models. Clinical trials are still required to evaluate systematically the beneficial and harmful effects of clinical hypothermia in different populations of head-injured patients. Because prolonged periods of hypothermia can create problems in terms of patient care, combination therapy including mild hypothermia and neuroprotective agents must be investigated in established models of TBI. The continued search for pharmacologic agents that reduce core and brain temperature when given systemically is also an exciting direction for research. The development of this class of drugs would allow emergency staff to administer agents at early periods after brain trauma. In this regard, additional studies are required to establish the therapeutic window for hypothermia under mild, moderate, and severe injury conditions.

References

1. Adams JH, Graham DI, Murray LS, Scott G (1982) Diffuse axonal injury due to nonmissle head injury in humans: An analysis of 45 cases. Ann Neurol 12:557–563
2. Adams JH, Doyle D, Ford I, Graham DI, McLellan D (1989) Diffuse axonal injury in head injury: Definition, diagnosis and grading. Histopathology 15:49–59
3. Baena RC, Busto R, Dietrich WD, Globus MY-T, Ginsberg MD (1997) Hyperthermia delayed by 24 hours aggravates neuronal damage in rat hippocampus following global ischemia. Neurology 48:768–773
4. Bramlett H, Green EJ, Dietrich WD, Busto R, Globus MY-T, Ginsberg MD (1995) Post-traumatic brain hypothermia provides protection from sensorimotor and cognitive behavioral deficits. J Neurotrauma 12:289–298
5. Bramlett HM, Dietrich WD, Green EJ, Busto R (1997) Chronic histopathological consequences of fluid-percussion brain injury: Effects of posttraumatic hypothermia. Acta Neuropath 93:190–199

6. Chan PH, Schmidley JW, Fishman RA, Longar SM (1984) Brain injury, edema, and vascular permeability changes induced by oxygen-derived free radicals. Neurology 34:315–320

7. Chatzipanteli K, Wada K, Busto R, Dietrich WD (1999) Effects of moderate hypothermia on constitutive and inducible nitric oxide synthase activities after traumatic brain injury. J Neurochem 72:2047–2052

8. Chatzipanteli K, Alonso O, Kraydieh S, Dietrich WD (2000) Importance of posttraumatic hypothermia and hyperthermia on the inflammatory response after fluid percussion brain injury. Biochemical and immunocytochemical studies. J Cereb Blood Flow Metab 20:531–542

9. Chen H, Chopp M, Welch KMA (1991) Effect of hyperthermia on the ischemic infarct volume after middle cerebral artery occlusion in the rat. Neurology 41:1133–1135

10. Clark RSB, Schiding JK, Kaczorowski SL, Marion DW, Kochanek PM (1994) Neutrophil accumulation after traumatic brain injury in rats: Comparison of weight drop and controlled cortical impact models. J Neurotrauma 11:499–506

11. Clifton GL, Jiang JY, Lyeth BG, Jenkins LW, Hamm RJ, Hayes RL (1991) Marked protection by moderate hypothermia after experimental traumatic brain injury. J Cereb Blood Flow Metab 11:114–121

12. Clifton GL, Allen S, Barrodale P, Plenger P, Berry J, Koch S, Fletcher J, Hayes RL, Choi SG (1993) A phase II study of moderate hypothermia in severe brain injury. J Neurotrauma 10:263–271

13. Clifton GL (1995) Systemic hypothermia in treatment of severe brain injury: a review and update. J Neurotrauma 12:923–927

14. Colbourne F, Sutherland G, Corbett D (1997) Postischemic hypothermia. A critical appraisal with implications for clinical treatment. Molec Neurobiol 14:171–201

15. Conti AC, Raghupati R, Trojanwski JQ, McIntosh TK (1998) Experimental brain injury induces regionally distinct apoptosis during the acute and delayed post-traumatic period. J Neurosci 18:5663–5672

16. Cortez SC, McIntosh TK, Noble LJ (1989) Experimental fluid percussion brain injury: Vascular disruption and neuronal and glial alterations. Brain Res 482:272–282

17. DeWitt DS, Prough DS, Tayor CT, Whitley JM (1992) Reduced cerebral blood flow, oxygen delivery, and electroencephalographic activity after traumatic brain injury and mild hemorrhage in cats. J Neurosurg 76:812–821

18. Dietrich WD, Busto R, Halley M, Valdes I (1990) The importance of brain temperature in alterations of the blood-brain barrier following cerebral ischemia. J Neuropathol Exp Neurol 49:486–497

19. Dietrich WD, Busto R, Valdes I, Loor Y (1990) Effects of normothermic versus mild hyperthermic forebrain ischemia in rats. Stroke 21:1318–1325

20. Dietrich WD, Busto R, Alonso O, Globus MY-T, Ginsberg MD (1993) Intraischemic but not postischemic brain hypothermia protects chronically following global forebrain ischemia in rats. J Cereb Blood Flow Metab 13:541–549

21. Dietrich WD, Alonso O, Busto R, Globus MY-T, Ginsberg MD (1994) Post-traumatic brain hypothermia reduces histopathological damage following concussive brain injury in the rat. Acta Neuropathol 87:250–258

22. Dietrich WD, Alonso O, Halley M (1994) Early microvascular and neuronal consequences of traumatic brain injury: A light and electron microscopic study in rats. J Neurotrauma 11:289–301

23. Dietrich WD, Alonso O, Busto R, Prado R, Dewanjee S, Dewanjee MK, Ginsberg MD (1996) Widespread hemodynamic depression and focal platelet accumulation after fluid percussion brain injury: A double-label autoradiographic study in rats. J Cereb Blood Flow Met 16:481–489

24. Dietrich WD, Busto R, Globus MY-T, Ginsberg MD (1996) Brain damage and temperature: Cellular and molecular mechanisms. In: Siesjo B, Wieloch T (eds) Cellular and Molecular Mechanisms of Ischemic Brain Damage. Lippincott-Raven Publishers, Philadelphia, PA, Advances in Nuerology 71:177–198

25. Dietrich WD, Alonso O, Halley M, Busto R (1996) Delayed posttraumatic brain hyperthermia worsens outcome after fluid percussion brain injury: A light and electron microscopic study in rats. Neurosurgery 38:533–541

26. Dietrich WD, Alonso O, Busto R, Dewanjee MK, Ginsberg MD (1998) Post-traumatic cerebral ischemia after fluid percussion brain injury: An autoradiographic and histopathological study in rats. Neurosurgery 43:585–594

27. Edwards AD, Uue X, Squier MV, Thoresen M, Cady EB, Penrice J, Cooper CE, Wyatt JS, Reynolds EOR, Mehmet H (1995) Specific inhibition of apoptosis after hypoxia-ischaema by moderate post-insult hypothermia. Biochem Biophys Res Comm 217:1193–1199

28. Gennarelli TA, Thibault LE, Adams JH, Graham DI, Thompson CJ, Marcincin RP (1982) Diffuse axonal injury and traumatic coma in the primate. Ann Neurol 12:564–574

29. Ginsberg MD, Zhao W, Alonso O, Loor-Estades JY, Dietrich WD, Busto R (1997) Uncoupling of local cerebral glucose metabolism and blood flow after acute fluid-percussion injury in rats. Am J Physiol 272:H2859–2868

30. Globus MYT, Alonso O, Dietrich WD, Busto R, Ginsberg MD (1995) Glutamate release and free radical production following brain injury: Effects of posttraumatic hypothermia. J Neurotrauma 65:1704–1711

31. Goss JR, Styren PO, Miller PO, Kochanek PM, Palmer DW, Marion DW, DeKosky ST (1995) Hypothermia attenuates the normal increase in interleukin-1beta RNA and nerve growth factor following traumatic brain injury in the rat. J Neurotrauma 12:159–167

32. Goss JR, O'Malley ME, Zou L, Styren SD, Kochanek PM, DeKosky ST (1998) Astrocytes are the major source of nerve growth factor upregulation following traumatic brain injury in the rat. Exp Neuropl 149:301–309

33. Hayashi N, Hirayama T, Ohata M (1993) The computed cerebral hypothermia management technique to the critical head injury patients. Adv Neurotrauma Res 5:61–64

34. Hayes RL, Yang K, Raghupathi R, McIntosh TK (1995) Changes in gene expression following traumatic brain injury. J Neurotrauma 12:779–790

35. Henker RA, Brown SD, Marion DW (1998) Comparisons of brain temperature with bladder and rectal temperature in adults with severe head injury. Neurosurg 42:1071–1075

36. Ishige N, Pitts LH, Berry I, Carlson SG, Nishimura MC, Moseley ME, Weinstein PR (1987) The effect of hypoxia on traumatic head injury in rats: Alterations in neurologic function, brain edema, and cerebral blood flow. J Cereb Blood Flow Metabol 7:759–767

37. Jiang JY, Lyeth BG, Kapasi MZ, Jenkins LW, Povlishock JT (1992) Moderate hypothermia reduces blood-brain barrier disruption following traumatic brain injury in the rat. Acta Neuropathol 84:495–500

38. Kamme F, Campell K, Wieloch T (1995) Biphasic expression of the Fos and Jun families of transcription factors following transient forebrain ischaemia in the rat: Effect of hypothermia. European J Neurosci 7:2007–2016

39. Koizumi H, Povlishock JT (1998) Posttraumatic hypothermia in the treatment of axonal damage in an animal model of traumatic axonal injury. J Neurosurg 89:303–309

40. Lyeth BG, Jiang JY, Shanliang L (1993) Behavioral protection by moderate hypothermia initiated after experimental traumatic brain injury. J Neurotrauma 10:57–64

41. Marion DW, Obrist WD, Carlier PM, Penrod LE, Darby JM (1993) The use of moderate therapeutic hypothermia for patients with severe head injuries: A preliminary report. J Neurosurg 79:354–362

42. Marion DW, Penrod LE, Kelsey SF, Obrist WD, Kochanek PM, Palmer AM, Wisniewki SR, DeKosky ST (1997) Treatment of traumatic brain injury with moderate hypothermia. N Eng J Med 336:540–546

43. Marion DW, White MJ (1996) Treatment of experimental brain injury with moderate hypothermia and 21-aminosteroids. J Neurotrauma 13:139–147

44. Miller JD (1985) Head injury and brain ischemia: Implication for therapy. Br J Anaesth 57:120–129

45. Palmer AM, Marion DW, Botsceller ML, Redd EE (1993) Therapeutic hypothermia is cytoprotective without attenuating the traumatic brain injury-induced elevations in interstitial concentrations of aspartate and glutamate. J Neurotrauma 10:363–372

46. Povlishock JT, Becker DP, Sullivan HG, Miller JD (1978) Vascular permeability alterations to horseradish peroxidase in experimental brain injury. Brain Res 153:223–239

47. Povlishock JT, Becker DP, Cheng CLY, Vaughan GW (1983) Axonal changes in minor head injury. J Neuropathol Exp Neurol 42:225–242

48. Povlishock JT, Dietrich WD (1992) The blood-brain barrier in brain injury: An overview. In: Globus MY-T, Dietrich WD (eds) The Role of Neurotransmitters in Brain Injury. Plenum Publishing, New York, pp 265–269
49. Povlishock JT (1992) Traumatically induced axonal injury: Pathogenesis and pathobiological implications. Brain Pathol 2:1–12
50. Raghupathi R, Welsh FA, Lowenstein DH, Gennarelli TA, McIntosh TK (1995) Regional induction of c-fos and heat shock protein 72 mRNA following fluid-pecussion brain injury in the rat. J Cereb Blood Flow Metab 15:467–473
51. Resnick DK, Marion DW, Darby JM (1994) The effect of hypothermia on the incidence of delayed traumatic intracerebral hemorrhage. Neurosurg 34:252–256
52. Rink A, Fung KM, Trojanowski JQ, Lee VM-Y, Neugbauer E, McIntosh TK (1995) Evidence of apoptotic cell death after experimental traumatic brain injury in the rat. Am J Pathol 147:1575–1583
53. Schoettle RJ, Kochanek PM, Magargee MJ, Uhl MW, Nemoto EM (1990) Early polymorphonuclear leukocyte accumulation correlates with the development of posttraumatic cerebral edema in rats. J Neurotrauma 7:207–217
54. Shiozaki T, Sugimoto H, Taneda M, Yoshida H, Iwai A, Yoshioka T, Sugimoto T (1993) Effect of mild hypothermia on uncontrollable intracranial hypertension after severe head injury. J Neurosurg 79:363–368
55. Shiozaki T, Sugimoto H, Taneda M, Oda J, Tanaka H, Hiraide A, Shimazu T (1998) Selection of severely head injured patients for mild hypothermia therapy. J Neurosurg 89:206–211
56. Smith DG, Chen X-H, Pierce ES, McIntosh TK (1997) Progressive atrophy and neuronal death for one year following brain trauma in the rat. J Neurotrauma 14:715–727
57. Smith SL, Hall ED (1996) Mild pre- and posttraumatic hypothermia attenuates blood-brain barrier damage following controlled cortical impact injury in the rat. J Neurotrauma 13:1–9
58. Steiger H-J, Asslid R, Stooss R, Seiler RW (1994) Transcranial Doppler monitoring in head injury: Relationship between type of injury, flow velocities, vasoreactivity and outcome. Neurosurgery 34:79–86
59. Sternau L, Thompson C, Dietrich WD, Busto R, Globus MY-T, Ginsberg MD (1991) Intracranial tempertuare: Observations in human brain. J Cereb Blood Flow Metab 11(2):S123
60. Tanno H, Nockels RP, Pitts LH, Noble LJ (1992) Breakdown of the blood-brain barrier after fluid percussion brain injury in the rat: Part 2: Effect of hypoxia on permeability to plasma proteins. J Neurotrauma 9:335–347
61. Toyoda T, Suzuki S, Kaddell NF, Lee KS (1996) Intraischemic hypothermia attenuates neurophil infiltration in the rat neocortex after focal ischemia-reperfusion injury. Neurosurg 39:1200–1205
62. Truettner J, Schmidt-Kastner R, Busto R, Alonso OF, Loor JY, Dietrich WD, Ginsberg MD (1995) Expression of brain-derived neurotrophic factor, nerve growth factor, and heat shock protein HSP70 following fluid percussion brain injury in rats. J Neurotrauma 16:471–486
63. Uhl MW, Biagas KV, Grundl PD, Barmada MA, Schiding JK, Nemoto EM, Kochanek PM (1994) Effects of neutropenia on edema, histology, and cerebral blood flow after traumatic brain injury in rats. J Neurotrauma 11:303–315
64. Wada K, Chatzipantelli K, Busto R, Dietrich WD (1998) The role of nitric oxide on the pathophysiology of traumatic brain injury in the rat. J Neurosurgery 89:807–818
65. Wada K, Chatzipantelli K, Busto R, Kraydieh S, Dietrich WD (1998) Inducible nitric oxide synthase activation after traumatic brain injury. Neurosurgery 43:1427–1436
66. Wada K, Chatzipantelli K, Busto R, Dietrich WD (1999) Effects of L-NAME and 7-NI on NOS catalytic activity and behavioral outcome after traumatic brain injury in the rat. J Neurotrauma 16:203–212
67. Yamamoto M, Marmarou CR, Stiefel MF, Beaumont A, Marmarou A (1999) Neuroprotective effect of hypothermia on neuronal injury in diffuse traumatic brain injury coupled with hypoxia and hypotension. J Neurotrauma 16:487–500
68. Young W (1988) Secondary CNS injury. J Neurotrauma 5:219–221
69. Zhao W, Alonso O, Loor J, Busto R, Ginsberg MD (1999) Influence of early posttraumatic hypothermia therapy on local cerebral blood flow and glucose metabolism after fluid-percussion brain injury. J Neurosurg 90:510–519

Mild Hypothermia Amelioration of Damage During Rat Spinal Cord Injury: Inhibition of Pathological Microglial Proliferation and Improvement of Hind-limb Motor Function

Tadanori Ogata[1], Tadao Morino[1], Jun Takeba[1], Yoshiro Matsuda[1], Hideo Okumura[1], Taihoh Shibata[1], Peter Schubert[2], and Kiyoshi Kataoka[3]

Summary. The effects of mild hypothermic treatment on motor functions and immunological changes were tested in rats after spinal cord injuries. To simulate spinal cord injury, the rat spinal cord was exposed at the 11th vertebra and compressed using 20 g of weight for 20 min. The temperature of the animals was fixed for 1 h from the beginning of the compression period at 33°C and 37°C for the mild hypothermic treatment and the control, respectively. At 24 h after injury, the frequency of vertical movement (standing) during a 1-h period, which reflected rat hind-limb function, of both the control animals and the hypothermia-treated animals was about 45% that of the sham animals, which had undergone laminectomy without compression. The hind-limb function of hypothermia-treated animals gradually increased and completely recovered at 72 h after injury, whereas the control animals showed little recovery. A marked proliferation of positive isolectin-staining microglia was observed in the control animals from 48 h after the injury. On the other hand, in both hypothermia-treated and sham animals, a small number of microglia were observed up to 72 h after the injury. These results suggest that mild hypothermia is an effective treatment for secondary neuronal damage after spinal cord injury, and inhibition of microglial proliferation may be one of the mechanisms of the mild hypothermic effect.

Key words. Mild hypothermia, Microglia, Spinal cord, Behavior, Animal model

Introduction

Treatment using mild hypothermia—temperatures of 33°–35°C—has been reported to be an effective therapeutic method for central nervous system damage such as brain trauma and ischemia. Using experimental brain neuron damage models for trauma [11] or ischemia [4], the efficacy of hypothermia has been clearly proven. The working mechanism of the neuroprotective hypothermic treatment has been believed to be complicated. Burger et al. [2]

[1] Department of Orthopaedic Surgery, Ehime University School of Medicine, Shitsukawa, Shigenobu-cho, Onsen-gun, Ehime 791-0295, Japan
[2] Max-Planck-Institute for Neurobiology, Department of Neuromorphology, Am Klopferspitz 18a, Martinsried 82152, Germany
[3] Department of Physiology, Ehime University School of Medicine, Shitsukawa, Shigenobu-cho, Onsen-gun, Ehime 791-0295, Japan

reported that hypothermic treatment decreased intracranial pressure and increased micro-circulation. Dietrich et al. [10] reported that hypothermic treatment effectively preserved the blood-brain barrier against ischemic damage. The ischemia-induced elevation of extracellular glutamate concentration has been believed to be one of the most dangerous triggers for neuronal damage. Busto et al. [5] reported that this ischemia-induced excitatory neurotransmitter release is temperature-dependent, so hypothermic treatment inhibits the elevation of extracellular glutamate. This may explain, at least partly, the working mechanism of hypothermic treatment.

Recently the inflammatory response has become a candidate for a determining factor of an injured neuron's fate after central nervous injury. Toyoda et al. [17] reported that intraischemic hypothermia decreased the neutrophil inflammatory response to transient focal ischemia in the rat neocortex. Microglia, immune cells in the central nervous system (CNS), mainly take charge of the inflammatory response against infections. Moreover in several CNS pathological conditions such as trauma [15] and ischemia [16], microglia have been reported to proliferate and be activated. Activated microglia seems to accelerate neuronal damage by release of nitric oxide, superoxide, and cytokines such as tumor necrosis factor-α (TNF-α). One study revealed a microglial contribution to the progress of Alzheimer's disease [13]. To clarify one of the working mechanisms of hypothermic treatment of spinal cord injury, we examined the effect of mild hypothermia on the proliferation of microglia in spinal cord tissue and on the behavioral activity of animals after compression injuries in the rat spinal cord.

Materials and Methods

Spinal Cord Mild Compression Model

The 250-g female Wistar rats were used for this study. Under general anesthesia using halothane, the rat spinal cord was carefully exposed by removing vertebral lamina at the 11th vertebra level. Direct compression was performed using a 20-g weight, of which the dura contact portion was made of soft, round silicone to prevent violent injury that might cause axonal tearing or hemorrhaging in the spinal cord. Using this model, we did not see any serious damage, such as hyperextension or paresis of hind-limbs or histological hemorrhaging with tissue destruction of the compressed portion. The weight was gently put on the dura mater of thoracic spinal cord for 20 min. The temperature of the animals was controlled for 1 h from the beginning of the compression period: 33°C and 37°C for the mild hypothermic treatment group and the controls, respectively. Temperature control was performed using a water-cooling mat and a small-animal body temperature controller by infrared irradiation (IFR-100; Unique Medical Co., Tokyo, Japan). The results were evaluated by comparison to sham animals, which underwent laminectomy without spinal cord compression. The histological and the behavioral changes of treated animals were observed 24, 48, and 72 h after compression.

Analysis of Animal Behavior

Animal behavior was analyzed using Scanet MV-10 (MATYS Toyo Sangyo, Japan). Infrared detector rays in a box ($50 \times 50 \times 35$ cm) recognized and recorded animal movement that passed through the rays. There were both lower and upper detectors in the machine. The horizontal movement was quantified using the lower detector. When the animals moved 6 mm, the machine recognized one "small movement." A 48-mm movement was recognized as one "large movement." The hind-limb function of the rat was evaluated by counting the frequency of vertical movements using the upper detector. Rats often take the position of lifting their fore-limbs and supporting their weight by only their hind-limbs. Here we call this vertical movement "standing." Rats usually take this standing posture about 50–60 times per hour. A decrease of the standing frequency should reveal the severity of the thoracic spinal cord injury. Rats often raised their head without lifting their fore-limbs. The upper detector was set high enough to prevent recognition of such small vertical movements. Behavioral analysis was performed in a dark, silent room to prevent any influence of environmental stimulation. Results were expressed as percentages of the average values in the sham animals.

Histological Examination

The animals were sacrificed by deep anesthesia and following decapitation. The spinal cord of the 11th vertebral level (compression part) was immediately removed, and coronal freezing microtome sections of 5 μm thickness were prepared. The proliferated microglia in spinal cord slices were stained with isolectin (*Griffonia simplicifolia* IB4). The sections were fixed on glass slides by 4% paraformaldehyde in phosphate-buffered saline (PBS) for 5 min. Then, after washing twice with PBS, endogenous peroxidase was blocked by treatment with 0.3% H_2O_2/methanol for 15 min. After pretreatment with 0.1% Triton-X (Wako Chemicals, Osaka, Japan) in PBS for 15 min, slices on the slides were exposed to peroxidase-labeled isolectin (L5391; Sigma, St. Louis, MO, USA). 0.1% Triton-X 5 μg/ml in PBS, overnight at 4°C. Sections were then color developed using diaminobenzidine (DAB; Wako Chemicals) substrate (0.02% H_2O_2 plus 0.1% DAB in 0.1 M Tris buffer) for 7 min and washed immediately with water for 20 min. Sections were dehydrated through graded alcohols and xylene and were then mounted in Harleco Synthetic Resin (HSR). To determine the specificity of the immunoreaction, control sections were processed as above without the presence of isolectin. To quantify microglia proliferation, fine photographs were taken and the lectin-positive cells in the gray matter were counted by three people who did not have any information about the pictures. The average of the three counts was employed, and data were expressed as the number of cells per area of gray matter. Area of gray matter was calculated from the picture using NIH Image software. The existence of neuronal cells was recognized by microtubule-associated protein 2 (Amersham). Activation of microglia was detected by OX42 staining (Serotec, Japan) which has been reported to recognize activated immune cells [9].

Results

In the normal (without treatment) or sham animals, only a few microglia were observed in one spinal cord slice (1–3 microglia per slice, data not shown). At 48 h after compression of the spinal cord by a 20-g weight for 20 min, a remarkable proliferation of microglia (Fig. 1a), detected by lectin-staining, was observed. This compression injury-induced microglia proliferation appeared mainly in gray matter (more than 90% of proliferated microglia). The hypothermic treatment at 33°C during the compression period and the following 40 min potently inhibited the microglial proliferation (Fig. 1b). Only a few lectin-positive cells were observed in injured spinal cord tissue.

Figure 2 shows the time course of microglial appearance after spinal cord injury. At 24 h after compression, the number of lectin-positive cells was low. During the following 24 h, a marked proliferation of microglia (more than 5 times higher than those in 24-h slices) was observed in normothermic (37°C) animals. At 72 h after compression a large number of the proliferated microglia were still seen in normothermic animals, but no increase was observed in hypothermic animals. In slices from normothermic animals at 48 and 72 h after injury, most of the proliferated microglia were positive to OX-42 staining (data not shown), which recog-

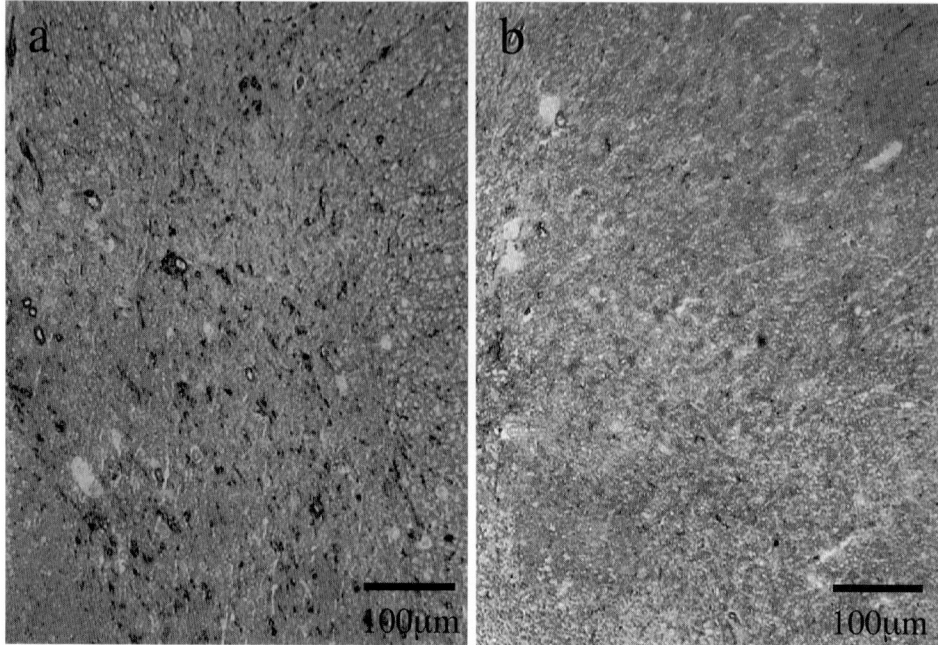

FIG. 1. Lectin staining of injured spinal cord gray matter. The spinal section was obtained 48 h after spinal cord injury from normothermic (**a**, 37°C) and hypothermic (**b**, 33°C) animals. It was stained with isolectin

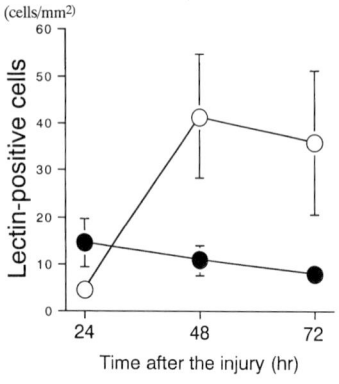

FIG. 2. Microglia proliferation after spinal cord injury. Spinal cord compression injury was performed in temperature-controlled animals. The temperature of animals was controlled for 1 h from the beginning of the compression period at 33°C (*closed circles*) and 37°C (*open circles*) for mild hypothermia and normothermia, respectively. The spinal cords were removed from the animals at 24, 48, and 72 h after spinal cord injury. The coronal slices were stained by lectin, and the positive cells were counted. Data are means ± SEM (*n* = 6–8)

nizes reactive immune cells, indicating that the proliferated microglia were activated. Most of the proliferated microglia in the injured spinal cord gray matter of normothermic animals had disappeared 7 days after compression (data not shown). Neuronal survival in the compressed part was evaluated 1 week after the spinal cord injury by microtubule-associated protein 2 staining (data not shown). The number of microtubule-associated protein 2-positive neurons was markedly decreased in the ventral horn of normothermic animals, whereas most of the neurons were preserved in hypothermic animals.

The animals' behavior after spinal cord compression was compared between normothermic and hypothermic animals (Fig. 3). Three behaviors were evaluated: frequency of small movement, large movement, and "standing." At 24 h after spinal cord injury, the frequency of

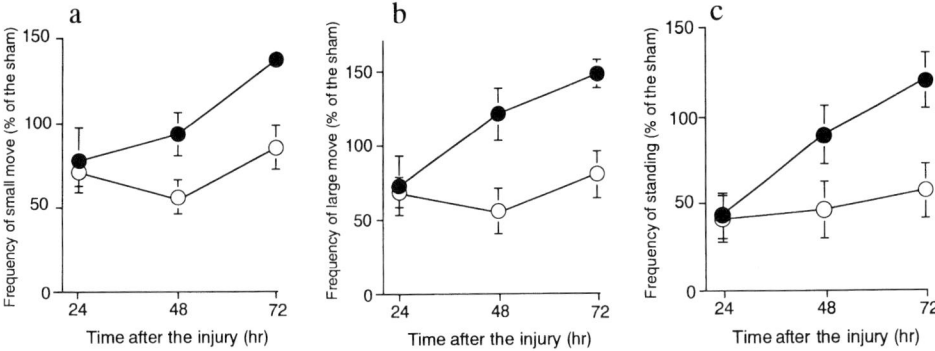

FIG. 3. Effect of hypothermic treatment on animal behaviour. Spinal cord compression injury was performed in temperature-controlled animals at 33°C (*closed circles*) and 37°C (*open circles*). The animal behavior was then analyzed using Scanet MV-10 at 24, 48, and 72 h after injury. Two horizontal movements (**a**, small movements; **b**, large movements) and one vertical movement (**c**, standing) were detected. Data are means ± SEM ($n = 6$–7)

small movements (Fig. 3a: one count per 6 mm horizontal movement) of both normothermic and hypothermic animals decreased to 70%–75% of that of sham animals. Small movement activity of hypothermia-treated animals increased with time and completely recovered by 72 h after the compression injury. In contrast, no significant recovery was detected in the normothermic group up to 72 h after the compression. The effect of hypothermia on large movements was more obvious (Fig. 3b: one count per 48 mm horizontal movement). Complete recovery of large movements was observed in the hypothermia-treated rats 48 h after the injury, whereas the normothermic groups showed no recovery. Because the spinal cord injury was to the thoracic spinal cord, the loss of motor function should occur only in the hind-limbs, with the activity of the fore-limbs intact. The frequency of vertical movement may reveal the severity of spinal cord injury most clearly in this experiment. Vertical movement means "standing" behavior; animals raised their heads and sustained their weight only by their hind-limbs. In normal rats the frequency of "standing" was about 50 to 60 times per hour. Twenty-four hours after spinal cord injury, the frequency in both normothermic and hypothermic groups was about 45% of that of the sham animals (Fig. 3c). The disturbance of vertical motor activity by thoracic spinal cord injury was more severe than that of horizontal motor activity (at 24 h: small movements 70%–80%, large movements 70%–75%). This seems reasonable, as horizontal motor activity is influenced by the "intact" fore-limbs. Vertical movement activity of hypothermia-treated animals increased with time and completely recovered at 72 h after the compression injury. In contrast, no significant recovery was observed in the normothermic group up to 72 h after spinal cord compression.

Discussion

There have been many trials to evaluate spinal cord injury. Disturbance of hind-limb motor ability has usually been used to analyze and evaluate thoracic spinal cord injury. In the present study, to quantify the severity of spinal cord damage in the compressed part we detected the frequency of the "standing" posture. Typical evaluation methods include Tarloph's score, the inclined plane test, and analysis of foot printing such as stride length and base of support.

Tarloph's score is not useful for quantifying motor ability. The inclined plane test and foot printing are influenced by intact fore-limb motor ability, such as "horizontal movement," in this study. We think that counting the standing frequency is the ideal method to quantify hind-limb ability because in this posture animals sustain their weight only by their hind-limbs.

The target of hypothermic treatments may be, at least in part, some delayed response after injury. Busto et al. [3] showed that even after ischemia and reperfusion the hypothermic treatment effectively diminished ischemic neuronal damage. This report encouraged the clinical possibility of hypothermic treatment after traumatic or ischemic CNS injury. Colbourne and Corbett [8] also showed the efficacy of posttraumatic hypothermia in the gerbil brain. These reports suggest that the hypothermic treatment may act by some delayed damage-progress mechanism. Microglial proliferation after the injuries may be one of the key events of the rather delayed neuronal damage processes. From our time-course data, microglial proliferation in the spinal cord gray matter was a rather delayed response. At 24 h after the compression injury, only a small number of microglia were observed in both hypothermic and normothermic animals. At 48 h after the injury, a large number of microglia appeared in the normothermic animals. Moreover, the difference of hind-limb motor activity between the normothermic and hypothermic animals emerged beginning at 48 h after the injury, the same time point as the increase of microglia. Hence these results suggest a possibility that one of the working mechanisms of hypothermic treatment is inhibition of microglial proliferation and the subsequent inflammatory responses. Several reports may support this idea.

Coimbra et al. [7] reported that an early and extended period of postischemic hypothermia provides powerful, long-lasting protection if followed by treatment with an anti-inflammatory/antipyretic drug. Goss et al. [12] reported that hypothermia diminishes the posttrauma inflammatory cascade in the brain as suggested by the decrease in interleukin-1β (IL-1β). After CNS ischemia or trauma, many events can take place during the early stages (i.e., increased extracellular glutamate, ATP failure, acidosis).

To prevent these early events, therapy should start immediately after the injury. If part of the neuronal damage is due to the microglia, this delayed onset may be clinically important. The "golden" time for therapy against the immune response may be at more than 24 h. It is enough time to prepare several therapies, including hypothermia.

Systemic hypothermic treatment under anesthesia has been introduced for heart and aortic surgery [18], and recently it has been introduced into the emergency clinical field [1,14]. The efficacy of this treatment has been established, although several serious side effects have been reported. Among them, sepsis induced by suppression of the immune system is one of the most serious and fatal. To avoid these serious systemic side effects, local cooling should be considered. However, regional hypothermic therapy of the brain is difficult because of anatomical reasons: The brain is covered with bone, which is continuously perfused with flesh blood and therefore effectively prevents brain cooling from the outside. Local cooling of the spinal cord may be anatomically and technically easier. Cambria and Davison [6] tried to cool the spinal cord (26°–28°C) during thoracoabdominal aortic surgery, which could induce ischemia of nervous tissue. They performed local cooling by an epidural perfusion system. Only 2.9% of the patients ($n = 70$) who were treated with epidural cooling revealed neurological deficits. On the other hand, 23% of control patients without the hypothermic treatment showed neurological deficits after the aortic cross-clamping. Another possibility is to put some cooling system beside the dura after removing the laminae. Operations to remove laminae are not difficult for orthopaedic surgeons or neurosurgeons. Local cooling of the spinal cord may even be possible for awake patients. Local hypothermic therapy is probably cost-effective after considering the nursing efforts necessary to control general conditions in the intensive care unit and the use of large amounts of expensive drugs against systemic side effects including sepsis.

Acknowledgments. The studies have been supported by Grant-in-Aids for Scientific Research 09771094 to T.O. from the Ministry of Education, Science, and Culture of Japan. We thank Dr. Miao Chuai, Mr. Yoshio Ohnishi, and Mr. Masahiro Tada for their excellent technical help.

References

1. Bernard S (1996) Induced hypothermia in intensive care medicine. Anaesth Intensive Care 24:382–388
2. Burger R, Vince GH, Meixensberger J, Roosen K (1998) Hypothermia influences time course of intracranial pressure, brain temperature, EEG and microcirculation during ischemia-reperfusion. Neurol Res 20(Suppl 1):s52–s60
3. Busto R, Dietrich WD, Globus MY-T, Ginsberg MD (1989) Postischemic moderate hypothermia inhibits CA1 hippocampal ischemic neuronal injury. Neurosci Lett 101:299–304
4. Busto R, Dietrich WD, Globus MY-T, Valdes I, Scheinberg P, Ginsberg MD (1987) Small differences in intraischemic brain temperature critically determine the extent of ischemic neuronal injury. J Cereb Blood Flow Metab 7:729–738
5. Busto R, Globus MY-T, Dietrich WD, Martinez E, Valdes I, Ginsberg MD (1989) Effect of mild hypothermia on ischemia-induced release of neurotransmitters and free fatty acids in rat brain. Stroke 20:904–910
6. Cambria RP, Davison JK (1998) Regional hypothermia for prevention of spinal cord ischemic complications after thoracoabdominal aortic surgery: experience with epidural cooling. Semin Thorac Cardiovasc Surg 10:61–65
7. Coimbra C, Drake M, Boris-Moller F, Wieloch T (1996) Long-lasting neuroprotective effect of postischemic hypothermia and treatment with an anti-inflammatory/antipyretic drug: evidence for chronic encephalopathic processes following ischemia. Stroke 27:1578–1585
8. Colbourne F, Corbett D (1994) Delayed and prolonged post-ischemic hypothermia is neuroprotective in the gerbil. Brain Res 654:265–272
9. Coyle DE (1998) Partial peripheral nerve injury leads to activation of astroglia and microglia which parallels the development of allodynic behavior. Glia 23:75–83
10. Dietrich WD, Busto R, Halley M et al. (1990) The importance of brain temperature in alternations of the blood-brain barrier following cerebral ischemia. J Neuropathol Exp Neurol 49:486–497
11. Dixon CE, Markgraf CG, Angileri F, Pike BR, Wolfson B, Newcomb JK, Bismar MM, Blanco AJ, Clifton GL, Hayes RL (1998) Protective effects of moderate hypothermia on behavioral deficits but not necrotic cavitation following cortical impact injury in the rat. J Neurotrauma 15:95–103
12. Goss JR, Styren SD, Miller PD, Kochanek PM, Palmer AM, Marion DW, DeKosky ST (1995) Hypothermia attenuates the normal increase in interleukin 1 beta RNA and nerve growth factor following traumatic brain injury in the rat. J Neurotrauma 12:159–167
13. Griffin WS, Sheng JG, Royston MC, Gentleman SM, McKenzie JE, Graham DI, Roberts GW, Mrak RE (1998) Glial-neuronal interactions in Alzheimer's disease: the potential role of a "cytokine cycle" in disease progression. Brain Pathol 8:65–72
14. Hayashi N, Hirayama T, Udagawa A, Daimon W, Ohata M (1994) Systemic management of cerebral edema based on a new concept in severe head injury patients. Acta Neurochir Suppl (Wien) 60:541–543
15. Holmin S, Soderlund J, Biberfeld P, Mathiesen T (1998) Intracerebral inflammation after human brain contusion. Neurosurgery 42:291–299

16. Morioka T, Kalehua AN, Streit WJ (1991) The microglial reaction in the rat dorsal hippocampus following transient forebrain ischemia. J Cereb Blood Flow Metab 11:966–973
17. Toyoda T, Suzuki S, Kassell NF, Lee KS (1996) Intraischemic hypothermia attenuates neutrophil infiltration in the rat neocortex after focal ischemia-reperfusion injury. Neurosurgery 39:1200–1205
18. Tsai TP, Nessim S, Kass RM, Chaux A, Gray RJ, Khan SS, Blanche C, Utley C, Matloff JM (1991) Morbidity and mortality after coronary artery bypass in octogenarians. Ann Thorac Surg 51:983–986

Local Cooling: Limits on Secondary Injury and Neuronal Death Following Spinal Cord Injury

Minoru Fujiki, Mitsuo Isono, and Shigeaki Hori

Summary. This study evaluates the effects of local cooling by irrigating artificial cerebrospinal fluid for mild hypothermia to spinal cord injury in rats. Crush injuries were produced at the T8 level using an extradural approach. Local hypothermia was established immediately after crush and maintained under several conditions (irrigation temperature, velocity, duration). Animals were allowed to survive 24 h and 1, 3, and 8 weeks postinjury, and spinal cords were prepared for histological evaluation using hematoxylin-eosin staining for general histopathology. DNA fragmentation following spinal cord crush were evaluated using TUNEL staining. The evolution of secondary injury following crush injury with local mild hypothermia decreased dramatically compared with that in rats treated without hypothermia, even though the primary lesions were statistically the same size. In particular, although there was complete destruction of neural tissue at the crush site, the area was filled in by other cells including neutrophils and connective tissue elements in both the hypothermia-treated and the untreated groups. These was a striking reduction in the progressive necrosis and cavitation that is characteristic of the response to spinal cord injury in the normothermic condition. Control and treated animals differed in terms of the appearance of the TUNEL-positive cell response to injury. In control animals, increases in TUNEL-positive cells 24 h after crush were most pronounced not at the crush site but in an area several millimeters distant from the crush edge. The control and hypothermia-treated animals did not differ in this regard. There were substantial increases in TUNEL-positive cells at the crush site and for some distance rostral and caudal to the injury, especially within the areas containing the long ascending and descending tracts that would contain myelinated axons undergoing Wallerian degeneration and the gray matter. In animals treated with hypothermia, however, there was little increase in TUNEL-positive cells at 24 h after crush, and the increase that was seen occurred primarily in the area immediately surrounding the wound cavity where the tissue had been damaged directly. Increases in apoptotic cells did not become prominent at the site of the crush and for some distance both rostral and caudal to the injury in animals treated with and without hypothermia until 24 h after injury. These results indicate that decreases in secondary injury comes not from suppression of apoptosis but from necrosis, especially at sites some distance rostral and caudal to the injury.

Department of Neurosurgery, Oita Medical University, 1-1 Idaigaoka, Hasamamachi, Oita 879-5593, Japan

55

Key words. Spinal cord injury, Hypothermia, Local cooling, Cell death, Secondary injury

Introduction

Spinal cord injury leads to a progressive series of cellular changes at the injury site that culminate in a tissue environment in which degenerative events predominate and growth and repair processes are minimally expressed. Presumably, the poor prognosis following spinal cord injury is in part due to the predominance of degenerative processes.

We have been interested in the effect of hypothermia following central nervous system (CNS) injury because it provides an interesting experimental setting in which to explore the mechanism of protection from cell death following CNS injury [5]. In particular, given that the hypothermia affects one of the potential triggers for cellular responses, the dependence of later events on this trigger can be ascertained. Moreover, it seems likely that hypothermia would lead to an experimental situation in which the entire cascade of injury-induced cellular responses may be different.

The goal of the present study was to compare the sequelae of spinal cord crush injury in control and animals treated with local hypothermia. We focused on the general histological appearance in the tissue treated with local hypothermia and the appearance of TUNEL-positive cells, especially apoptotic cells. Our reasoning was that if the reactive response of cell death following spinal cord injury was triggered by apoptosis or necrosis, this process of cell death may be reduced in the animals treated with local hypothermia.

Materials and Methods

Experimental animals were young adult female rats (7–8 weeks of age, weighing about 180–200 g). Crush injuries of the spinal cord were produced using an extradural approach [3]. The spinal cord was then crushed for 1 s between the blades of a No. 5 Dumont Jewler's forceps. Local hypothermia was induced by irrigation of artificial cerebrospinal fluid (CSF) under several conditions (irrigation temperatures 4°, 21°, 37°C; velocities 5, 10, 25, 50, 100 m/s; duration 1, 2, 4, 8, 12, 24 h).

Rats were allowed to survive after the crush injury for 24 h and 1, 3, and 8 weeks ($n = 3$ animals per time point). The spinal cords were prepared for histological evaluation using hematoxylin-eosin (H-E), Bodian, and OX42 stains. Alternate sections were stained with the trichrome stain for general histology and connective tissue, with protargol impregnation (Bodian) for nerve fibers, and with TUNEL stain for DNA fragmentation.

Results

We analyzed sections from animals killed at 24 h and at 1, 3, and 8 weeks after injury. The temperature profiles of the hypothermia group and the normothermia group indicated a significant difference, with a small fluctuation in the hypothermia group and moderate increases in the normothermia group. The histological appearance in animals treated with local hypothermia differed in some important respects from what has been treated without hypothermia. In particular, there was little evidence of progressive necrosis or cavitation in the treated group.

Histopathology After Spinal Cord Injury in Control Animals

Basic Histopathology Revealed by H-E

By 24 h after the lesion, the H-E sections from control animals revealed that erythrocytes in the tissue appeared dramatically not only at the crush site but in the area several millimeters distant from crush edge. The areas previously occupied by erythrocytes were instead populated with neutrophils and a small number of large cells that had the histological appearance of large macrophages (foamy granular cytoplasm) surrounded by connective tissue and fibroblasts identified by their fusiform cell body and elongated nucleus. The progression of secondary injury appeared several millimeters distant from the crush edge, corresponding to the distribution of erythrocytes.

TUNEL Staining

TUNEL-positive cells began to increase at the edge of the crush 12 h after the crush, although staining was not prominent at this point. The number of TUNEL-positive cells at the crush site increased steadily over time and appeared to reach a peak at about 24 h. A large number of TUNEL-positive cells also appeared along the dorsal column 24 h after the crush. No apoptotic cells with darkly stained condensed nuclei appeared at the edge of the crush, but they were seen at the dorsal column several millimeters distant from the crush edge.

Histopathology After Spinal Cord Injury in Local Hypothermia-Treated Animals

In most ways the histopathological changes after crush injury were similar in local hypothermia-treated animals. There were some important differences, however.

First, even at 24 h after crush there appeared to be more intact axons and fewer degenerating axons in the ascending dorsal columns, consistent with the suppressed extent of secondary injury with hypothermia treatment (55%) in the injured spinal cord. Second, the increases in TUNEL-positive cells appeared with a different distribution. In particular, although TUNEL-positive cells at the lesion margin were increased at 24 h after crush in the hypothermia-treated animals, they were seen to the same extent in the normothermia group. Fewer TUNEL-positive cells appeared in the dorsal column of hypothermia-treated animals than in the normothermia group. No apoptotic cells with darkly stained condensed nuclei appeared at the edge of the crush but only at the dorsal column several millimeters distant from the crush edge. Thus, the avoidance of secondary injury correlates well with the suppression of increases in TUNEL-positive cells at the area several millimeters distant from the crush edge.

Limitation of secondary injury was altered by irrigating conditions. Among the combinations of conditions (irrigation temperatures 4°, 21°, and 37°C; velocities 5, 10, 25, 50, 100 m/s; duration 1, 2, 4, 8, 12, 24 h), 21°C and 50 m/s for 4 h were the optimal conditions for this treatment (Figs. 1, 2, 3).

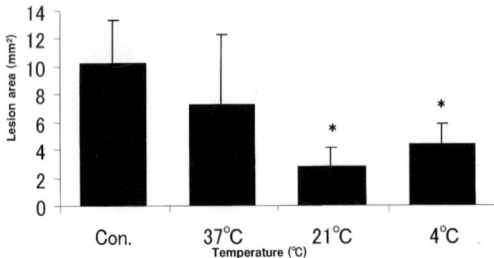

FIG. 1. Comparison of lesion area in animals treated with hypothermia at various cerebrospinal fluid (CSF) temperatures

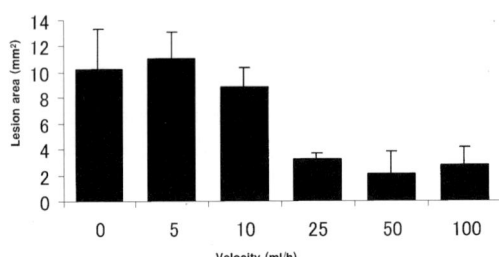

FIG. 2. Comparison of lesion area in animals treated with hypothermia at various CSF irrigation velocities

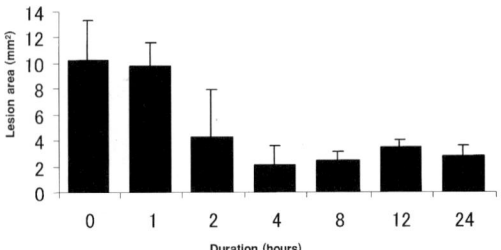

FIG. 3. Comparison of lesion area in animals treated with hypothermia at various irrigation durations

Discussion

In general, the nature and time course of the initial cellular response to spinal cord crush injury in control animals were compatible to what has been described previously [2,4]. The progression of secondary injury of the spinal cord that would contain degenerating axons was also comparable to what has been described in a previous report [2].

There were dramatic increases in TUNEL-positive cells in the dorsal columns that peaked at about 24h. Intensely stained TUNEL-positive cells were also evident in other portions of the spinal cord parenchyma that would contain degenerating axons, but not to the same extent as in the dorsal columns.

Previous authors have noted that a prominence of TUNEL-positive cells is associated with both necrosis and apoptosis activation in the dorsal columns versus other areas that contain degenerating axons (e.g., the corticospinal tract) [2]. Previous authors have suggested that the appearance of apoptotic cells may be especially prominent not in areas in which axons have already died but in areas that contain both oligodendroglia and degenerating myelinated fibers. (Axons in the dorsal columns of rodents are heavily myelinated, whereas axons in the corticospinal tract are lightly myelinated.) The present observations are consistent with this proposal.

Progressive cavitation after spinal cord injury is also prominent in other species, including humans. Progressive cavitation even within 24 h was suppressed in the local hypothermia-treated animals.

There is no obvious explanation why progressive necrosis and cavitation should be inhibited in hypothermia-treated animals. Among the hypotheses to account for the secondary degeneration and cavitation are that: (1) activated macrophages/microglia release toxic cytokines that destroy neural tissue; and (2) secondary degeneration is due to excitotoxic cell death. In support of the former hypothesis, it has been shown that treatments that modify macrophage/microglial function can reduce cavitation [1]. In support of the latter hypothesis is the fact that much of the neural injury appears to occur before the macrophages invade the tissue [2]. In both cases, cavitation presumably occurs as the dead neural tissue is removed.

The present study indicated local cooling by irrigating artificial CSF limited progressive secondary injury. Among the combination of the conditions (irrigation temperature, velocity, and duration), the optimal combination was 21°C and 50 m/s for 4 h. The temperature of the injured spinal cord surface was optimum at an irrigating CSF temperature of 21°C. The meaning of each parameter is still uncertain. Further studies are required for answers to this question.

References

1. Blight AR (1994) Effects of silica on the outcome from experimental spinal cord injury: implication of macrophages in secondary tissue damage. Neuroscience 60:263–273
2. Dusart I, Schwab ME (1994) Secondary cell death and the inflammatory reaction after dorsal hemisection of the rat spinal cord. Eur J Neurosci 6:712–724
3. Guth L, Barrett CP, Donati EJ, Anderson FD, Smith MV, Lifson M (1985) Essentiality of a specific cellular terrain for growth of axons into a spinal cord lesion. Exp Neurol 88:1–12
4. Reier PJ, Stensaas LJ, Guth L (1983) The astrocytic scar as an impediment to regeneration in the central nervous system. In: Kao CC, Bunge RP, Reier PJ (eds) Spinal cord reconstruction. New York: Raven
5. Steward O (1992) Signals that induce sprouting in the central nervous system: sprouting is delayed in a strain of mouse exhibiting delayed axonal degeneration. Exp Neurol 118:340–351

Effect of Intraischemic Hypothermia on Expression of c-Fos, c-Jun, and HSP72 After Transient Focal Cerebral Ischemia in Rat Brain

Kazunori Akaji*, Sadao Suga, Keita Mayanagi, Joji Inamasu, Takashi Horiguchi, Shuzo Sato, and Takeshi Kawase

Summary. Male Wistar rats underwent right middle cerebral artery occlusion for 1 h with the intraluminal suture method. During ischemia, animals were assigned to either a normothermic (NT) or a hypothermic (HT) group. In the NT group the animals were left at ambient temperature (21°C), and the brain temperature was elevated to 40°C during ischemia. In the HT group the animals were put into a cold room (1°C), and the brain temperature was decreased to 30°C. In both groups the animals ($n = 4$) were sacrificed 48 h after reperfusion, and %infarct volume were calculated after 2,3,5-triphenyltetrazolium hydrochloride (TTC) staining. In rat striatum there was no significant difference of %infarct volume between the NT and HT groups. In contrast, the %infarct volume of the cortex was decreased in the HT group compared with that in NT group. To evaluate the effect of hypothermia on gene expression after transient focal ischemia, animals (n = 5 per time point) were sacrificed at 3, 6, and 24 h after reperfusion. Immunohistochemistry was performed at each time point with c-Fos, c-Jun, and HSP72 antibody. Our results revealed that increased c-Fos immunoreactivity in the cortex was observed at 3 h after reperfusion in the NT group but not in HT group, c-Jun expression was not affected by HT treatment, and HSP72 expression in the cortex was decreased in the HT group compared to that in the NT group. In conclusion, hypothermia suppressed aggravation of cerebral infarction, and c-Fos expression in the periinfarct area of cortex might play a crucial role in cell survival.

Key words. Hypothermia, c-Fos, c-Jun, HSP72, Focal cerebral ischemia

Introduction

The neuroprotective effect of intraischemic hypothermia is widely accepted, and several mechanisms (e.g., reduced cerebral metabolism, decreased excitatory neurotransmitter release, and protection of the blood–brain barrier) are suggested. Gene expression after transient cerebral ischemia is also known to play a cardinal role in cell survival or death, and some immediate early genes (IEGs) are supposed to be candidates for mediating cell injury. The

---

Department of Neurosurgery, Keio University School of Medicine, Shinanomachi 35, Shinjuku-ku, Tokyo 160-8582, Japan
* Present address: Department of Neurosurgery, Mihara Memorial Hospital, 366 Otamachi, Isesaki, Gunma 372-0006, Japan

aim of this study was to examine the effect of hypothermia on the expression of c-Fos, c-Jun, and heat shock protein 72 (HSP72) after transient focal cerebral ischemia in the rat brain and clarify the role of IEGs and HSP72 after insults.

Materials and Methods

Animal Preparation

Male Wistar rats weighing 300–320 g were given free access to food and water prior to the surgery. Anesthesia was induced with a mixture of 30% O_2, 68.5% N_2O, 1.5% halothane. The animals underwent right middle cerebral artery occlusion for 1 h with the intraluminal suture method [7]. The brain temperature was monitored using a probe of the telemeter system (Asahi Biomed, Kanagawa, Japan), which had been placed in the left occipital lobe at the day before the surgery. During ischemia, animals were assigned to either a normothermic (NT) group or a hypothermic (HT) group. In the NT group, animals were left at ambient temperature (21°C). In HT group, animals were put into a cold room (1°C). During ischemia animals were awake, and those that presented left hemiparesis were subjected to the experiment. After reperfusion, animals were awake in the ambient temperature (21°C) and were given free access to food and water. Sham-operated normothermic and hypothermic animals were also included in the study.

Infarct Volume Measurement

In both groups the animals ($n = 4$) were sacrificed 48 h after reperfusion, and brains were cut into 2 mm thick sections from the frontal pole to posterior; six slices were obtained. After 2,3,5-triphenyltetrazolium hydrochloride (TTC) staining, each slice was scanned by a digital camera, and the image was transferred to a Macintosh 8600 computer; the infarct area of the slice was measured by NIH image 1.60. The infarct volume was calculated as an infarct area by 2 mm, and the ratio of the infarct volume/unaffected side volume was reported as the %infarct volume. The hemispheric volume was estimated by the sum of the six slices; and the cortical or striatum volume was estimated by the sum of all the slices.

Immunohistochemistry

In both groups the animals ($n = 5$ per time point) were sacrificed at 3, 6, and 24 h after reperfusion and were perfused with 4% paraformaldehyde in 0.1 M PBS, pH 7.4. Vibratome sections of 50 μm thickness were cut, and sections at the level of striatum (bregma 1.2 mm anterior) and hippocampus (bregma 2.3 mm posterior) were used for immunoreaction, as described by Vass [6]. The sections were left in ammonium chloride solution for 1 h and left in Triton solution for 1 h. They were then blocked with normal goat serum (NGS) for 4 h in the refrigerator. A rabbit IgG polyclonal antibody to c-Fos (cat. no. PC05, PC05L; Oncogene Research Products), a rabbit IgG polyclonal antibody to c-Jun (cat. no. PC06, PC06L; Oncogene Research Products), and a mouse IgG monoclonal antibody to HSP72 (RPN1197; Amersham) was diluted 1:400, 1:40, and 1:200 in 10% NGS, respectively. The sections were incubated in the diluted primary antibody in the refrigerator after agitation overnight. After several washes, they were incubated in a biotin-labeled anti-rabbit IgG (176-15-06; Kirkegaar & Perry Laboratories) at 1:200 dilution for c-Fos and c-Jun or a biotin-labeled anti-mouse IgG (16-18-06; Kirkegaar & Perry Laboratories) at 1:200 dilution for HSP at ambient temperature for 3 h. The sections were soaked in 3% hydrogen peroxide solution for 20 min and then incubated for

1 h in peroxidase-labeled streptavidin (14-30-00; Kirkegaar & Perry Laboratories). They were finally stained in diaminobenzidine 1 mg/m1. Control sections were run without primary antibodies to exclude nonspecificity and cross-reactivity with the secondary antibodies.

Results

Changes of Brain Temperature

In the NT group the brain temperature increased up to 40°C during ischemia (Fig. 1). In the HT group the brain temperature decreased to 30°C (Fig. 2). After reperfusion, the brain temperature returned to the preischemic temperature of around 38°C in both groups.

Infarct Volume

Infarct volume in several lesions were examined at 48 h of recirculation. The infarct volumes of the hemisphere were $32.8 \pm 8.4\%$ and $14.5 \pm 6.1\%$ in the NT and HT groups, respectively; thus hypothermia significantly reduced the %infarct volume compared with that in the NT group (Fig. 3) ($P < 0.05$). In the cortex the infarct volumes of the NT and HT groups were 36.3

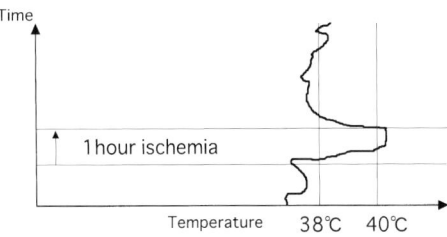

FIG. 1. Representative recording of brain temperature in the normothermic group. Note that the brain temperature elevated to 40°C during ischemia

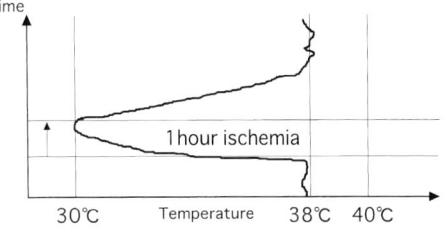

FIG. 2. Representative recording of brain temperature in the hypothermic group. Note that the brain temperature reduced to 30°C during ischemia

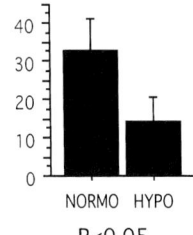

FIG. 3. Percent infarct volume in the hemisphere. Hypothermia reduced the percent infarct volume compared with that in the normothermic group ($P < 0.05$). *NORMO*, normothermic group; *HYPO*, hypothermic group

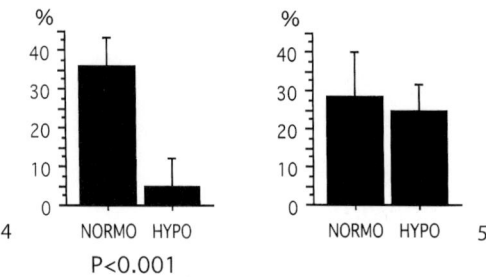

Fig. 4. Percent infarct volume in the cortex. Hypothermia significantly reduced the percent infarct volume compared with that of the normothermic group ($P < 0.001$)

Fig. 5. Percent infarct volume in the striatum. Hypothermia gave no significant protection

± 7.0% and 4.8 ± 6.5%, respectively; thus hypothermia significantly reduced the %infarct volume compared with that in the NT group (Fig. 4) ($P < 0.001$). In the striatum the infarct volumes of the NT and HT groups were 28.8 ± 11.5% and 24.8 ± 6.9%, respectively; hence hypothermia showed no significant protection here (Fig. 5) ($P > 0.05$).

IEGs and HSP Expression

We focused the IEGs and HSP expression in the cortex because the protective effect of hypothermia was shown in the cortex. C-Fos immunoreactivity (CFI) was detected in the nucleus of cortical neurons. CFI in the cortex was not observed in the controls and increased moderately at 3–6 h; it was not detected 24 h after reperfusion in the NT group, whereas strong expression was noted at 3 h into the recirculation period in the HT group (Fig. 6, Table 1). C-Jun immunoreactivity was also detected constitutively in the nucleus of cortical neurons and was not affected during the 24-h recirculation period by hypothermic treatment. HSP72 immunoreactivity was present only in the NT group during the 24-h recirculation period in the cortex. In contrast, HSP72 immunoreactivity was not present in the HT group (Fig. 7, Table 1).

TABLE 1. Time course of c-Fos, c-Jun, and HSP72 expression in the cortex

Protein expression	Temperation	3 Hours	6 Hours	24 Hours
c-Fos	Normothermic	+	+	—
c-Fos	Hypothermic	+++	—	—
c-Jun	Normothermic	++	++	++
c-Jun	Hypothermic	++	++	++
HSP72	Normothermic	++	++	++
HSP72	Hypothermic	—	—	—

+++, strong expression; ++, moderate expression; +, weak expression; —; no expression

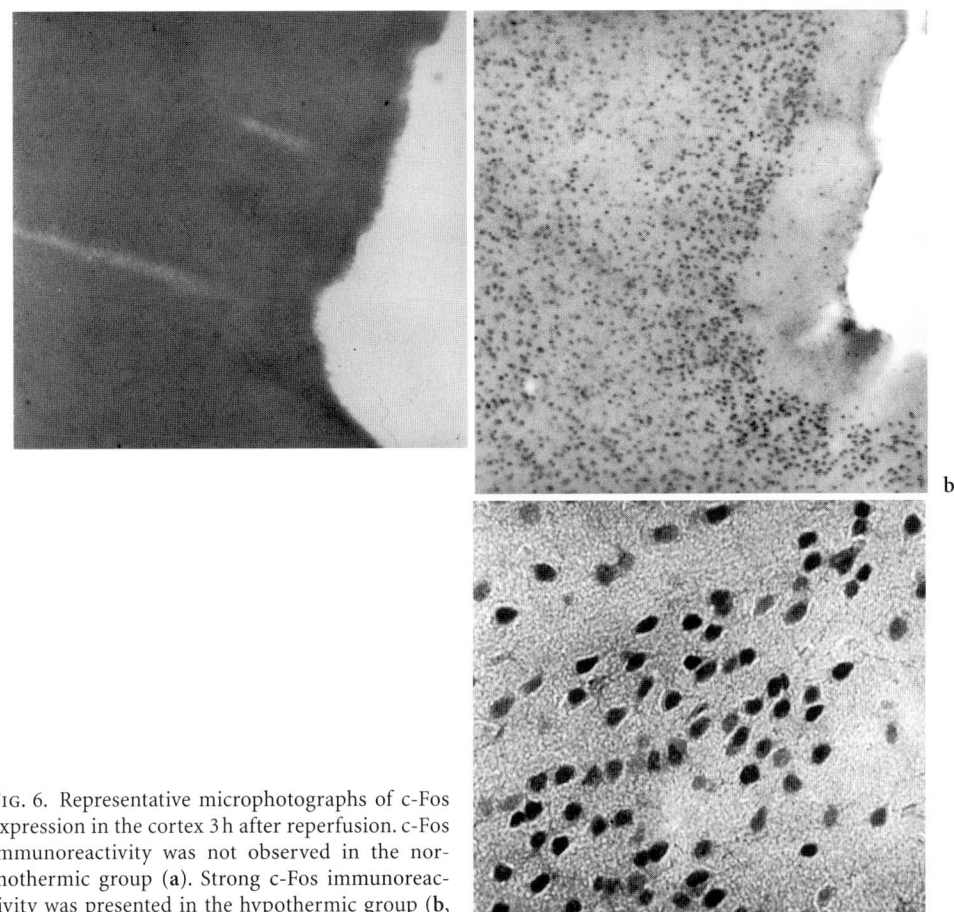

FIG. 6. Representative microphotographs of c-Fos expression in the cortex 3 h after reperfusion. c-Fos immunoreactivity was not observed in the normothermic group (a). Strong c-Fos immunoreactivity was presented in the hypothermic group (b, low magnification; c, high magnification)

Discussion

Many authors have reported that intraischemic hypothermia reduced the infarct volume during global or focal ischemia [1,4,5]. Our results also showed that intraischemic hypothermia reduced the infarct volume not in the striatum but in the cortex. In our model the striatum is the ischemic core, and hypothermia did not have a beneficial effect on it. In contrast, the periischemia area, the so-called ischemic penumbra, was rescued by hypothermia.

Several mechanisms for the protective effect of intraischemic hypothermia on the ischemic penumbra have been documented. Energy metabolism suppression, decreased intracellular calcium influx, and inhibited glutamate release have been suggested.

The IEGs are called "third messengers" and act as transcriptional factors that transcribe target genes. Although the paradigms of IEG expression have been uncertain, expression of

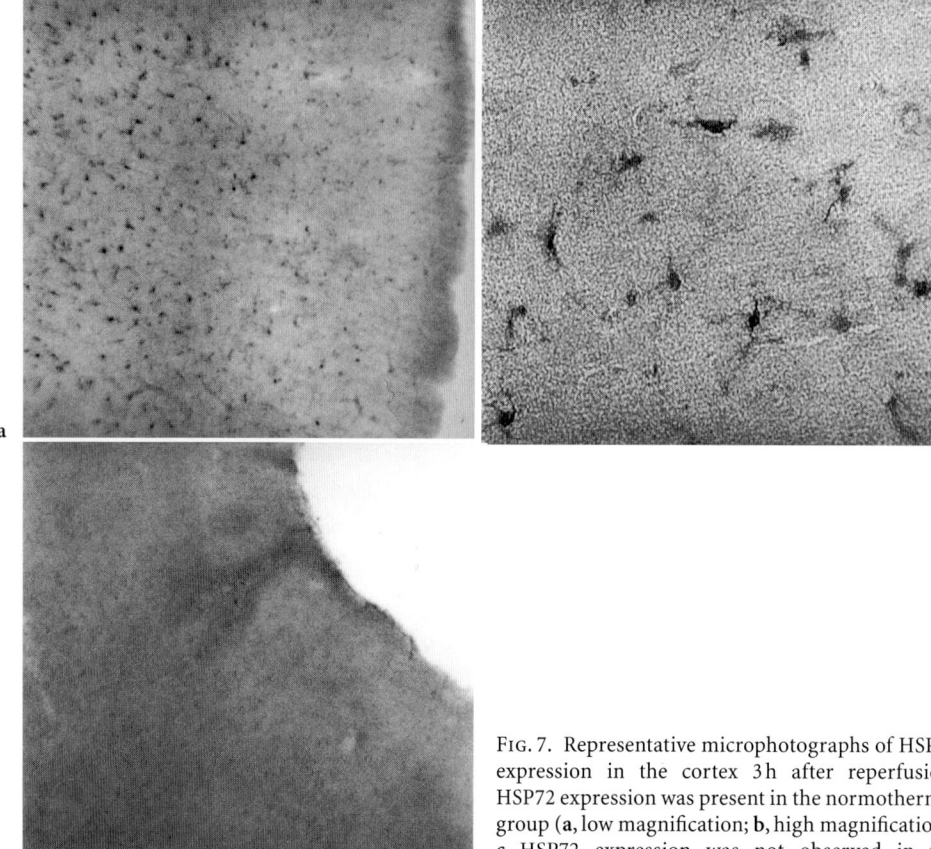

FIG. 7. Representative microphotographs of HSP72 expression in the cortex 3h after reperfusion. HSP72 expression was present in the normothermic group (**a**, low magnification; **b**, high magnification). **c** HSP72 expression was not observed in the hypothermic group

IEGs has been demonstrated to induce cell survival or apoptosis. In the gerbil, after 2 or 5 min of forebrain ischemia, c-fos mRNA was expressed in the CA1, CA3, and dentate gyrus, but c-Fos protein was expressed not in the CA1 but in CA3 and the dentate gyrus where neurons survived. In the rat focal ischemia model, c-Fos was expressed in the periinfarct area, and spreading depression was supposed to be the mechanism [2]. Our results demonstrated that c-Fos was induced strongly in the hypothermic penumbra area where neurons survived but was induced weakly in the NT group. This suggests that strong c-Fos expression may contribute to cell survival in the periinfarct area.

The HSP has been a stress marker after several stimuli (e.g., heat, ischemia, and expression of HSP) induced ischemic tolerance and cell survival. Our results demonstrated that HSP expression was observed in the periinfarct area in the normothermic animals not in the hypothermic animals. This indicates that hypothermia suppressed the stress response in the penumbra, and cells could be protected from stress. The minute mechanism of HSP induction has not been clear, but similar results were seen in gerbil hippocampal neurons after transient forebrain ischemia, and the effect of hypothermia on protein synthesis, especially of HSP72 had been investigated [3,5]. It has been shown that intraischemic hypothermia diminished HSP72 expression throughout the hippocampus. Our results clarify that intraischemic hypothermia also suppressed HSP72 expression in the cortex after transient focal cerebral ischemia in rat brain. Hypothermia can suppress increased extracellular glutamate and intracellular Ca^{2+} elevation, so HSP72 synthesis might decrease.

Conclusions

Increased c-Fos expression in the cortex during the early stage could be one of the protective mechanisms or survival markers affected by hypothermia against neuronal death. Hypothermia, which suppresses HSP72 expression in the cortex, reduced the stress response after ischemia. Such harmonization of gene expressions may play a paramount role in the signal transduction cascade after insults.

References

1. Inamasu J, Suga S, Horiguchi T, Sato S, Akaji K, Kawase T (1998) Evaluation of neuroprotective effect of post-ischemic hypothermia using transient focal ischemia model in rats. In: Yamashima T (ed) Ischemic neuronal death. pp 162–173, Psymed, Japan
2. Jari H, Bradly AS, Philip RW, Jose E, Frank RS (1997) Expression of zinc finger immediate early genes in rat brain after permanent middle cerebral artery occlusion. J Cereb Blood Flow Metab 17:636–646
3. Kumar K, Wu X, Evans AT, Marcoux F (1995) The effect of hypothermia on induction of heat shock protein (HSP)-72 in ischemic brain. Metab Brain Dis 10:283–291
4. Miyazawa T (1996) Effect of mild hypothermia on focal brain ischemia: review of experimental studies. Jpn J Stroke 18:263–273
5. Ogino M (1995) The effect of hypothermia on gene expression after transient cerebral ischemia. Keioigaku 72:441–453
6. Vass K (1988) Localization of 70-kDa stress protein induction in gerbil brain after ischemia. Acta Neuropathol (Berl) 77:128–135
7. Zea Longa E, Weistein PR, Carlson S, Cummins R (1989) Reversible middle cerebral artery occlusion without craniectomy in rats. Stroke 20:80–91

Neuroprotective Effect of Mild Hypothermia in Experimental Brain Ischemia

Hisato Yanase and Kiyoshi Kataoka

Summary. Modern hypothermia therapy has a history of more than a half century. However, this therapy was not commonly accepted as a treatment for cerebral damage because of its harmful complications and the lack of basic knowledge of its beneficial effects. In 1987, it was shown in animal experiments that lowering brain temperature only by a few degrees Celsius during ischemia could protect central neurons against ischemic damages. Since then, widespread basic experiments have started, providing useful information for the clinical application of hypothermia. The extent of neuronal protection by postischemic hypothermia depends on the time of introduction, the duration and the depth of hypothermia, and the degree of ischemic damages. In our gerbil models, hippocampal CA1 neurons were definitely protected against damage by hypothermia, initiated several hours after 5-min forebrain ischemia and maintained for 24 h. In a focal ischemia model of the rat, hypothermia at 33°C for 24 h, which was introduced several hours after ischemia, decreased the infarct volume of the ischemic hemisphere. The mechanism underlying the protective effect of postischemic hypothermia is not clear yet. A growing body of evidence has indicated that lowering temperature depresses ischemia-induced glutamate release, intracellular calcium mobilization, and microglial activation along with the production of NO and superoxides. This lowering of temperature also restores postischemic protein synthesis, permeability of vessels, and the function of the blood-brain barrier, and obviously induces transcription factors like AP1, which may be linked to the synthesis of cytokines. Thus, the mode of action of hypothermia is broad and nonspecific and may be greatly advantageous in regard to cerebral protection against ischemic damage.

Key words. Hypothermia, Neuroprotection, Ischemia, Excitotoxicity, Microglia

Introduction

Mild hypothermia is becoming a focus of countermeasures against ischemic neuronal death, particularly for patients at the very acute stages of stroke, cerebral trauma, or cardiopulmonary resuscitation. These clinical trials have been based on recent animal experiments in which lowering body temperature by only several degrees Celsius definitely resuscitates

Department of Physiology, Ehime University School of Medicine, Shitsukawa, Shigenobu-cho, Onsen-gun, Ehime 791-0295, Japan neurons after ischemic damage [1]. Resuscitation occurs even at late introduction, such as starting 5–6h after reperfusion following transient ischemic insult [11]. This beneficial finding of postischemic hypothermia is important, because this means that in patients transported to an emergency hospital after onset, there still exists time for the introduction of hypothermia with therapeutic efficacy. Indeed, certain institutions have reported unexpected beneficial effects of mild hypothermia on patients with cerebral trauma or stroke [10,23].

The application of whole body hypothermia for ischemic brain diseases is not a new treatment, but has a history of more than a half century. In earlier periods, few basic animal experiments had been carried out. Thus, there was no knowledge available regarding when and how body temperature should be lowered and at what degree and for how long body temperature could be maintained. Furthermore, negative effects including severe infection such as pneumonia or cardiovascular dysfunction such as arrhythmia were frequently seen during longstanding and deeply maintained hypothermia. Therefore, hypothermia therapy was not readily accepted. Busto et al. reported that mild hypothermia down to 33°C was effective enough to resuscitate dying neurons in ischemic rodents [1]. Since then, widespread basic experiments have started, providing useful information for the clinical application of hypothermia. This chapter will summarize the historical background of hypothermia therapy for brain ischemia, and will repeat findings of our recent research on hypothermia and its possible mechanism underlying ischemic cellular processes.

Historical Background of Hypothermia Study for Neuronal Protection or Resuscitation

Local cooling has long been performed as a folk remedy, known for its beneficial effect as early as Hippocrates' time. Human refrigeration was first introduced by Temple Fay about 60 years ago, which is the actual dawn of hypothermia therapy for brain protection or resuscitation [7]. He introduced whole body cooling principally for the purpose of pain killing or the inhibition of metastasis in patients with malignant cerebral neoplasm, and recognized beneficial effects of hypothermia on head trauma patients, albeit the number of the latter cases was limited [8]. Fay's methods of whole body cooling were essentially identical with those used today. Although not recognized at that time, Fay's pioneering work is greatly appreciated in retrospective considerations. Rosomoff and Holaday indicated in experiments using dogs that cerebral blood flow and oxygen consumption decreased linearly by 6.7% per 1°C drop in temperature, which is still central in the contemporary understanding of the efficacy of hypothermia on ischemic neurons [24]. The same authors reported that the sizes of cerebral infarction in dogs following ischemic insult at 30°C were definitely smaller than those at 37°C [25]. As far as we are aware, this is the first description of the beneficial effect of hypothermia in an animal stroke model.

Animal Models for Study of Brain Hypothermia

For the study of brain ischemia, many animal models have been developed, including forebrain and focal ischemia models. In both models, the effects of hypothermia on ischemic neuronal damage have been clarified. Accumulating evidence has indicated that in forebrain ischemia models, hypothermia produces beneficial effects on damaged neurons following ischemia. Herewith, we describe our recent data from related research.

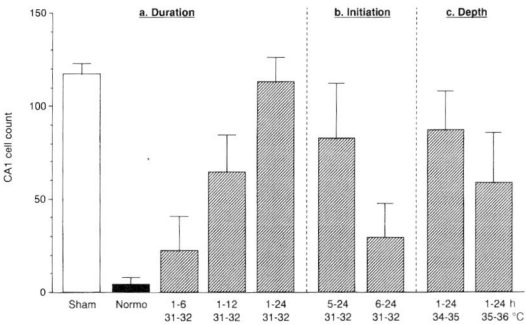

FIG. 1. Effects of postischemic hypothermia on the extent of damage in hippocampal CA1 neurons. *White, black,* and *hatched columns* represent sham-operated (*Sham*), normothermia (*Normo*), and hypothermia groups, respectively. *Numerals on the ordinate* represents the number of survived CA1 neurons within $100 \times 500\,\mu m$ grid. *Numerals on the abscissa* represent the periods of postischemic hypothermia (in hours) and brain temperature (°C). (**a**) Hypothermia at 31°–32°C was initiated 1 h after ischemia and maintained for different durations. (**b**) Long-duration hypothermia (18–19 h) at 31°–32°C was initiated various times after the ischemia. (**c**) Hypothermia lasting 23 h was initiated 1 h after ischemic insult at varying brain temperatures

Forebrain Ischemia Models

Confirming data from other investigations, our experimental paradigm has indicated that postischemic hypothermia rescues neurons from transient ischemic damage. The extent of neuronal protection depends on the time of introduction, the duration, and the depth of hypothermia, as well as the degree of ischemic damage. We evaluated the neuroprotective effects of postischemic hypothermia on ischemic damage in a transient forebrain ischemia model of the gerbil.

Male Mongolian gerbils were used. Under halothane anesthesia, a brain temperature probe (XM-FH, Mini-Mitter, Sunriver, OR, US) was inserted into the right striatum (2 mm ventral to the cortical surface, 2 mm anterior and lateral to the bregma) and was attached to the skull with anchoring screws and dental cement. The position of the probe tip was approximately at the same depth as the hippocampus. Animals were subjected to 5-min forebrain ischemia by the occlusions of bilateral common carotid arteries. Brain temperature during ischemia was maintained around 37.5°C. Brain temperature after reperfusion was measured by using a brain temperature control system (AQTEMP-20 software, Furusawa Lab, Saitama, Japan) [36]. A postoperative gerbil was placed in a Plexiglass box (31 × 18 × 13 cm) resting on a telemetry receiver, which was placed in an incubator box. The telemeter was devised so that changes in brain temperature could be converted into changes in frequency of electric pulses. Such electric pulses were received by the telemetry receiver, modified into electric pulses, and interfaced to a computer through an interface board. Temperature data were recorded and analyzed using a brain temperature control system (see the following section on the detailed method of induction and maintaining hypothermia). Thirty days later, the animals were anesthetized with pentobarbital. Brains were perfusion-fixed by 10% formalin and embedded in paraffin wax. Sections (4 μm) of gerbil hippocampus were stained with cresyl-violet, and the extent of CA1 neuronal damage in the middle hippocampus was assessed by counting normal-appearing neurons in a $100 \times 500\,\mu m$ grid.

Three separate studies were conducted. The first one was designed to define the optimal duration of postischemic hypothermia (Fig. 1a). Hypothermia was initiated 1 h after ischemia and was maintained for different amounts of time. Hypothermia at 31°–32°C for 11 h resulted in significant protection of CA1 neurons. However, its efficacy was half that for 23 h, which yielded almost full resuscitation of CA1 neurons at the same degree of temperature. Hypothermia for 5 h seemed too short to cause a significant beneficial effect. The second study was designed to determine the effects of different starting times of postischemic hypothermia (Fig. 1b). Long-standing hypothermia (18–23 h) at 32°C was initiated at various times after reperfusion. In the first study, hypothermia of 31°–32°C initiated 1 h after ischemia and lasting for 23 h greatly prevented ischemic neuronal damage. A marked protection of CA1 neurons was still observed even when hypothermia was initiated up to 5 h after ischemia and concluded 24 h after insult. However, no significant protection was detected in 6-h-delayed postischemic hypothermia. When the length of hypothermia, which was initiated 6 h after ischemia, lasted for 24 or 48 h, the number of surviving CA1 neurons increased (data not shown). The third study was designed to define the optimal depth of postischemic hypothermia (Fig. 1c). Hypothermia lasting for 23 h was introduced 1 h after the ischemic insult at varying brain temperatures. Hypothermia maintained at temperatures below 35°C was significantly neuroprotective against ischemic damage; lower temperatures resulted in higher rates of neuronal survival. Even in a mild hypothermia group at 35°–36°C, almost half of the CA1 neurons apparently remained intact 30 days after ischemia.

Multiple mechanisms of postischemic hypothermia for neuronal protection have been identified, namely, reducing metabolic rate, decreasing excitatory transmitter release, suppressing intracellular calcium mobilization, and reducing vascular permeability, edema, and blood-brain barrier (BBB) disruption. Our results indicated that these postischemic phenomena leading to cell death are reversible until 6 h after reperfusion in a transient forebrain ischemia model.

Focal Ischemia Models

Little is known about possible neuronal protection by postischemic hypothermia in focal cerebral ischemia. Therefore, we tried to evaluate whether or not postischemic hypothermia would affect the infarct volume produced after middle cerebral artery occlusion (MCAO). Reversible MCAO was performed using a suture technique in male Sprague–Dawley rats weighing 280–380 g. The right common carotid artery (CCA), external carotid artery (ECA), internal carotid artery (ICA), and the pterygopalatine artery (PPA) were exposed. The ECA was dissected and the CCA, ICA, and PPA were temporarily occluded with arterial clips. Monofilament nylon line, 0.148 mm in diameter (with a silicone-coated tip, 0.3 mm in diameter and 5 mm in length), was inserted into the ECA stump and was extended through the ICA 18–23 mm beyond the bifurcation. At this point, the intraluminal nylon line reached the opening of the middle cerebral artery (MCA) and was kept in place for 2 h. Reperfusion was achieved by the removal of the nylon line after ischemia. The rats were divided into two groups— normothermia and hypothermia. A brain temperature probe was inserted into the left striatum (3.5 mm ventral to the cortical surface, 1.5 mm posterior, and 3 mm lateral to the bregma). Brain temperature was monitored and regulated using the brain temperature control system during the ischemia and following 27 h reperfusion in conscious and freely moving rats. Hypothermia was introduced 1 h after reperfusion. In the hypothermia group, total body cooling was started by spraying water onto the animal surface under a blowing fan and by reducing the temperature of the incubator box to about 10°C. Brain temperature was regulated at 33 ± 1.0°C by using a feedback system of the brain temperature control system, where a heating fan was turned on automatically when the brain temperature fell below 32.5°C, and was turned off immediately when brain temperature reached 32.5°C. Figure 2 is a long-term

Fig. 2. A long-term recording of brain temperature of a rat from the hypothermia group. Brain temperatures before ischemia were in the range of 37°–37.5°C. During the occlusion and the release of the right middle cerebral artery (MCA), the rat was removed from a brain temperature control system. After the occlusion of the right MCA, brain temperature increased up to 39°C (so-called postischemic hyperthermia). Two hours after reperfusion, hypothermia was initiated and kept for 24 h at around 33°C

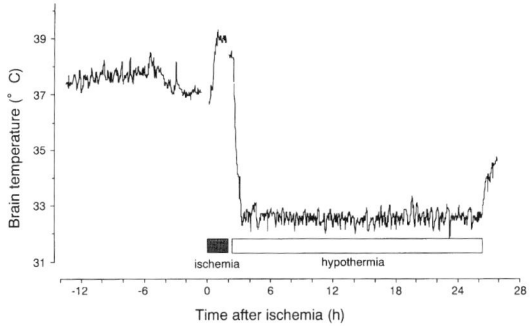

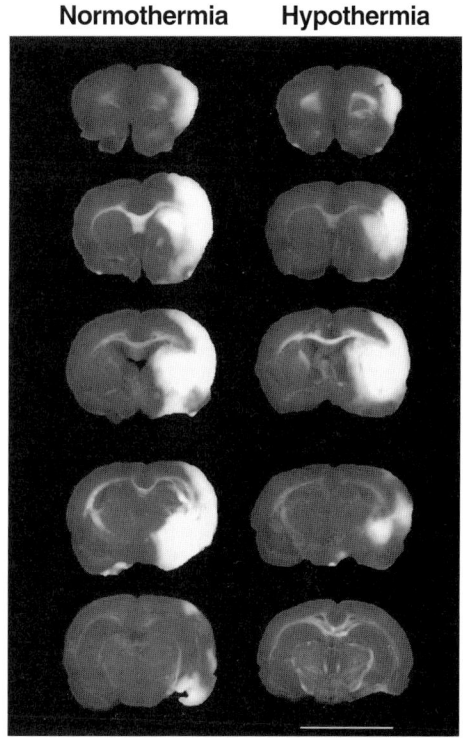

Fig. 3. TTC-stained brain slices (coronal sections) obtained 28 h after the occlusion of the right middle cerebral artery (MCA) in the normothermia (*left*) and hypothermia groups (*right*). The *white areas* indicate infarction. *Bar* = 10 mm

recording of the changes of brain temperature in a hypothermic rat. Then rats were anesthetized with pentobarbital after 28 h of reperfusion. Brains were removed and slices (2 mm) were obtained. Morphometric measurements for infarct volume were performed using 2,3,5-triphenyltetrazolium chloride (TTC) staining (Fig. 3). Both sides of TTC-stained slices were scanned with an image scanner, and infarct areas were measured with an image analysis system (NIH Image 1.61). Infarct volume was corrected for edema ([corrected infarct volume] = [volume of contralateral hemisphere] − [noninfarct volume of ipsilateral hemisphere]). The corrected infarct volume of the ischemic hemisphere in the hypothermia group was significantly smaller than that in the normothermia group, namely, 123.3 ± 39.4 mm^3 (mean ± SD, $n = 6$) and 194.8 ± 45.0 mm^3 ($n = 6$), respectively (Fig. 4a). The direct measurement of the

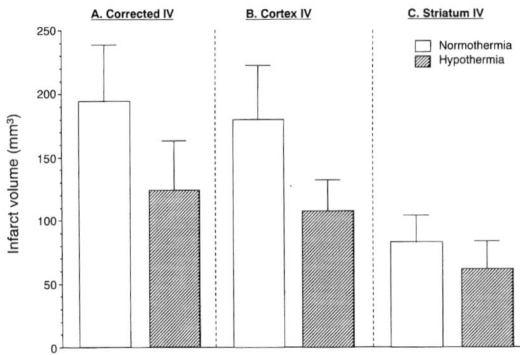

FIG. 4. Effects of postischemic hypothermia on infarct volume (*IV*). Brain specimens were prepared 28 h after ischemia. *White and hatched columns* represent the infarct volume (mm³) in the normothermia and hypothermia groups, respectively. (a) The corrected infarct volume in the ischemic hemisphere; (b) the uncorrected infarct volume in the cerebral cortex; (c) the uncorrected infarct volume in the striatum

infarct volume (uncorrected infarct volume) in the cerebral cortex in the hypothermia group was also significantly smaller than that in the normothermia group, namely, 106.9 ± 24.5 mm³ ($n = 6$) and 179.2 ± 42.9 mm³ ($n = 6$), respectively (Fig. 4b). However, there was no significant difference in the direct measurement of the infarct volume in the striatum between the normothermia and the hypothermia groups (82.5 ± 21.2 mm³ vs 61.0 ± 22.6 mm³) (Fig. 4c). These data suggest that postischemic hypothermia is a beneficial means for neuronal protection against ischemic damage, at least in the cerebral cortex.

Many reports indicated that the therapeutic time window of hypothermia is within 1 h after insult in focal ischemia models. Zhang et al. reported that hypothermia at 30°C for 3 h, initiated 1 h after reperfusion and following 2-h MCAO, reduced infarct volume [37]. Yanamoto et al. reported that hypothermia in the range of 31°–35°C for 21 h, initiated just after reperfusion and following 3-h MCAO, provided neuronal protection [31]. Our data also suggest that the allowed delay of hypothermia is at least within 3 h after reperfusion. In the focal ischemia model, it has been recognized that the extent of neuronal protection by postischemic hypothermia is greater in the cerebral cortex than in the striatum.

Mode of Action of Hypothermia

The mechanisms of neuroprotection by postischemic hypothermia are not yet clear. In hypothermic animals and hibernating animals, metabolic rate and oxygen consumption are remarkably reduced as temperature lowers. The demand for oxygen and glucose should always be lower than the supply at any temperature during hypothermia. This may explain why at lower body temperatures there are more neurons resistant to ischemia. Although the knowledge at hand of the cellular processes after ischemia, particularly those of the late phenomena after excitotoxicity, is still only fragmentary, it is very likely that in and around ischemic neurons there is a multiplicity of cascade reactions that dynamically proceed in both temporal and spatial ranges. At the present stage, it is assumed that the mode of action of mild to moderate hypothermia is nonspecific and multifocal suppressions of widely progressing cascade reactions after ischemia.

Excitotoxicity

At the very initial stage of ischemia, excitotoxicity plays a pivotal role, when a large-scale glutamate surge occurs. Such a sustained overflow of glutamate continuously stimulates neuronal glutamate receptor channels, which induce vivid in-and-out flow of sodium and potassium ions with markedly enhanced ATP expenditure to pump these monovalent ions back. Severe

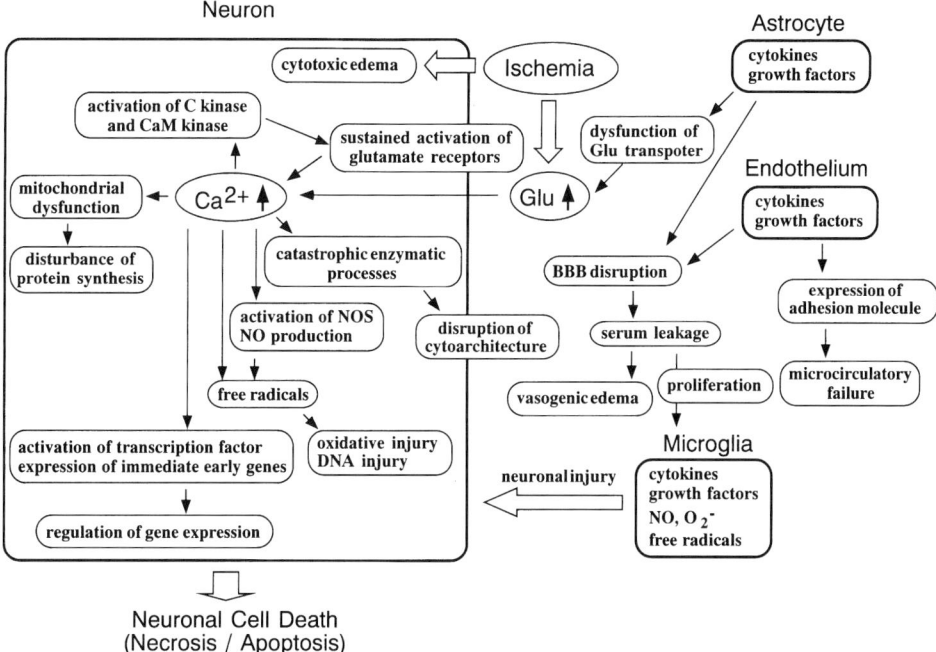

FIG. 5. Illustration of a pathway leading to ischemic neuronal death. When the brain is exposed to ischemia, glutamate (*Glu*) release occurs immediately from presynaptic neurons followed by postsynaptic neurons and astroglial cells by dysfunction of the glutamate transporter. The extracellular glutamate surge induces a marked Ca^{2+} mobilization in neurons through glutamate receptors. An augmented intracellular Ca^{2+} induces various cascade reactions such as activation of proteinase enzyme activities, sustained activation of glutamate receptors, dysfunction of mitochondrial energy production, activation of nitric oxide synthesis (*NOS*), production of free radicals, and change of gene expression, all of which lead to neuronal death. Not only neurons, but also astroglial cells, endothelium cells, and microglial cells are profoundly affected by ischemic insult, which results in the disruption of the blood-brain barrier (*BBB*), microcirculatory failure, and the activation of both astroglial cells and microglial cells. Microglial cells produce plenty of superoxide anions (O_2^-) and nitric oxide (*NO*), which may strongly damage neurons. CaM kinase, calcium/calmodulin-dependent protein kinase

ischemia, however, decreases the ATP supply within a few minutes, inhibiting the cell's capability of maintaining the transmembrane ion gradient and simultaneously induces neuronal depolarization and large accumulations of extracellular potassium ions and intracellular hydrated sodium. Thus, cytotoxic edema occurs in the early stage of ischemia.

A microdialysis study, using a transient ischemia model of the gerbil, revealed that the glutamate surge began within 20–30 s after the start of the ischemic insult in the hippocampal CA1 [15]. At 5 and 10 min after the start of the ischemic insult, the extracellular glutamate level sometimes exceeded 20 and 100 times the basal preischemic level, respectively. It was confirmed that in the CA1 region of the gerbil hippocampus, the ischemic glutamate surge starts first from the presynaptic region, followed by the postsynaptic region, and finally from astrocytes [19]. The glutamate surge in an ischemic condition is an outward flow of this amino acid into the extracellular space, which is induced by dysfunction of glutamate transporter molecules owing to the lack of ATP supply after ischemia and the release from highly concentrated intracellular glutamate pools (mM concentrations).

In the studies of Ca^{2+} microfluorometry imaging on slices from gerbil hippocampi, intracellular calcium mobilization is induced within 2–3 min after the start of in vitro ischemic simulations. Calcium mobilization exclusively occurs in the CA1 region, more significantly in the stratum radiatum and the stratum oriens than in the stratum pyramidale, leaving the CA3 region little affected [18]. The increase in intracellular calcium concentration ($[Ca^{2+}]_i$) by ischemia comes partly from outside the cell through voltage-dependent Ca^{2+} channels and through glutamate receptor channels, such as N-methyl-D-aspartate (NMDA)-type, α-amino-3-hydroxy-5-methyl-4-isoxazolepropionic acid (AMPA)-type and kainate-type. The $[Ca^{2+}]_i$ also originates from intracellular Ca^{2+} stores mediated by ryanodine-type receptors or inositol trisphosphate (IP_3)-type receptors. Calcium permeability of AMPA-type receptors is intrinsically small compared with that of NMDA-type receptors. However, the permeability increases after ischemic conditions in vivo [9] and in vitro [33], because a new subtype lacking Glu R2 appears, through which more Ca^{2+} passes than through a receptor subtype containing Glu R2. Sustained Ca^{2+} mobilization is lethal when it exceeds a certain level, because Ca^{2+} damages mitochondrial respiration and induces uncontrolled Ca^{2+}-dependent cascade reactions.

When ischemic insults were performed at lower temperatures, the degree of the glutamate surge was largely depressed [2,16] and the onset of Ca^{2+} mobilization was significantly delayed [17]. While excitotoxicity is considered to be completely finished within 1 or 2 h after the ischemic insult [5], postischemic hypothermia introduced some hours after insult still significantly resuscitates hippocampal neurons [3]. It therefore appears that other processes should follow the excitotoxicity, which are also highly temperature-sensitive. In other words, the excitotoxicity may play a role as a necessary condition, which triggers the initial processes to death, but by itself it cannot complete the whole process unless it is followed by succeeding events. One of the processes leading to cell death may be the postischemic, sustained activation of glutamate receptors [20]. Additionally, intraischemic hypothermia, which totally resuscitated the ischemic neurons, apparently prevented this phenomenon [32].

Mechanisms Involving Functions of Cell Nuclei

It is well known that protein synthesis is almost totally and irreversibly depressed in the CA1 sector after an ischemic insult, which suggests a key phenomenon in explaining the mechanism of delayed neuronal death [30]. We measured [^{14}C]leucine protein incorporation in the CA1, CA3, and dentate gyrus of ischemic gerbils by quantitative autoradiography. In the normothermia animals after 5-min ischemia, protein synthesis rates returned to normal after 1 day in all regions except in the CA1 sector, whereas the rate in the CA1 sector did not recover to normal. When hypothermia for 24 h was induced 3 h after transient forebrain ischemia, the protein synthesis rate in the CA1 sector recovered to a normal level 2 days after ischemia at the latest (unpublished data).

In the cell nuclei of ischemic neurons, dramatic changes develop in limited numbers of genes. A growing body of evidence indicates that a number of immediate early genes such as Fos and Jun families and many different kinds of transcription factors encoded by the immediate early genes are induced in cerebral tissues after ischemic insults. A marked enhancement of the DNA binding ability of a transcription factor, AP-1, in the gerbil hippocampus and other central areas has been reported [34]. The time course for the activity enhancement was prolonged from 1 to 9 h in the CA3 and the dentate gyrus, both comparatively resistant to ischemia, while a rather short-lived enhancement was observed in the CA1, the area extremely vulnerable to ischemia. However, gerbils with prior ischemic insults at 32°C showed a prolonged period of binding activation in the CA1, which was closer to the profiles for the

CA3 and dentate gyrus. Similar prolongation was seen in gerbils, which were rendered resistant to ischemic insult by a prior loading with a short ischemic insult for 2 min [35]. Although the peptide that is synthesized after AP-1 and binds to an upstream region of the corresponding gene is still unidentified, it is probably related to the protection or resuscitation of neurons.

Several lines of evidence point to a functional significance of specific genes, which are apparently activated in ischemic conditions to synthesize their respective peptides. It is likely that these genes are involved in accelerating or protecting the mechanisms of apoptosis [13]. Thus, it is not known whether apoptosis or necrosis operates independently on specified neurons, or whether both can take place at the same time in a single neuron. On the basis of ample findings in animal experiments that mild hypothermia protects neurons on a large scale against ischemic damage, it is speculated that mild hypothermia, as well as neuronal death through necrosis, may prevent neuronal death through apoptosis. Although no evidence is available at present, lowering body temperature will most likely interact with mechanisms that facilitate survival or that inhibit the death processes.

Microglial Cell Activation

Among the late-appearing cellular events in ischemic conditions, the responses of glial cells should be very important. One is astroglial activation. It seems that such responses help to protect neurons against damage. The other important glial response occurs in microglial cells. The proliferation of microglial cells was observed in hippocampal CA1 shortly after the ischemic insult, reaching its peak 4 days later [22]. There has been a general notion that microglia appear in the later stage of cerebral injuries to scavenge damaged neurons; then astrocytes occupy the space, and this is known as gliosis. However, Morioka's report indicated the appearance of microglial cells before neurons were damaged. According to recent findings, it appears that the central nervous system intimately cooperates with the immune system. Microglial cells, often called brain macrophages, have many different surface antigens common to those on peripheral macrophages. Cultured microglia are similar in shape to macrophages. Other common features of microglial cells are the production and release of superoxide anions (O_2^-) and nitric oxide (NO). Although it is still controversial whether NO molecules are actually toxic to neurons, O_2^- molecules are obviously toxic. Moreover, O_2^- and NO easily react to produce the highly toxic molecule peroxynitrite ($ONOO^-$).

The production of O_2^- in cultured microglial cells after protein kinase C activation by phorbol 12-myristrate 13-acetate (PMA) was so highly temperature-dependent that the product at 30°C was significantly lower than that at 37°C [26]. Lipopolysaccharide (LPS) induces the inducible NO synthesis (iNOS) enzyme in microglial cells, which produce NO molecules. At 30°C, the production of NO was reduced to one fifth of that at 37°C [26]. When evaluated by the [³H]thymidine uptake rate, the proliferation rate of microglial cells at 30°C was as low as 16% of that at 37°C, which was significantly lower in comparison to the proliferation of astroglial cells and fibroblasts at 30°C [26]. Thus, these phenomena all appear to be extremely temperature-dependent, and are significantly suppressed by lowering the temperature. This leads to the notion that neuron-aggravating characteristics of microglial cells, such as their proliferation and the production of O_2^- and NO, are significantly depressed by mild hypothermia, and that this may be a rational basis for neuronal resuscitation by postischemically introduced mild hypothermia. We examined the time course of microglial proliferation after 5-min forebrain ischemia in gerbils. Lectin-positive microglial cells first appeared 6 h after ischemia in the normothermia group, and the strongest microglial reactions were observed 4 days after ischemia. In the 23-h postischemic hypothermia group, the microglial reactions were continually reduced throughout until 30 days after ischemia (unpublished data).

Endothelial cells as well as glial cells, both astroglial and microglial cells, are included in the ischemic pathophysiological processes. In connection with this, a recent report described a functional involvement of albumin in the ischemic responses of microglial cells. When cultured microglial cells were exposed to a minute concentration of albumin, the cells remarkably proliferated, significantly increasing both PMA-induced production of O_2^- and LPS-induced formation of NO molecule [27]. Thus, it may be possible that when albumin leaks out through the postischemically deteriorated BBB, it begins to stimulate microglial cells to proliferate in the brain parenchyma, which then induces the production of O_2^- and NO in these cells, causing damage to ischemic neurons. These findings suggest that microglial cells in ischemic conditions play a role in inducing damage to neurons, although they behave as scavengers after neurons die.

Cerebral Edema

As noted previously, cytotoxic edema occurs shortly after ischemia because of an insufficient ATP supply along with excitotoxic processes. In the later stage after ischemia, vasogenic edema occurs where water moves across the dysfunctional BBB into the interstitial space. The disruption of the BBB can be demonstrated by observing extravasation of injected horseradish peroxidase or albumin as stated above, and such BBB deterioration was reduced in hypothermic rats [6]. Leukotriene B_4, an arachidonic metabolite produced by ischemic degradation of a membrane lipid, reportedly has been linked to the development of ischemia-induced vasogenic edema. The postischemic production of leukotriene B_4 was decreased by mild hypothermia [4]. Amelioration of cytotoxic edema by mild hypothermia is very likely when hypothermic reduction of the glutamate surge, calcium mobilization, and ATP expenditure are taken into consideration. It is worth nothing here that clinical institutions believe that mild hypothermia has a significant effect in reducing cerebral edema in ischemic or traumatic brain injury.

Hyperthermia

Previously, much evidence indicated that long-time exposure to heat induced cerebral injuries, implying that hyperthermia would have been detrimental to brain tissue. Experimental evidence has indicated that mild intraischemic hyperthermia significantly enhanced damage to ischemic rat brain [14]. It was shown in the rat that delayed postischemic hyperthermia, introduced 24h after 3-h transient ischemia, provided worse results in terms of the infarct size [12]. Such postischemic hyperthermia, probably due to dysfunction of the temperature regulation center in the hypothalamus, is not uncommon for stroke patients and may exacerbate serious complications. An enhanced glutamate release was postulated in hyperthermic ischemia more than in normothermic ischemia in a transient MCAO model of rats [28]. These findings suggest that brain temperature after cerebral ischemia should be kept at least at normothermic range.

A Brief Summary of the Research Project in Japan

A research project entitled, "Mild hypothermia for a treatment of stroke—basic investigations and clinical studies" (Chairperson: K.K. of the present authors), was organized for 3 fiscal years, 1994–1996, under the support of the Ministry of Health and Welfare in Japan. At the end of the

TABLE 1. Mild hypothermia for the treatment of stroke and head injury

Anesthesia
general anesthetics
muscle relaxant (pancuronium), tranquilizers (GABA agonist: midazolam, α-blocker: droperidol), analgetics (fentanyl)

Cooling methods
use of a cooling blanket (occasionally with intragastric or surface alcohol cooling)
stop cooling at 34°–35°C (step down)

Time window
3 h (head injury), 3–6 h (SAH), 6 h (cerebral infarction)

Extent
32°–34°C (head injury), 33°–34°C (SAH), 33°–34°C (cerebral infarction)
35°C (less-experienced institutions)

Duration
case by case
<6 days (head injury), 3–12 days (SAH), 3–7 days (cerebral infarction)

Criteria for physical management
BPs > 100 mmHg, ICP < 20 mmHg, CPP > 80 mmHg, $SjvO_2$ = 70–75%, Hb > 12 g/dl, CO > 3 l/min/m^2

Monitoring
temperature of intrajugular vein (additionally tympanitic membrane, urinary bladder or pulmonary vein), Swan–Ganz catheter

Rewarming
slow rewarming (0.1°C/h), stop rewarming at 34°–35°C (step up)

For complications
supplementation of platelets, K$^+$, growth hormone and/or L-arginine, colon preparation, enteric nutrition

GABA, γ-aminobutylic acid; SAH, subarachnoidal hemorrhage; BPs, systolic blood pressure; ICP, intracranial pressure; CPP, cerebral perfusion pressure; $SjvO_2$, internal jugular venous oxygen saturation; Hb, hemoglobin; CO, cardiac output

project, a consensus was reached on the basic methods of hypothermia treatment, which is shown in Table 1. Hypothermia can be applied to patients with brain injury, cerebral infarction, subarachnoidal hemorrhage (after clipping), and transient cardiopulmonary resuscitation at their acute stages. The methods of hypothermia, such as extent and duration, are slightly different among these diseases. Essentially, it is important that a sufficient oxygen supply to the brain is provided with intensive control of general and cerebral circulation. Consequently, it is necessary to monitor the movement of general and cerebral circulation and oxygen supply and consumption by systolic blood pressure (BPs), internal jugular venous oxygen saturation ($SjvO_2$), cardiac output (CO), intracranial pressure (ICP), and cerebral perfusion pressure (CPP). Mild hypothermia treatment has indicated a good neurological outcome in some institutions. However, several side effects of mild hypothermia were pointed out: a rise in viscosity of circulating blood, hypovolemic circulation, reduction in cardiac function with arrhythmias, pulmonary edema, platelet dysfunction with poor coagulative activity, immunologic depression with severe infection such as pneumonia, shivering, and changes in hormonal conditions. Mechanisms of these complications are not fully understood; however, precautions against and proper treatments for these adverse phenomena are urgent problems to be solved in order to attain potential benefits and low risk application of mild hypothermia.

Although a positive efficacy of mild hypothermia on brain injury at acute stages can be deduced, no objective evaluation of hypothermia treatment has been made. One of the problems to be pointed out is that the methods of hypothermia such as depth, duration, rewarming, and medications are independently employed. A large-scale randomized multicenter study is urgently needed to investigate the proper techniques of mild hypothermia in stroke, injury, or other disease involving cerebral ischemia and also to find ways to minimize unfavorable complications.

Perinatal Cerebropathy and Hypothermia

Hypoxia by asphyxia or fatal ischemic cerebropathy (leucomalacia, pontosubicular degeneration, etc.) is serious matter, so that elucidation of their pathogenesis is urgent. Recently, it was clarified in neonatal rats, corresponding to 30 weeks postgestational stage in humans, the NMDA receptor subunit NR2C, which is less susceptible to magnesium block, was temporally expressed. This finding indicates involvement of excitotoxic mechanism in the pons degeneration [21]. This process is theoretically sensitive to hypothermia. On the other hand, in neonate swines, postasphyxic cerebral edema developed slowly in the course of more than 10h, and this edema was markedly depressed by hypothermia [29]. In general, body temperature of neonates, particularly immature babies, easily falls because of prematurity of their temperature control center in the hypothalamus, so that it is actually not simple but difficulty to maintain or control body temperature in a normal range. Nevertheless, some groups try to apply hypothermia therapy to encephalopathic infants.

References

1. Busto R, Dietrich WD, Globus MY-T, Valdés I, Scheinberg P, Ginsberg MD (1987) Small differences in intraischemic brain temperature critically determine the extent of ischemic neuronal injury. J Cereb Blood Flow Metab 7:729–738
2. Busto R, Globus MY-T, Dietrich WD, Martinez E, Valdés I, Ginsberg MD (1989) Effect of mild hypothermia on ischemia-induced release of neurotransmitters and free fatty acids in rat brain. Stroke 20:904–910
3. Colbourne F, Corbett D (1994) Delayed and prolonged post-ischemic hypothermia is neuroprotective in the gerbil. Brain Res 654:265–272
4. Dempsey RJ, Combs DJ, Maley ME, Cowen DE, Roy MW, Donaldson DL (1987) Moderate hypothermia reduces postischemic edema development and leukotriene production. Neurosurgery 21:177–181
5. Deshpande JK, Siresjö BK, Wieloch T (1987) Calcium accumulation and neuronal damage in the rat hippocampus following cerebral ischemia. J Cereb Blood Flow Metab 7:89–95
6. Dietrich WD, Busto R, Halley M, Valdes I (1990) The importance of brain temperature in alterations of the blood-brain barrier following cerebral ischemia. J Neuropathol Exp Neurol 49:486–497
7. Fay T, Henny GC (1938) Symposium on cancer. Correlation of body segmental temperature and its relation to the location of carcinomatous metastasis. Clinical observations and response to methods of refrigeration. Surg Gynecol Obstet 66:512–524
8. Fay T (1959) Early experiences with local and generalized refrigeration of the human brain. J Neurosurg 16:239–260
9. Gorter JA, Petrozzino JJ, Aronica EM, Rosenbaum DM, Opitz T, Bennett MVL, Connor JA, Zukin RS (1997) Global ischemia induces downregulation of Glur2 mRNA and increases AMPA receptor-mediated Ca^{2+} influx in hippocampal CA1 neurons of gerbil. J Neurosci 17: 6179–6188

10. Hayashi N (1997) Prevention of vegetation after severe head trauma and stroke by combination therapy of cerebral hypothermia and activation of immune-dopaminergic nervous system. Soc Treat Coma Pro 6:133–145
11. Kataoka K, Yanase H (1998) Mild hypothermia—a revived countermeasure against ischemic neuronal damages. Neurosci Res 32:103–117
12. Kim Y, Busto R, Dietrich WD, Kraydieh S, Ginsberg MD (1996) Delayed postischemic hyperthermia in awake rats worsens the histopathological outcome of transient focal cerebral ischemia. Stroke 27:2274–2280
13. MacManus JP, Linnik MD (1997) Gene expression induced by cerebral ischemia: An apoptotic perspective. J Cereb Blood Flow Metab 17:815–832
14. Minamisawa H, Smith M-L, Siesjö BK (1990) The effect of mild hyperthermia and hypothermia on brain damage following 5, 10, and 15 minutes of forebrain ischemia. Ann Neurol 28:26–33
15. Mitani A, Kubo H, Iga K, Imon H, Kadoya F, Kataoka K (1990) A new enzymatic cycling technique for glutamate determination in brain microdialysates. J Neurochem 54:709–711
16. Mitani A, Kataoka K (1991) Critical levels of extracellular glutamate mediating gerbil hippocampal delayed neuronal death during hypothermia: Brain microdialysis study. Neuroscience 42:661–670
17. Mitani A, Kadoya F, Kataoka K (1991) Temperature dependence of hypoxia-induced calcium accumulation in gerbil hippocampal slices. Brain Res 562:159–163
18. Mitani A, Yanase H, Sakai K, Wake Y, Kataoka K (1993) Origin of intracellular Ca^{2+} elevation induced by in vitro ischemia-like condition in hippocampal slices. Brain Res 601:103–110
19. Mitani A, Andou Y, Matsuda S, Arai T, Sakanaka M, Kataoka K (1994) Origin of ischemia-induced glutamate efflux in the CA1 field of the gerbil hippocampus: An in vivo brain microdialysis study. J Neurochem 63:2152–2164
20. Mitani A, Namba S, Ikemune K, Yanase H, Arai T, Kataoka K (1998) Postischemic enhancements of N-methyl-D-aspartic acid (NMDA) and non-NMDA receptor-mediated responses in hippocampal CA1 pyramidal neurons. J Cereb Blood Flow Metab 18:1088–1098
21. Mitani A, Watanabe M, Kataoka K (1998) Functional change of NMDA receptors related to enhancement of susceptibility to neurotoxicity in the developing pontine nucleus. J Neurosci 18:7941–7952
22. Morioka T, Kalehua AN, Streit WJ (1991) The microglial reaction in the rat dorsal hippocampus following transient forebrain ischemia. J Cereb Blood Flow Metab 11:966–973
23. Naritomi H, Shimizu T, Oe H, Kinugawa H, Sawada T, Hirata T (1996) Mild hypothermia therapy in acute embolic stroke: A pilot study. J Stroke Cerebrovasc Dis 6 (Suppl 1):193–196
24. Rosomoff HL, Holaday DA (1954) Cerebral blood flow and cerebral oxygen consumption during hypothermia. Am J Physiol 179:85–88
25. Rosomoff HL (1956) Hypothermia and cerebral vascular lesions. I. Experimental interruption of the middle cerebral artery during hypothermia. J Neurosurg 13:332–343
26. Si Q-S, Nakamura Y, Kataoka K (1997) Hypothermic suppression of microglial activation in culture: Inhibition of cell proliferation and production of nitric oxide and superoxide. Neuroscience 81:223–229
27. Si Q-S, Nakamura Y, Kataoka K (1997) Albumin enhances superoxide production in cultured microglia. Glia 21:413–418
28. Takagi K, Ginsberg MD, Globus MY-T, Martinez E, Busto R (1994) Effect of hyperthermia on glutamate release in ischemic penumbra after middle cerebral artery occlusion in rats. Am J Physiol 266:H1770–H1776
29. Thoresen M, Wyatt J (1997) Keeping a cool head, post-hypoxic hypothermia—an old idea revisited. Acta Paediatr 86:1029–1033
30. Widmann R, Kuroiwa T, Bonnekoh P, Hossmann K-A (1991) [^{14}C]Leucine incorporation into brain proteins in gerbils after transient ischemia: Relationship to selective vulnerability of hippocampus. J Neurochem 56:789–796
31. Yanamoto H, Hong S-C, Soleau S, Kassell NF, Lee KS (1996) Mild postischemic hypothermia limits cerebral injury following transient focal ischemia in rat neocortex. Brain Res 718:207–211
32. Yanase H, Mitani A, Kataoka K (1995) Post-ischemic enhancement of calcium mobilization to NMDA, and the effect of hypothermia. J Neurochem 65:17

33. Ying HS, Weishaupt JH, Grabb M, Canzoniero LMT, Sensi SL, Sheline CT, Monyer H, Choi DW (1997) Sublethal oxygen-glucose deprivation alters hippocampal neuronal AMPA receptor expression and vulnerability to kainate-induced death. J Neurosci 17:9536–9544

34. Yoneda Y, Ogita K, Inoue K, Mitani A, Zhang L, Masuda S, Higashihara M, Kataoka K (1994) Rapid potentiation of DNA binding activities of particular transcription factors with leucine-zipper motifs in discrete brain structures of the gerbil with transient forebrain ischemia. Brain Res 667:54–66

35. Yoneda Y, Azuma Y, Inoue K, Ogita K, Mitani A, Zhang L, Masuda S, Higashihara M, Kataoka K (1997) Positive correlation between prolonged potentiation of binding of double-stranded oligonucleotide probe for the transcription factor AP1 and resistance to transient forebrain ischemia in gerbil hippocampus. Neuroscience 79:1023–1037

36. Zhang L, Mitani A, Yanase H, Kataoka K (1997) Continuous monitoring and regulating of brain temperature in the conscious and freely moving ischemic gerbil: effect of MK-801 on delayed neuronal death in hippocampal CA1. J Neurosci Res 47:440–448

37. Zhang R-L, Chopp M, Chen H, Garcia JH, Zhang ZG (1993) Postischemic (1 hour) hypothermia significantly reduces ischemic cell damage in rats subjected to 2 hours of middle cerebral artery occlusion. Stroke 24:1235–1240

4. Clinical Studies of Brain Hypothermia

                     a. Mechanism
                     b. Diagnosis
                     c. Treatment

Spontaneous Cerebral Hypothermia After Severe Head Injury: Relation with Brain Chemistry and Cerebrovascular Parameters

Michael M. Reinert, Jens Soukop, Alois Zauner, Egon Doppenberg, and M.R. Ross Bullock

Summary. Secondary ischemic events are one of the major causes of bad outcome in patients with severe traumatic brain injury (TBI). Multiple clinical trials testing diverse neuroprotective compounds have so far failed to provide new therapies. Nevertheless, multiple studies using hypothermia have shown evidence of benefit, and the latest results of a U.S. multicenter hypothermia trial are awaited. Meanwhile hypothermia is being used in many neurosurgical centers all over the world and especially in Japan. We therefore retrospectively analyzed patients suffering from TBI with a Glasgow Coma Scale (GCS) score of 8 or less. We studied brain temperature using a multiparameter sensor, brain chemistry using microdialysis, intracranial pressure (ICP) using a ventriculostomy, and cerebral blood flow (CBF) using stable-xenon CT. Patients were retrospectively separated into four temperature cohorts according to their brain temperature. Patients with spontaneous hypothermia (Tbr < 36°C) significantly differed from the other cohorts. The mean ICP ($P < 0.01$), cerebral perfusion pressure (CPP) ($P < 0.001$), and glutamate $P < 0.0004$) were significantly higher, whereas the CBF ($P < 0.05$) and brain glucose were lower. A negative brain temperature–rectal temperature (Trect) difference (ΔTbr–Trect) was correlated with a bad outcome as observed in the patients with spontaneous brain hypothermia and those with therapeutic cooling. When monitoring severely brain-injured patients, spontaneous brain hypothermia and a negative brain to rectal temperature difference (ΔTbr–Trect) represents an indicator of bad outcome and brain chemistry derangement (glutamate, lactate, glucose) and CBF.

Key words. Severe head injury, Hypothermia, Spontaneous, Outcome, Brain microdialysis, Neuromonitoring

Introduction

Hypothermia may be defined as mild (32°–36°C), moderate (28°–32°C), deep (15°–25°C), or profound (<15°C) [21,36]. Although the current literature supports a good general correlation between brain and body temperature [9,24,26,42], previous data have also demonstrated that monitoring body temperature alone is not sufficient to allow conclusions regarding the actual temperature status of the brain or the efficiency of cooling therapy [24–27,39]. Many experi-

Division of Neurosurgery, Medical College of Virginia, Virginia Commonwealth University, PO Box 989631, Richmond, VA 23298, USA

mental and clinical studies have been undertaken to devise a reliable technique for obtaining useful brain temperature measurement during treatment. Mild to moderate variations in brain temperature have been shown to have significant consequences on pathological and functional outcome in various models of brain injury [10,11,14,20]. The oxygen transport to cerebral tissue is influenced by temperature changes due to changes in the oxygen dissociation curve and in the affinity for hemoglobin, which is shifted to the left at lower temperatures and implies that oxygen is liberated less from red blood cells at lower temperatures. However the solubility for gases (CO_2 and O_2) increases at lower temperatures.

The biosynthesis and uptake of neurotransmitters are temperature-dependent as well. Intracellular Ca^{2+} exchange is also decreased during hypothermia, and it may thus protect cells from membrane breakdown [29,41]. Hypothermia has also been shown to reduce intracranial pressure (ICP) and cerebral blood flow after severe human head injury [23,28] and has been claimed to improve outcome [7,22]. Fluctuations in brain temperature may also be an indication of changes in brain metabolism, cerebral blood flow (CBF), neuronal damage, and brain function [4]. Hence a reduction in cellular metabolism has been suggested as a main mechanism for hypothermic protection. A decline in the metabolic rate of oxygen and glucose and a decrease in high-energy phosphates, accompanied by low CO_2 and lactate production, are seen during hypothermia [3,5,15,17].

Hagerdal et al. demonstrated in 1975 that CBF in rats was much more sensitive to hypocapnia in hypothermic rats (22°C) compared to that in normothermic rats (37°C). Thus at a $PaCO_2$ of 15 mmHg the CBF was only about 25% of normal at 22°C body temperature when compared to CBF values at 37°C. It has also been shown that the cerebral metabolic rate of oxygen is depressed by about 5% for each degree reduction in body temperature [16]. Further data support the idea that there is a comparable reduction in the cerebral metabolic rate for glucose (CMRG).

Independent of these temperature effects, studies in animal trauma models and head-injured humans have demonstrated that after posttraumatic injury there is an increase in transmembrane ionic shifts via several mechanisms: neuroexcitation, leaky ion channels, or membrane disruption by microporation. If the magnitude of the ionic shift surpasses a certain level, an irrecoverable ionic imbalance results that may consume energy metabolites in excess of supply [18,19]. Pellerin and Magistretti have shown in vitro that glutamate drives glycolysis, leading to an increase in lactate [34]. Such an elevation in lactate can also be due to an overload of the malate-aspartate transporter as a result of a massive sudden demand in energy-rich phosphates. This in turn leads to the depletion of cytosolic NAD, which is then provided by lactate dehydrogenase, which converts pyruvate to lactate [2,40]. This might be one of the several mechanisms responsible for increased extracellular lactate after traumatic brain injury (TBI).

To learn more about the effect of brain temperature on brain biochemistry, the present study examined the correlation between brain (Tbr) and rectal (Trect) temperature and the time course of both measurements, as well as their relation to ICP, cerebral perfusion pressure (CPP), CBF, brO_2, $brCO_2$, and extracellular glucose lactate and glutamate in four retrospectively defined patient temperature cohorts after severe human head injury.

Patients and Methods

Patients

The study was approved by the Committee for Conduct of Human Research at the Virginia Commonwealth University. Informed consent was obtained from family members upon arrival of the patient.

Patients suffering from TBI who were older than 16 years with a Glasgow Coma Score (GCS) of 8 or less were admitted to the neuroscience intensive care unit (NICU) at the Medical College of Virginia (MCV). Only patients who underwent ventriculostomy for ICP monitoring and treatment were included in this analysis. All 58 patients were treated by an ICP-directed management protocol as used at MCV. Measures included intermittent cerebrospinal fluid (CSF) drainage, sedation, systemic neuromuscular paralysis, mild hyperventilation (arterial $PaCO_2$ 32–34 mmHg), intravenous mannitol (0.5–1.0 mg/kg), and mild hypothermia in selected cases when the ICP did not respond to other measures. Care was taken to keep the arterial partial oxygen pressure (P_aO_2) above 100 mmHg, the hemoglobin concentration above 10 g/dl, and the CPP above 70 mmHg. If necessary, blood pressure was supported with vasopressor therapy. Mild therapeutic hypothermia was induced for a variable time in 33 patients, with a sustained increased ICP above 20 mmHg. The outcome of all patients was measured 3 months after injury according to the Glasgow Outcome Scale (GOS).

Therapeutic Cooling

The rectal core temperature was measured continuously with a thermocouple (HP21075A, Hewlett Packard). The thermocouple accuracy was ±0.1°C. Commercially available water cooling blankets, ice packs, and gastric ice water lavage were used for surface cooling in selected patients with a progressive ICP increase during the ICP-directed management, for the first 48 hours after injury and continued as long as needed. All febrile patients (Trect > 38.5°C) were cooled as well to try to achieve normothermia. All cooled patients were sedated, pharmacologically paralyzed, and ventilated. In addition, paracetamol (600 mg every 4–6 hours, if needed) was given to patients with a Trect > 38.5°C, independent from ICP management.

Neuromonitoring

The hemodynamic monitoring included continuous measurements of arterial blood pressure (ABP), peripheral oxygen saturation (SO_2) and central venous pressure (CVP) in selected patients. A three-lumen transcranial bolt was placed either on arrival at the NSICU or in the operating room after evacuation of a hematoma, as described by Zauner et al. [43]. Its purpose was to grip and immobilize the intraventricular catheter, the multiparameter sensor, and the microdialysis probe. The experimental and clinical validation of these techniques in brain tissue have been described [43]. The ICP was continuously measured using an intraventricular catheter or an intraparenchymal ICP sensor (Codman, Randolph, MA, USA).

The miniaturized multiparameter probe (Paratrend 7-Neurotrend; Diametrics Medical, Roseville, MN, USA) was used for continuous measurement of brain tissue oxygen tension ($pbrO_2$), carbon dioxide ($pbrCO_2$), pH, and temperature. The oxygen sensor consisted of a miniaturized Clark electrode (in the Paratrend 7) or an optical fiber containing a photosensitive dye, ruthenium red, sensitive to oxygen, as in the "Neurotrend." The thermocouple in the Paratrend 7 was located at the tip of the probe, whereas in the Neurotrend the thermocouple was located 1.5 cm from the tip of the probe. An accuracy of ±0.02°C was given by the manufacturer for the probes.

Microdialysis

Microdialysis was performed using a 56 mm long flexible probe with a 10 mm long collecting membrane, with a cutoff level of 20 kD (CMA, Acton, MA, USA). The probe was continuously perfused at a flow rate of 2 μl/min with sterile 0.9% saline. Sixty microliter Dialysates (60 μl) were collected every 30 min into sealed glass vials stored at 4°C into a refrigerated collector

(Honeycomb, BAS, Bioanalyticalsystems). To measure glucose and lactate, an enzymatic technique was used (YSI 2700 Select, Yellow Springs Instrument Co., OH, USA). The analysis of the excitatory amino acids (EAAs) was performed via high-performance liquid chromatography (HPLC) using an electrochemical detection system [35]. Samples were analyzed and time-linked to the continuously measured parameters.

Data Acquisition and Parameter Analysis

All clinical parameters (ABG, SO_2, ICP, CPP) from each patient were transferred from the bedside monitor every 3 s to a VAX mainframe computer for the entire monitoring period. Data from the Paratrend-Neurotrend systems were time-locked and loaded into a separate computer (Apple Computers, Cuppertino, CA, USA).

The mean values of all continuously measured parameters were averaged over a period of 30 min and compared to each other and to neurochemical analytes. Each parameter was analyzed based on four brain temperature cohorts that became apparent during data analysis.

Normothermic	Tbr between 36.0°C and 37.5°C
Hyperthermic	Tbr > 37.5°C
Therapeutic cooling	Tbr < 36.0°C due to mild hypothermia
Spontaneous hypothermic	Tbr < 36°C

Further analysis was done using the temperature difference (ΔTbr-Trect) between Tbr and Trect and classified as positive (ΔTbr-Trect > 0°C) or negative (ΔTbr-Trect < 0°C).

Cerebral Blood Flow Measurements

In 56 patients the stable xenon technique (XeCT Enhancer 3000 DDP, Houston, TX, USA) was used to measure CBF both shortly after admission and on the third or fourth day. The measurement was done by repeated CT scanning with a gas mixture of 30% xenon and 30%–60% oxygen, with the remaining gas room air. The regional CBF was calculated using a 20 mm cir-

ROI

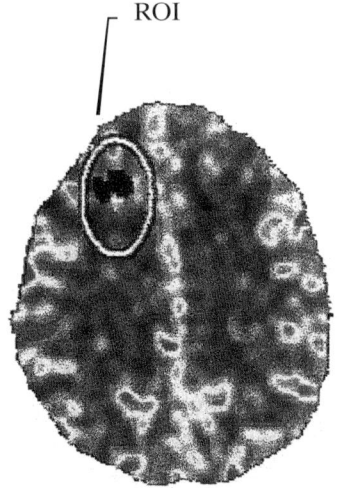

Fig. 1. Cerebral blood flow (CBF) study [xenon computed trmography (CT)] of patient, demonstrating the technique of regional CBF measurement (*white circle*) around the multiparameter sensor and microdialysis probe. *ROI*, region of interest

cular region of interest (ROI), drawn around the multiparameter and microdialysis probes, on the xenon scan (Fig. 1). For technical reasons we did not cool patients during xenon CBF studies, but measurements were correlated with the immediate pre- and postxenon CT temperatures.

Statistical Analysis

All physiological parameters were presented as means ± standard error of the mean (SEM). For calculating correlations between the various measurements, Pearson's coefficient or a simple regression analysis was applied. Analyzing the effect of different brain temperatures and the temperature difference (Tbr-Trect) on the continuously measured parameters, a factorial analysis of variance (ANOVA) and the Fisher's PLSD were used unless specified otherwise. All statistical tests were analyzed with significance assumed at 0.05. The software package Stat View 4.0 (Abacus Concepts, Berkeley, CA, USA) was used for all statistical calculations.

Results

Fifty-eight patients were included in the analysis. There were no significant differences between cohorts regarding the initial GCS, start time of monitoring, surgery, and CT diagnosis.

Relation Between Brain Temperature and Rectal Temperature

The Tbr and Trect correlated strongly ($r^2 = 0.725$). When analyzing the temperature difference (Tbr-Trect) an interesting observation was made. The spontaneously hypothermic cohort was characterized by a large negative temperature difference (ΔTbr-Trect) of −0.8 ± 1.4°C. During mild hypothermia (therapeutic cooling) patients had a negative ΔTbr-Trect, of −0.2 ± 0.6 as well. A minimal positive ΔTbr-Trect was found in the normothermic cohort (0.0 ± 0.5°C) and in the hyperthermic cohort (0.3 ± 0.5°C). Table 1 shows the significant intrapatient relation of Tbr, Trect, and ΔTbr-Trect for all four cohorts.

TABLE 1. Temperature cohorts and their brain temperatures, rectal temperatures, and brain-rectal temperature difference; their respective significances compared with each other

Condition	Tbr*	Trect**	ΔTbr-Trect
Normothermic (n = 2525)	36.9 ± 0.4	36.9 ± 0.6	0.0 ± 0.5
Hyperthermic (n = 3979)	38.2 ± 0.5	37.9 ± 0.5	0.3 ± 0.5
Therapeutic cooling (n = 1072)	35.3 ± 0.5	35.5 ± 1.0	−0.2 ± 0.6
Spontaneously hypothermic (n = 145)	34.4 ± 1.5	35.0 ± 0.8	−0.8 ± 1.4

Results are the mean ± SEM
n, number of observation points; Tbr, brain temperature; Trect, rectal temperature
*Significant difference between all groups ($P < 0.0001$); **significant difference within each group ($P < 0.0001$)

TABLE 2. Temperature cohorts and their respective brain tissue oxygen and brain tissue carbon dioxide; their significances compared with each other

Condition	$PbrO_2$	$PbrCO_2$
Nomothermic	35 ± 25*†	46 ± 11*†
Hyperthermic	34 ± 19*†	48 ± 9*†
Therapeutic cooling	31 ± 22**	40 ± 4*
Spontaneously hypothermic	25 ± 33	74 ± 46

$PbrO_2$, brain tissue oxygen; $PbrCO_2$, brain tissue carbon dioxide
* Versus spontaneously hypothermic, $P < 0.0001$; ** versus spontaneously hypothermic, $P < 0.05$; † versus therapeutic cooling, $P < 0.0001$

Relation Between Brain Temperature and Brain Oxygenation

Normothermic patients had the highest brain tissue oxygen values (35 ± 25 mmHg), compared to all other cohorts. In patients who underwent therapeutic cooling (Tbr < 36°C) for ICP control, the $P_{br}O_2$ was significantly lower (31 ± 22 mmHg) than in patients with Tbr > 36°C. The lowest $P_{br}O_2$ was measured in the spontaneously hypothermic cohort (Table 2).

Brain $P_{br}CO_2$ was significantly different in all four cohorts as well (Table 1). In nomothermic patients the $PbrCO_2$ was 46 ± 11 mmHg, whereas mild therapeutic hypothermia decreased the $P_{br}CO_2$ by 13% (40 ± 3 mmHg, $P < 0.0001$). However in spontaneously hypothermic patients a CO_2 accumulation took place (74 ± 46 mmHg) (Table 2).

Relation Between Temperature Cohorts and ICP and CPP

The mean ICP in the normothermic cohort was 14.9 ± 1 mmHg. In the therapeutic cooling cohort the ICP was 13.5 ± 2.3 mmHg and in the hyperthermic cohort 14.6 ± 0.8 mmHg. The mean ICP did not increase above 20 mmHg when mild therapeutic hypothermia was in use. In the spontaneously hypothermic cohort the ICP was significantly higher (25.1 ± 8.3 mmHg; $P < 0.01$) compared to all other cohorts.

The CPP for the normothermic cohort was 81.2 ± 2.5 mmHg. The lowest CPP was seen in the spontaneously hypothermic cohort (50.6 ± 60.23 mmHg). All cohorts were significantly different ($P < 0.001$) compared to the spontaneously hypothermic cohort. The mean ICP and CPP values are shown in Fig. 2.

Relation Between Temperature Cohorts and Dialysate Glucose, Lactate, and EAA

Forty-eight patients underwent microdialysis studies. Few microdialysis data were available for the hyperthermic cohort and therefore are not reported. Dialysate glucose was lower in the spontaneously hypothermic cohort compared to all other cohorts ($P < 0.01$). There was a trend to lower glucose in patients who underwent therapeutic cooling (564 ± 79 μmol/l) compared to normothermic patients (671 ± 289 μmol/l) (Fig. 3).

Lactate was lower during therapeutic cooling (1041 ± 343 μmol/l) than in all other cohorts. Patients in the spontaneously hypothermic cohort had the highest lactate levels ($1649 \pm$

Mean ICP versus Temperature Cohort

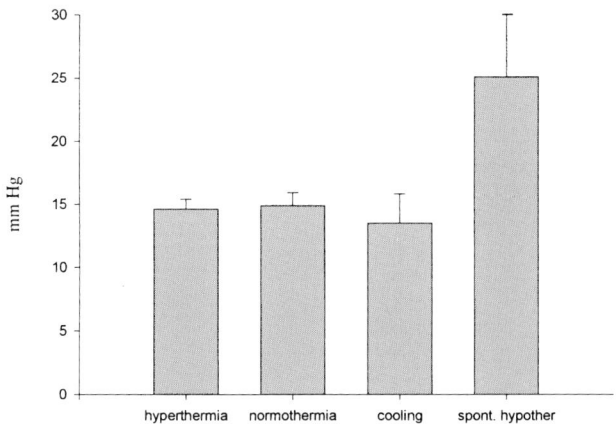

Mean CPP versus Temperature Cohort

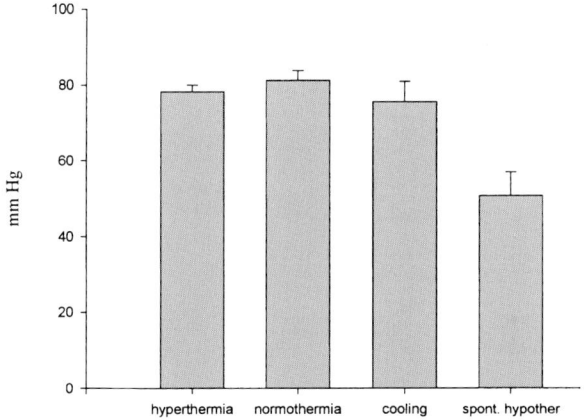

FIG. 2. Intracranial pressure (*ICP*) and cerebral perfusion pressure (*CPP*) in the four study cohorts (mean ± SEM). ICP is significantly higher in the spontaneous hypothermia cohort compared to the others ($P < 0.01$). CPP is significantly lower in spontaneous hypothermia cohort compared to the others ($P < 0.001$)

450 µmol/l) (Fig. 3). No significant difference was found upon analyzing the relation between lactate and glucose and ∆Tbr-Trect.

Glutamate was lowest during mild therapeutic hypothermia (6.7 ± 2.3 µmol/l) and highest in the spontaneously hypothermic cohort (130 ± 92 µmol). The difference was significant compared to all groups ($P < 0.0004$) (Fig. 3).

Therapeutic hypothermia was thus associated with a significant decrease of dialysate glutamate and lactate compared to that at higher temperature levels. The highest lactate and glutamate levels were obtained in the spontaneously hypothermic cohort, whereas brain pH and pO_2 were lowest compared to all other patients.

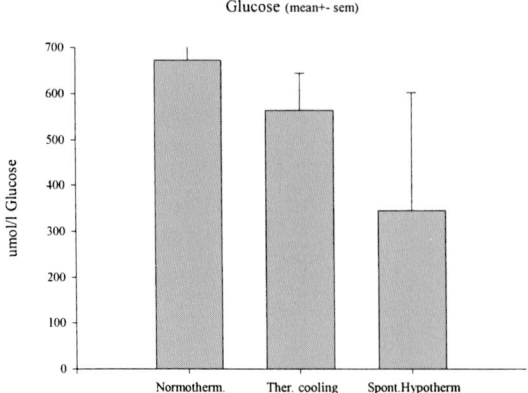

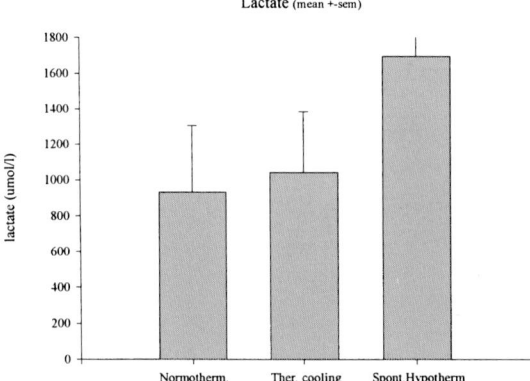

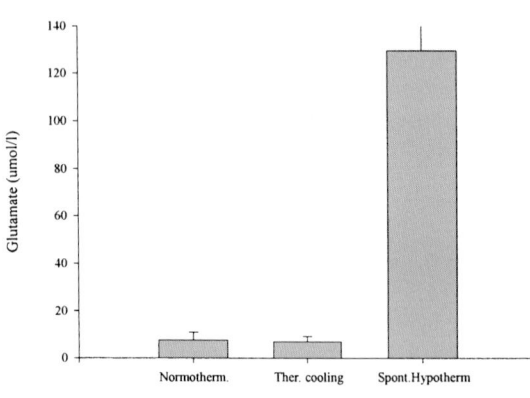

FIG. 3. Glucose, lactate, and glutamate in the study cohorts (mean ± SEM). Few data were available for the hyperthermia cohort and are therefore not shown. Glucose was lower in the spontaneous hypothermia cohort compared to the others. Lactate was higher and glutamate was significantly higher ($P < 0.0004$) in the spontaneous hypothermia cohort compared to the others

Fig. 4. Cerebral blood flow (CBF) measured by stable xenon CT, showing significantly ($P < 0.05$) lower flow values in
the spontaneous hypothermia cohort
compared to the others

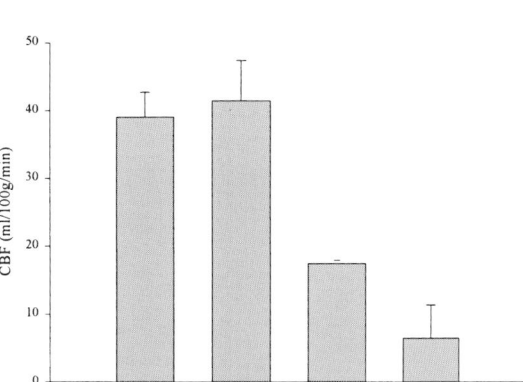

CBF (Mean +- SEM) Versus Temperature Cohort

Relation Between Temperature Cohorts and CBF

Fifty-six CBF studies were analyzed on 41 patients for studying the relation between temperature and CBF. The CBF values were the lowest in the spontaneous hypothermia and therapeutic cooling cohorts (17.1 ± 14.0 ml/100 g/min). Thus in patients with a negative temperature
difference (ΔTbr-Trect) the CBF was significantly lower (31.4 ± 14.8 ml/100 g/min) than in
patients with a positive difference (40.5 ± 16.9 ml/100 g/min) ($P < 0.05$) (Fig. 4).

Relation Between Temperature Cohort and GCS and Outcome

The Tbr was significantly lower in patients with a GCS of 3–4 ($37.1° \pm 2.1°$C) than in patients
with a GCS of 7–8 ($38.2° \pm 1.2°$C) ($P < 0.05$) during the first 6h of monitoring.

The outcome after 3 months (GOS-3) was analyzed in 51 patients. Performing a chi-square
test for the various temperature management conditions, there was no significant difference
across the temperature cohorts for outcome. However, death (GOS-4) was significantly more
frequent in the spontaneous hypothermic cohort (Fig. 5).

Discussion

The application of hypothermia has long been thought to improve outcome after both brain
trauma and aneurysm surgery [1,8,13]. Promising effects for mild hypothermia in severely
head-injured patients have been demonstrated by several authors [6,22,23]. Recently a large
U.S. multicenter trial designed to test the effect of early mild hypothermia on outcome after
severe head injury was prematurely terminated. The results are not yet available at the time
of writing. Therefore at present severe head injury continues to represent the commonest indication for inducing mild and moderate hypothermia, especially in Japan [30–33,38]. In many
neurosurgical centers application of mild hypothermia has become standard practice after
severe head injury. In our institution, we have been impressed with the ability of hypothermia to reduce ICP and improve CPP when brain swelling is present. Accordingly, we have
incorporated mild hypothermia (33°C) into our "therapeutic staircase" approach to control
ICP. We have modified the protocols of Clifton, Hayashi, and Marion, for use at MCV.

Over the last few years, we have perfected new techniques for multimodality neurochemical and substrate monitoring that allow continuous brain temperature monitoring, and thus

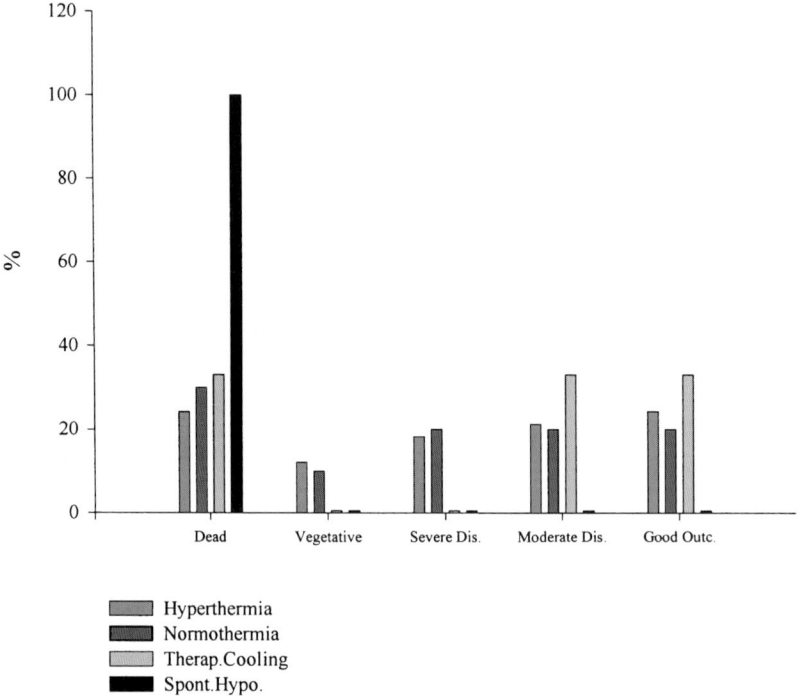

Fig. 5. Outcome as measured by Glasgow Outcome Score (GOS-3 months) shows no clear distribution for the temperature cohorts, except for the spontaneous hypothermia cohort, for which all patients had GOS-4 (death)

cross-correlation between these parameters and brain temperature in the same region. Newly developed technologies have now made multimodal brain monitoring possible, allowing better understanding of the pathophysiological events after TBI and thus possibly accelerating the necessary therapeutic modulations for improving outcome [12].

Spontaneously Hypothermic Patients

Brain temperature is mainly dependent on cerebral blood flow. Local brain metabolism is a much less important determinant of local temperature. The present study demonstrates that brain temperature and especially a negative Tbr-Trect gradient is an index for bad outcome (Table 2, Fig. 5). When analyzing the CBF in relation to temperature, the lowest CBF values were observed in the spontaneously hypothermic cohort. CPP, brain tissue oxygen, and glucose were the lowest in this cohort as well, whereas the ICP, lactate, and glutamate were the highest. We hypothesize that these data chiefly reflect a state of reduced CBF as a consequence of the traumatic injury in the spontaneously hypothermic patients. The *negative* gradient (ΔTbr-Trect) represents a predictor for hypoperfusion and thus bad outcome.

Therapeutic Cooling

Patients in the therapeutic cooling cohort initially had increased ICP, similar to the patients in the spontaneously hypothermic cohort. However, their response to mannitol and initiation of mild hypothermia was more favorable, and so their outcome was significantly better. These patients demonstrated higher brain oxygen values, higher CPPs, and lower ICP values than the spontaneously hypothermic patients. Nevertheless, their outcome as demonstrated in Fig. 5 was not significantly different from the other temperature cohorts, except the spontaneous hypothermia. The microdialysis analysis (Fig. 3) showed higher glucose and lower glutamate and lactate levels, suggesting a more favorable metabolic condition in these therapeutic cooling patients. The CBF was increased compared to that in the spontaneously hypothermic patients, but it was lower than in the normothermic and hypothermic cohorts. This reduction in CBF might be explained in part by the possible CBF decreasing effect of induced mild hypothermia.

Normothermia

Normothermia patients demonstrated higher CBF values, higher oxygenation, and higher glucose and lower glutamate and lactate microdialysis values than those in the other temperature cohorts.

Comment

We have shown that patients who are spontaneously hypothermic as measured by brain temperature, and a *negative* Tbr-Trect have a worse outcome. Our biochemical data suggest that we may advance the following hypothesis: a more severe injury may induce more glutamate release, with consequent cell swelling, more lactate release, and low glucose. These events, in turn, lead to reduced local CBF, possibly due to astrocyte swelling, which compresses the local microvasculature [37]. These events, if they overshoot certain thresholds, probably lead to a point of no return, where cells swell further and thus compromise local CBF. We hypothesize that when the tissue reaches this point the CBF is severely compromised, and the temperature gradient (Tbr-Trect) tends to become negative.

Conclusions

Multiparameter monitoring is safe. Brain temperature monitoring is important and may in the future have the potential to improve outcome, especially if the brain-rectal gradient (Tbr-Trect) is analyzed continuously. Patients with a clear negative Tbr-Trect, as represented by our spontaneously hypothermic cohort, have increased glutamate and lactate, reduced glucose, and lowered CBF—and thus a uniformly bad outcome. Future analysis might demonstrate that rigorous and early application of mild hypothermia, before ICP increases, might have a beneficial effect on outcome.

Acknowledgments. Ross Bullock is supported by the Reynolds Foundation, and Michael Reinert is supported by NIH NINDS grant 12587 and the Novartis Foundation.

References

1. Adams J, Wylie E (1959) Value of hypothermia and arterial occlusion in the treatment of intracranial aneurysms. Surg Gynecol Obstet 108:631–635

2. Bittar P, Charnay Y, Pellerin L, Bouras C, Magistretti P (1996) Selective distribution of lactate dehydrogenase isoenzymes in neurons and astrocytes of human brain. J Cereb Blood Flow Metab 16:1079
3. Brunberg J, Reilly E, Doty D (1974) Central nervous system consequences in infants of cardiac surgery using deep hypothermia and circlatory arrest. Circulation 50:60–68
4. Busto R, Dietrich W, Globus M, Valdes I, Schienberg P, Ginsberg M (1987) Small differences in intraischemic brain temperature critically determine the extent of ischemic neuronal injury. J Cereb Blood Flow Metab 7:729–738
5. Busto R, Globus M, Dietrich D, Martinez E, Valdes I, Ginsberg M (1989) Effect of mild hypothermia on ischemia-induced release of neurotransmitters and free fatty acids in rat brain. Stroke 20:904–910
6. Clifton G, Allen S, Barrodale P (1993) A phase II trial of systemic hypothermia in severe head injury. J Neurotrauma 10:263–271
7. Clifton G, Jiang J, Lyeth B, Jenkins L, Hamm R, Hayes R (1991) Marked protection by moderate hypothermia after experimental traumatic brain injury. J Cereb Blood Flow Metab 11:114–121
8. Connolly J, Boyd R, Calvin J (1962) The protective effect of hypothermia in cerebral ischemia: experimental and clinical application by selective brain cooling in the human. Surgery 51:15–23
9. Crowder M, Tempelhoff R, Theard A, Cheng M, Todorov A, Dacey R (1996) Jugular bulb temperature: comparison with brain surface and core temperature in neurosurgical patients during mild hypothermia. J Neurosurg 85:98–103
10. Dietrich W (1992) The importance of brain temperature in cerebral injury. J Neurotrauma 9:476–485
11. Dietrich W, Busto R, Globus M, Ginsberg M (1996) Brain damage and temperature: cellular and molecular mechanisms. In: Wieloch BSAT (ed) Cellular and molecular mechanisms of ischemic brain damage. Philadelphia: Lippincott-Raven
12. Doppenberg E, Zauner A, Bullock R, Ward J (1998) Correlation between brain tissue oxygen tensiom, carbon dioxide, pH and cerebral blood flow: a better way of monitoring the severely injured brain? Surg Neurol (in press)
13. Drake C, Barr W, Coles S (1964) The use of extracorporeal circulation and profound hypothermia in the treatment of ruptured intracranial aneurysm. J Neurosurg 21:575–581
14. Ginsberg M, Sternau L, Globus W, Dietrich W, Busto R (1992) Therapeutic modulation of brain temperature: relevance to ischemic brain injury. Cerebrovasc Metab Rev 4:189–225
15. Globus M, Alonso O, Dietrich W, Busto R, Ginsberg M (1995) Glutamate release and free radical production following brain injury: effects of posttraumatic hypothermia. Neurochemistry 65:1704–1711
16. Hagerdal M, Harp J, Nilsson L, Siesjo B (1975) The effect of induced hypothermia upon oxygen consumption in the rat brain. J Neurochem 24:311–316
17. Hovda D, Lee S, Smith M, Stuck M, Bergsneider M, Kelly D, Shalmon E, Martin N, Caron M, Mazziotta J, Pheleps M, Becker D (1995) The neurochemical and metabolic cascade following brain injury: moving from animal models to man. J Neurotrauma 12:903–906
18. Katayama Y, Becker D, Tamura T, Hovda D (1990) Massive increases in extracellular potassium and the indiscriminate release of glutamate following concussive brain injury. J Neurosurg 73:889–900
19. Katayama Y, Cheung M, Alves A (1989) Ion fluxes and cell swelling in experimental traumatic brain injury: the role of excitatory amino acids. In: Hoff AB JT (ed) Intracranial pressure VII. Berlin: Springer, pp 584–588
20. Lucas J, Emery D, Wang G, Rosenberg L, Jordan R, Gross G (1994) In vivo investigations of the effects of nonfreezing low temperatures on lesioned and uninjured mammalian neurons. J Neurotrauma 11:35–61
21. Marion D, Leonov Y, Ginsberg M (1996) Resuscitative hypothermia. Crit Care Med 24: s81–s89
22. Marion D, Obrist W, Carlier P, Penrod L, Darby J (1993) The use of moderate therapeutic hypothermia for patients with severe head injuries: a preliminary report. J Neurosurg 79:354–362

23. Marion DW, Penrod LE, Kelsey SF, Obrist WD, Kochanek PM, Palmer AM, Wisniewski SR, DeKosky ST (1997) Treatment of traumatic brain injury with moderate hypothermia. N Engl J Med 336:540–546
24. Mellergard P (1992) Changes in human intracerebral temperature in response to different methods of brain cooling. Neurosurgery 31:671–677
25. Mellergard P, Nordstrom C (1990) Epidural temperature and possible intracerebral temperature gradients in man. Br J Neurosurg 4:31–38
26. Mellergard P, Nordstrom C (1991) Intracerebral temperature in neurosurgical patients. Neurosurgery 31:709–713
27. Mellergard P, Nordstrom C, Christensson M (1990) A method for monitoring intracerebral temperature in neurosurgical patients. Neurosurgery 27:654–657
28. Metz C, Holzschuh M, Bein T, Woertgen C, Frey A, Frey I, Taeger K, Brawanski A (1996) Moderate hypothermia in patients with severe head injury: cerebral and extracerebral effects. J Neurosurg 85:533–541
29. Mitani A, Kadoya F, Kataoka K (1991) Temperature dependence of hypoxia induced calcium accumulation in gerbil hippocampal slices. Brain Res 562
30. Mori K, Maeda M, Miyazaki M, Iwase H (1998) Effects of mild (33°C) and moderate (29°C) hypothermia on cerebral blood flow and metabolism, lactate, and extracellular glutamate in experimental head injury. Neurol Res 20:719–726
31. Mori K, Maeda M, Miyazaki M, Iwase H (1998) Effects of mild and moderate hypothermia on cerebral metabolism and glutamate in an experimental head injury. Acta Neurochir Suppl 71:222–224
32. Nakamura T, Nagao S, Kawai N, Honma Y, Kuyama H (1998) Significance of multimodal cerebral monitoring under moderate therapeutic hypothermia for severe head injury. Acta Neurochir Suppl 71
33. Nara I, Shiogai T, Hara M, Saito I (1998) Comparative effects of hypothermia, barbiturate and osmotherapy for cerebral oxygen metabolism, intracranial pressure and cerebral perfusion pressure in patients with severe head injury
34. Pellerin L, Magistretti P (1994) Glutamate uptake into astrocytes stimulates aerobic glycolisis: a mechanism coupling neuronal activity to glucose utilization. Neurobiology 91:10625–10629
35. Person L, Hillered L (1992) Chemical monitoring of neurosurgical intensive care patients using intracerebral microdialysis. J Neurosurg 76:72–80
36. Safar P, Bircher N (1988) Cardiopulmonary cerebral resucitation: an introduction to resuscitation medicine. In: Guidelines of the World Federation of Societies of Anaesthesiologists, 3rd edn. London: Saunders
37. Schroeder M, Muizelaar J, Fatouros P, Kuta A, Choi S (1998) Regional cerebral blood volume after severe head injury patients with regional cerebral ischemia. Neurosurgery 42:1276–1279
38. Shiozaki T, Sugimoto H, Taneda M, Oda J, Tanaka H, Hiraide A, Shimazu T (1009) Selection of severely head injured patients for mild hypothermia therapy. J Neurosurg 89:206–211
39. Shiraki K, Sagawa S, Tajima F, Yokota A, Hashimoto M, Brengelmann G (1988) Independence of brain and tympanic temperature in unanaesthesized humans. J Appl Physiol 65:482–486
40. Siesjo B (1978) Brain energy metabolism. New York, Wiley
41. Siesjo B (1981) Cell damage in the brain: a speculative synthesis. J Cereb Blood Flow Metab 1:1981
42. Weisend M, Feeney D (1994) The relationship between traumatic brain injury induced changes in brain temperature and behavioural and anatomic outcome. J Neurosurg 80:120–132
43. Zauner A, Doppenberg E, Woodward J, Allen C, Gebrailli S, Young H, Bullock R (1997) Multiparametric continuous monitoring of brain metabolism and substrate delivery in neurosurgical patients. Neurol Res 19:265–273

Effect of Therapeutic Moderate Hypothermia on Extracellular and CSF Intermediates of Secondary Brain Injury

Donald W. Marion

Summary. In a group of 82 patients entered into our single-center therapeutic moderate hypothermia trial, we found significant improvement in 6-month outcome in those with an admission Glasgow Coma Scale score of 5–7 who were treated with therapeutic moderate hypothermia. We also found a significant decrease in intracranial pressure among those patients during the period of cooling. Of the molecular intermediates of secondary brain injury that we studied, we found that therapeutic moderate hypothermia caused a significant reduction in extracellular and CSF levels of glutamate during the period of cooling, and a significant and sustained reduction in the CSF levels of IL-Iβ. Extracellular levels of this cytokine could not be measured because of the technical limitations of the dialysis catheter (molecular weight cutoff too small for this larger molecule).

Key words. Hypothermia, Secondary brain injury, Traumatic brain injury, Glutamate

Introduction

Moderate hypothermia has been shown to reduce extracellular levels of excitatory amino acids, free radicals, nerve growth factor, and microtubule-associated protein in animal models of traumatic brain injury [1,7,11,12,15]. It also has been shown to reduce the volume of brain tissue damaged as a result of controlled cortical contusion and to preserve the integrity of the blood-brain barrier [4,5,8,14]. Most important, this therapy has been found to reduce significantly the functional and behavioral deficits caused by controlled cortical contusion and fluid percussion injuries [3,6]. During the last 10 years numerous clinical trials of therapeutic moderate hypothermia have been reported [2,9,10,13]. Most have documented either significant neurologic improvement or a trend toward improvement at 6 months following injury in patients treated with therapeutic moderate hypothermia as compared with those kept normothermic. Most of the clinical trials have found a significant reduction of intracranial pressure as a result of therapeutic moderate hypothermia, although this beneficial effect is not sustained once the patients are rewarmed. In addition, most trials have not found benefit from therapeutic moderate hypothermia for patients with the most severe brain injuries (initial Glasgow Coma Scale [GCS] score of 3 or 4). The slight benefit from hypothermia observed

University of Pittsburgh Medical Center, 200 Lothrop Street, Suite B400, Pittsburgh, PA 15213, USA

with the large recently completed United States multicenter trial of hypothermia also was seen only in those with a higher GCS score.

From 1991 through 1994 we conducted a controlled prospective randomized trial of therapeutic moderate hypothermia for 24 hr in a group of patients with severe traumatic brain injury (TBI) cooled to 32°–33°C as soon as possible after admission, and compared their outcomes with those of a similar group of patients who were kept normothermic during this time [9]. We used a block randomization scheme in which those patients assigned to the hypothermia and normothermia groups who had an admission GCS score of 3 or 4 were randomized separately from those patients with an admission GCS score of 5–7. Only adults were entered into this trial. At 6 months following injury, neurologic outcome was assessed using the Glasgow Outcome Scale (GOS) score. We determined that those patients who had an admission GCS score of 5–7 and were randomized to the hypothermia group had a significantly better outcome than patients who were assigned to the normothermia group. Hypothermia did not benefit those patients who had an admission GCS score of 3 or 4.

We attempted to determine the effect of therapeutic moderate hypothermia on the molecular intermediates of secondary brain injury. Indeed, the primary rationale for initiating cooling as quickly as possible after the injury, and limiting cooling to the first 24 hr after injury, was based on the hypothesis that hypothermia would limit secondary brain injury. Laboratory investigations have suggested that the most important molecular cascades are initiated during the first few minutes and hours after the traumatic insult. Our hope was that hypothermia would either inhibit or limit these toxic cascades, thereby reducing post-traumatic brain swelling, intracranial hypertension, and ischemia.

To investigate the molecular changes after traumatic brain injury and effects of hypothermia on these secondary molecular cascades, we placed in vivo microdialysis probes into the brain tissue and collected dialysate samples every 30 min. All patients also had external ventricular drainage catheters placed into the right lateral ventricle and CSF was sampled every 4 hr. All patients who required a craniotomy for evacuation of a post-traumatic intracranial mass lesions (contusions, subdural hematomas, and intraparenchymal hematomas) were candidates for the microdialysis portion of the study. Following evacuation of the mass lesion a relatively normal-appearing gyrus adjacent to the contusion or underlying the evacuated clot was selected. A small hole was made in the pia mater, and the microdialysis probe was inserted obliquely into the brain such that the entire active end of the probe was within the brain and was estimated to lie primarily within the cortex. The microdialysis probes, pumps, and refrigerated automated fraction collector were supplied by CMA Microdialysis (Boston, MA, USA) with the following specifications: microdialysis probes, CMA-20, 10 mm active end, 20 kd molecular weight pore size of membrane. The infusion pump was a CMA-102, infusion rate of 2 μl per minute with sterile normal saline solution without preservatives. The refrigerated automated fraction collector we used was the CMA-170, with a sample rate of every 30 min, chamber temperature of 4°C. Dialysate specimens were collected for a maximum of 5 days or less if the patient regained consciousness during that time. Cerebrospinal fluid (CSF) specimens were passively withdrawn from the external ventricular drainage catheter and sampled every 6 hr for a maximum of 5 days.

Previous animal studies suggested that hypothermia was very effective in suppressing extracellular excitatory amino acid levels, particularly glutamate and aspartate. Those studies also suggested a significant suppression of cytokine levels. In addition, we were interested in the effect of hypothermia on extracellular and CSF lactate levels. However, we were concerned about interpretation of the absolute levels of all of these molecules because of the changes in extracellular water associated with cerebral edema during the first 24–48 hr after severe traumatic brain injury. Therefore, we also looked at the lactate/pyruvate ratio as a way to determine relative lactate levels that was a immune to changes in extracellular fluid concentrations.

Effect of Hypothermia on Extracellular Levels of Glutamate, Aspartate, and the Lactate/Pyruvate Ratio

Hypothermia led to a suppression of extracellular levels of glutamate during the period of cooling. Mean glutamate values for five patients who were cooled from 32°–33°C was 40% less than the glutamate levels in the dialysate fluid for five normothermia patients. Hypothermia had no effect on extracellular aspartate levels, the absolute lactate or pyruvate concentrations, or the lactate/pyruvate ratio.

We also performed a logistic regression analysis assessing the influence of time after injury, initial GCS score, 6-month GOS score, anatomic type of intracranial injury, intracranial pressure, and CPP on the levels of these compounds. None of these factors was significantly related to the absolute levels or trends in extracellular excitatory amino acids or the lactate/pyruvate ratio with the single exception of time after injury. The extracellular levels of all of these molecules were highest during the first 24 hr after injury.

Effect of Hypothermia on CSF Levels of These Molecules

Hypothermia caused a significant suppression of CSF glutamate levels and interleukin-1β (IL-Iβ) levels in the subpopulation of patients with an admission GCS of 5–7, though not in those with a GCS score of 3 or 4, as compared with normothermia patients. During the period of cooling in those with an initial GCS score of 5–7, the mean glutamate level in the hypothermia group was 0.04 ± 0.02 mg/dl, while in the normothermia patients it was 0.071 ± 0.05 mg/dl. This significant difference was not sustained once the hypothermia patients were rewarmed. In the patients with an initial GCS score of 5–7, the mean IL-Iβ level in hypothermia patients was 3.1 ± 3.5 picograms/ml, and 21.5 ± 3.9 picograms/ml for the normothermia patients. A significant suppression of CSF IL-Iβ levels in the hypothermia group was observed even after these patients were rewarmed.

We were also interested in how well CSF levels of glutamate, aspartate, lactate and the lactate/pyruvate ratio reflected the extracellular levels of these neurochemicals. Analysis of variance was performed comparing dialysate levels with CSF levels of these compounds for the 5 days after injury and there was no correlation observed. This was true in both the hypothermia and normothermia groups as well as those with the lower and higher admission GCS scores.

References

1. Boris-Moller F, Wieloch T (1998) Changes in the extracellular levels of glutamate and aspartate during ischemia and hypoglycemia. Effects of hypothermia. Exp Brain Res 121:277–284
2. Clifton GL, Allen S, Barrodale P, Plenger P, Berry J, Koch S, Fletcher J, Hayes RL, Choi SC (1993) A phase II study of moderate hypothermia in severe brain injury. J Neurotrauma 10:263–271
3. Clifton GL, Jiang JY, Lyeth BG, Jenkins LW, Hamm RJ, Hayes RL (1991) Marked protection by moderate hypothermia after experimental traumatic brain injury. J Cereb Blood Flow Metab 11:114–121
4. Dietrich WD (1992) The importance of brain temperature in cerebral injury. J Neurotrauma 9 Suppl 2:S475–485

5. Dietrich WD, Alonso O, Busto R, Globus MY, Ginsberg MD (1994) Post-traumatic brain hypothermia reduces histopathological damage following concussive brain injury in the rat. Acta Neuropathol 87:250–258

6. Dixon CE, Markgraf CG, Angileri F, Pike BR, Wolfson B, Newcomb JK, Bismar MM, Blanco AJ, Clifton GL, Hayes RL (1998) Protective effects of moderate hypothermia on behavioral deficits but not necrotic cavitation following cortical impact injury in the rat. J Neurotrauma 15:95–103

7. Globus MY, Alonso O, Dietrich WD, Busto R, Ginsberg MD (1995) Glutamate release and free radical production following brain injury: Effects of posttraumatic hypothermia. J Neurochem 65:1704–1711

8. Koizumi H, Povlishock JT (1998) Posttraumatic hypothermia in the treatment of axonal damage in an animal model of traumatic axonal injury. J Neurosurg 89:303–309

9. Marion DW, Penrod LE, Kelsey SF, Obrist WD, Kochanek PM, Palmer AM, Wisniewski SR, DeKosky ST (1997) Treatment of traumatic brain injury with moderate hypothermia. N Engl J Med 336:540–546

10. Metz C, Holzschuh M, Bein T, Woertgen C, Frey A, Frey I, Taeger K, Brawanski A (1996) Moderate hypothermia in patients with severe head injury: Cerebral and extracerebral effects. J Neurosurg 85:533–541

11. Mori K, Maeda M, Miyazaki M, Iwase H (1998) Effects of mild and moderate hypothermia on cerebral metabolism and glutamate in an experimental head injury. Acta Neurochir Suppl (Wien) 71:222–224

12. Sakamoto KI, Fujisawa H, Koizumi H, Tsuchida E, Ito H, Sadamitsu D, Maekawa T (1997) Effects of mild hypothermia on nitric oxide synthesis following contusion trauma in the rat. J Neurotrauma 14:349–353

13. Shiozaki T, Sugimoto H, Taneda M, Yoshida H, Iwai A, Yoshioka T, Sugimoto T (1993) Effect of mild hypothermia on uncontrollable intracranial hypertension after severe head injury. J Neurosurg 79:363–368

14. Smith SL, Hall ED (1996) Mild pre- and posttraumatic hypothermia attenuates blood-brain barrier damage following controlled cortical impact injury in the rat. J Neurotrauma 13:1–9

15. Taft WC, Yang K, Dixon CE, Clifton GL, Hayes RL (1993) Hypothermia attenuates the loss of hippocampal microtubule-associated protein 2 (MAP2) levels following traumatic brain injury. J Cereb Blood Flow Metab 13:796–802

Significance of Electrophysiologic Studies in Brain Hypothermia

Takashi Moriya, Atsushi Sakurai, Koichi Mera, Eiichiro Noda,
Kenji Okuno, Akira Utagawa, Kosaku Kinoshita,
and Nariyuki Hayashi

Summary. To evaluate the significance of an electrophysiologic monitoring system during brain hypothermia, we measured the brainstem auditory evoked potentials (BAEPs), somatosensory evoked potentials (SEPs), and topographic electroencephalography (EEG) in 29 critically ill patients (15 with severe head injury and 14 with encephalopathy following cardiopulmonary resuscitation). When the temperature measured in the internal jugular vein fell from 36°C to 33°C, the prolongation of latency in BAEPs was 0.1 ± 0.06 ms in wave I, 0.5 ± 0.23 ms in wave III, and 0.92 ± 0.86 ms in wave V. In addition, the prolongation of latency in SEPs was 1.2 ± 0.2 ms in N13 and 2.1 ± 0.4 ms in N20. The bifrontal fast wave responses, except for those of primary injured lesions, in the topographic EEG were recognized in 9 of 13 patients within 30 min after the injection of midazolam which was used as a sedative. When the temperature fell from 36°C to 33°C, the ratio of the delta and theta waves to the alpha waves recorded from 12 scalp electrodes increased. An electrophysiologic evaluation in critically ill patients should thus be considered an effective real-time monitoring system in patients experiencing brain hypothermia.

Key words. Brain hypothermia, Brainstem auditory evoked potentials, Somatosensory evoked potentials, Topographic electroencephalography, Latency

Introduction

There have recently been a number of reports about the resuscitation of traumatic brain injury [6,9] and ischemic-hypoxic encephalopathy [4] following cardiopulmonary arrest due to the development of monitoring systems in the intensive care unit (ICU). At our institution, we also measure the intracranial pressure (ICP), especially in cases of severe head injury and jugular venous oxygen saturation (SjO_2); and we evaluate cardiovascular function (cardiac index, pulmonary artery wedge pressure, delivery oxygen index, consumption oxygen index) using the Swan-Ganz catheter in a continuous monitoring system [7]. The most valuable prognostic indicators for this monitoring system and the best type of realtime monitoring system have not yet been elucidated in critically ill patients. As a first step, we measure and evaluate the electrophysiologic changes induced by a decreased

Department of Emergency and Critical Care Medicine, Nihon University School of Medicine, 30-1 Oyaguchi Kami-machi, Itabashi-ku, Tokyo 173-8610, Japan

temperature. In addition, various aspects regarding the use of a real time monitoring system for maintaining neurological function during brain hypothermia are herein described and discussed.

Material and Methods

The families of all patients were given informed consent for this study. The subjects consisted of 29 critically ill patients admitted to the ICU of the Emergency and Critical Care Center at the Nihon University School of Medicine from January 1997 to February 1998. Another patients, ranging in age from 17 to 72 years and including 12 males and 17 females, were randomly selected for this study. They all had severe head injury, no complicated injuries, a Glasgow Coma Scale (GCS) score of 3–7, and hypoxic-ischemic encephalopathy following cardiopulmonary arrest.

The systolic pressure without vasoactive agents was continuously maintained at more than 90 mmHg, and wave V in the brainstem auditory evoked potentials (BAEPs) was recorded. No severe complications were recognized.

To cool the body temperature, gastric lavage and a water cooling system blanket were utilized within 30 min following insertion of the internal jugular vein catheter. The BAEPs were recorded at 100 dB click, 9.5 Hz, 1000 addition; and the somatosensory evoked potentials (SEPs) were stimulated at the right median nerve with 15 mA, 2 Hz, 500 addition (NEC Synax 1100; NEC Tochigi, Utsunomiya, Japan). SEPs was recorded from four channels (CH 1: C4-A2, CH2: C4-Erb2, CH3: C5s-Fz, CH4: Erb1-Erb2). Each examination was carried out at temperatures of 36°, 35°, 34°, and 33°C in the internal jugular vein twice each. Topographic electroencephalography (EEG Telemeter; Nihon Koden Tomioka, Tokyo, Japan) was recorded from 16 spectra representing electrodes (Fp1, Fp2, F3, F4, F7, F8, C3, C4, T3, T4, T5, T6, P3, P4, O1, O2) of the 10–20 system. The spectra were displayed topographically so their position reflects that of the electrodes on the head. At 36°C the topographic EEG was recorded before and after injection of midazolam (0.1 mg/kg), at 34°C, and after the rewarming topographic EEG was done. Finally, the 29 critically ill patients who showed a complete recovery in the latencies of SEPs and BAEPs following rewarming were entered into this study.

Results

BAEP Recordings During Brain Hypothermia

When the temperature measured in the internal jugular vein fell from 36°C to 33°C, the prolongation of the latency was 0.1 ± 0.06 ms in wave I, 0.5 ± 0.23 ms in wave III, and 0.92 ± 0.86 ms in wave V. The prolongation of the interpeak latency was also 0.49 ms in waves I–III, 0.33 ms in waves III–V, and 0.82 ms in waves I–V (Figs. 1, 2).

SEP Recordings During Brain Hypothermia

When the temperature measured in the internal jugular vein fell from 36°C to 33°C the prolongation of latency in SEPs was 0.1 ms in wave I, 0.59 ms in wave III, and 0.92 ms in wave V. The prolongation of the interpeak latency was also 0.49 ms in waves I–III, 0.33 ms in waves III–V, and 0.82 ms in waves I–V (Figs. 3, 4).

FIG. 1. Representative case 1: a 25-year-old woman with cardiopulmonary arrest (CPA) due to upper airway obstruction postoperatively. When the temperature measured in the internal jugular vein fell from 36°C to 33°C within a few hours, the prolongation of latency in brainstem auditory evoked potentials (BAEPs) was recognized. *Up arrows*, wave I; *down arrows*, wave V. Glasgow Outcome Scale (GOS) showed moderate disability 3 months later

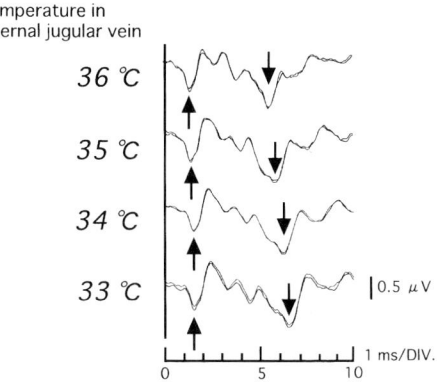

FIG. 2. Changes of latency (**left**) and interpeak latency (**right**) in BAEPs in 29 critically ill patients when the temperature measured in the internal jugular vein fell from 36°C to 33°C within a few hours. **Left** *x*, latency of wave V; *filled triangles*, latency of III; *filled squares*, latency of wave I. **Right** *x*, interpeak latency of wave I–V; *filled squares*, interpeak latency of wave I–III; *open circles*, latency of wave III–V

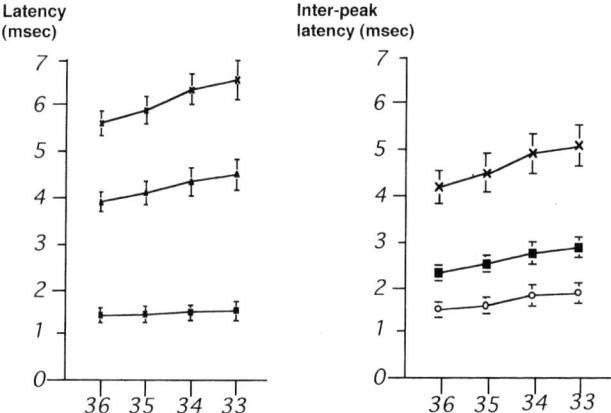

Topographic EEG Recordings During Brain Hypothermia

The topographic EEG at 36°C was recorded before and within 30 min after the injection of midazolam (0.1 mg/kg) and thus demonstrated the appearance of bilateral fast waves in 9 of 13 cases (69%). On the other hand, only 1 of 12 cases that resulted in a vegetative state and death showed bilateral fast waves after injection of midazolam (not shown). The topographic EEG recorded at 34°C during the cooling phase was predominantly comprised of slow waves compared to that at 36°C during the rewarming phase, where the fast wave ratio significantly decreased to less than 20%.

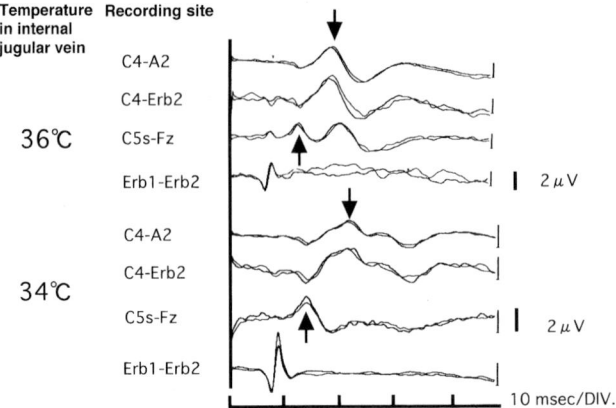

FIG. 3. Representative case 2: a 41-year-old woman with a CPA due to asphyxia. When the temperature measured in the internal jugular vein fell from 36°C to 33°C within a few hours, the prolongation of latency in somatosensory evoked potentials (SEPs) was recognized. *Up arrows*, N13; *down arrows*, N20. GOS showed good recovery 3 months later

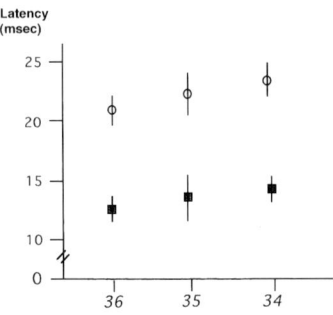

FIG. 4. Changes of latency and interpeak latency in SEPs in 17 critically ill patients, when the temperature measured in the internal jugular vein fell from 36°C to 34°C within a few hours. *Circles,* latency of N20 ($m = 17$); *squares,* latency of N13 ($m = 17$)

Discussion

The management of intracranial pressure to maintain intracranial homeostasis is well known to play an important role not only in severe head injury [10,12] and cerebrovascular disease but also in ischemic-hypoxic encephalopathy following cardiac arrest [15]. Grenvik and Safar [5] recently reported the importance of monitoring systems, although such procedures are still in the experimental stage [11,14].

Electrophysiological studies, especially a computed analysis of the EEG, should be used to evaluate comatose patients even in the ICU, where it is normally difficult to record the electrical activities of the cerebral cortex without some artifacts. In our study, when the temperature fell from 36°C to 33°C, the ratio of delta and theta waves to alpha waves recorded from 12 scalp electrodes naturally increased. Amrein et al. [1] expected that the rhythmic fast wave induced by diazepam might be recognized in all mentally handicapped patients. The appearance of bifrontal fast waves, except for primary injured lesions, upon topographic EEG mapping were temporarily recognized in 9 of 13 patients within 30 min after injection of midazolam, which was used as a sedative at the beginning of the hypothermia cooling stage.

On the other hand, some patients showed no bifrontal fast wave responses and thus demonstrated a persistent vegetative state and death (not shown). These facts suggest that the bifrontal changes on the topographic EEG induced by a sedative might thus be an effective early diagnostic tool for prognosis.

The importance of SEPs and BAEPs have been clinically postulated as well. The prolongation of the latencies in SEPs correlated closely with neurological deficits [8], which in BAEPs also lead to mortality [3]. In our study, the disappearance of SEPs and BAEPs resulted in a persistent vegetative state and death (not shown). In contrast, Schwarz et al. [13] reported that four adult patients showing bilateral loss of SEPs had a favorable recovery. They concluded that patients with hypothermia, deep sedation, or intoxication should be carefully observed, although bilateral loss of SEPs is a strong predictor of unfavorable outcome. Their experiences suggest that BAEPs may be a more important, effective diagnostic tool than SEPs. The mechanism of latency prolongation—whether the cause of prolongation is a depression of synapse conduction or axonal conduction—has yet to be evaluated. In the future, we need to establish the various conditions for stimulation when performing electrophysiologic studies.

Conclusions

To evaluate the significance of an electrophysiologic monitoring system during brain hypothermia, we measured BAEPs, SEPs, and topographic EEGs in 29 critically ill patients. Such evaluation should thus be considered an effective real-time monitoring system in patients experiencing brain hypothermia. BAEPs and SEPs may be especially effective if there are doubts about intracranial complications during hypothermia. On the other hand, the topographic EEG may be useful for the predicted clinical prognosis based on the findings of the EEG responses after injecting drugs.

References

1. Amrein R, Hetzel W, Harmann D, Lorscheid T (1988) Clinical pharmacology of flumazenil. Eur J Anesthesiol 2:65–80
2. Benita M, Conde H (1972) Effects of local cooling upon conduction and synaptic transmission. Brain Res 36:133–151
3. Garcia-Larrea A, Artru F, Garcia-Larrea L, Bertrand O, Pernier J, Mauguiere F (1992) The combined monitoring of brain stem auditory evoked potentials and intracranial pressure in coma: a study of 57 patients. J Neurol Neurosurg Psychiatry 55:792–798
4. Gisvold SE, Sterz F, Abramson NS, Bar-Joseph G, Ebmeyer U, Gervais H, Ginsberg M, Katz LM, Kochanek PM, Kuboyama K, Miller B, Obrist W, Roine RO, Safar P, Sim KM, Vandevelde K, White RJ, Xiao F (1996) Cerebral resuscitation from cardiac arrest. Crit Care Med 24:69–80
5. Grenvik A, Safar P (eds) Brain failure and resuscitation. In: Clinics in Critical Care Medicine. Churchill Livingstone, New York
6. Hayashi N, Hirayama T, Utagawa A (1994a) The cerebral thermo-pooling and hypothermia treatment of critical head injury patients. In: Nagai O et al (eds) Intracranial pressure. IX. Springer, Tokyo, pp 589–599
7. Hayashi N, Hirayama T, Utagawa A, Daimon W, Ohata M (1994b) Systemic management of cerebral edema based on a new concept in severe head injury patients. Acta Neurochir Suppl (Wien) 60:541–543
8. Hume AL, Cant BR, Shaw NA (1979) Central somatosensory conduction time in comatose patients. Ann Neurol 5:379–384

9. Marion DW, Obrist WD, Kochanek PM, Palmer AM, Wisniewski SR, DeKosky ST, Penrod LE, Kelsey SF (1997) Treatment of traumatic brain injury with moderate hypothermia. N Engl J Med 336:540–546
10. Millar JD, Becker DP, Ward JD, et al (1977) Significance of intracranial hypertension in severe head injury. J Neurosurg 47:503
11. Prior PF (1985) EEG monitoring and evoked potentials in brain ischemia. Br J Anaesth 57:63–81
12. Saul TG, Ducker TB (1982) Effect of intracranial pressure monitoring and aggressive treatment on mortality in severe head injury. J Neurosurg 56:498–503
13. Schwarz S, Schwab S, Aschoff A, Hacke W (1999) Favorable recovery from bilateral loss of somatosensory evoked potentials. Crit Care Med 27:182–187
14. Sclabassi RJ, Hinman CL, Kroin JS, Risch HA (1985) A non-linear analysis of affrent modulatory activity in the cat somatosensory system. Electroencephalogr Clin Neurophysiol 60:444–454
15. Nemoto EM, Snyder JV, Carroll RG, Morita H (1975) Global ischemia in dogs: intracranial pressures, brain blood flow and metabolism. Stroke 6:21–27

Mapping Analysis of Brain Tissue Temperature by Magnetic Resonance Imaging

T.A.D. Cadoux-Hudson

Summary. Head injury remains a common cause of long-term disability. Although some of this disability is due to the primary impact, much is due to secondary damage that is potentially reversible. Brain tissue temperature may contribute to this secondary damage, and hypothermia is an inexpensive and direct way of reducing tissue temperature. Thermocouples are an inexpensive and direct but invasive and inflexible method for measuring tissue temperature. There is a need for a noninvasive and flexible method for measuring brain tissue temperature from acute injury to long-term follow up. Magnetic resonance technology may be able to provide an accurate measure of brain tissue temperature and simultaneously co-correlate with other important variables such as regional cerebral blood flow and metabolism. The early application of this technology to acute human brain injury is described in this chapter.

Key words. MRI, MRS, Brain tissue temperature (BTT), Uncoupling protein, Phosphorus spectroscopy

Introduction

Magnetic resonance technologies [imaging (MRI) and spectroscopy (MRS)] can give us unique insights into the structure (MRI), regional cerebral blood flow [8], metabolism, function, and more recently regional brain tissue temperature [2]. Brain tissue temperature has a profound effect on the ability of the injured tissue to recover from trauma in animal models [9]. Increased tissue temperature above 38°C appears to adversely affect the ability of traumatized brain to recover in a histological [5] and functional sense. In addition to this observation, reduction of brain tissue temperature (brain hypothermia) improves the outcome after injury [6].

In human studies there are two separate but related strategies to improve outcome from brain injury. The first strategy is based on the hypothesis that a brain tissue temperature above 38°C adversely affects the brain injury outcome. Therapeutic intervention is then aimed at normalization of the brain tissue temperature (e.g., <38°C but > 35°C. There are no comparisons of this therapy versus standard head injury management.

Department of Neurosurgery, The Radcliffe Infirmary, Oxford OX2 6HE, UK
Department of Biochemistry, MRC Biochemical and Clinical Magnetic Resonance Unit, John Radcliffe Hospital, Oxford OX2 6HE, UK

The second strategy is to actively cool the brain to achieve mild (≥34°C), moderate (32°–34°C), or severe (<32°C) brain tissue temperatures. This hypothesis assumes that hypothermia reduces secondary tissue damage via such mechanisms as reduction of metabolic rate, reduced ion flux, and reduced free radical production.

Adverse effects of these strategies are possible. The brain has powerful autoregulatory mechanisms that have been reset to maintain an abnormally high temperature. Artificial attempts at temperature reduction may stimulate additional energy expenditure. The thalamus has the ability to release uncoupling protein [7] usually released by brown fat to maintain body temperature. Release of such compounds during brain injury may lead to further energy expenditure on cooling. Any mammalian system that has been artificially cooled must be rewarmed. Increasing the brain tissue temperature may cause additional injury. Vascular smooth muscle constricts during rewarming, particularly severely in the presence of subarachnoid haemorrhage. Vascular luminal narrowing during rewarming may lower the regional cerebral blood flow during a period of metabolic acceleration, resulting in tissue infarction.

Despite these conflicts, benefits have been demonstrated in rodents recovering from brain trauma when treated with tissue hypothermia. As a result of these and many other studies, brain hypothermia treatment has been applied to traumatic brain-injured patients. Early studies were performed in Stockholm during the 1960s following the introduction of whole-body hypothermia for cardiac and then cerebral aneurysm surgery. Prolonged (>48 h) whole-body hypothermia was associated with a disappointing systemic complication rate, with bronchopneumonia and pancreatitis leading a considerable list of problems.

Initial results of the effect of whole body hypothermia (<48 h) have suggested that the reduction of brain tissue temperature following brain injury may have a beneficial effect [3], and a randomized hypothermia study will be reported soon (NABISH II).

The thermistor has been the preferred method for measuring brain tissue temperature. Although it is an inexpensive and accurate (±0.1°C SD) the thermistor reports only on a small region of brain and can be placed for only relatively short periods of time (<5 days). More commonly primary brain injury causes a wide, poorly defined region of brain injury. Spatial and temporal distribution of injury have also been demonstrated to vary. Several researchers have therefore looked for a noninvasive and spatially flexible technique for measuring brain tissue temperature.

Magnetic resonance spectroscopy and imaging have been proposed as possible candidates. Evidence that the various magnetic resonance parameters first varied with temperature were reported in 1966 [4], and the biological implications were seen in 1985 [1]. These authors demonstrated a linear relation between temperature and proton chemical shift due to changes in the equilibrium between hydrogen-bound and monomeric water. By MRI parameters, it alters the T1 signal, apparent diffusion constant (ADC), and phase of the water signal. As a result, these parameters can be accurately imaged, producing a brain temperature map [10]. However, the techniques usually require a control image (at normal temperature) and a perturbed image, when the temperature is changed and a further image is acquired. The brain temperature map is produced from the difference of the two acquired images. These techniques are excellent for physiological perturbations but are not appropriate for most clinical situations. In addition, we know that both the phase and T1 of the water signal can be altered by other pathological processes following brain injury.

In addition to alteration in T1, phase, and ADC, temperature alters the chemical shift of the proton signal. Other chemical species in the proton magnetic resonance spectra of the human brain, such as the methyl signal of N-acetyl aspartate (NAA), are not involved in such an exchange of protons, experiencing no chemical shift with temperature. The chemical shift of water protons with temperature is relatively insensitive to pHi and physiological ionic fluctuations. We do not know whether other brain injury pathological processes can alter this chemical shift. The water proton chemical shift is small in the physiological range (0.08 ppm per 1°C change). The first step was to test the repeatability and reliability of this technique on a control population and then test the robustness of the technique in a brain-injured group, focusing on traumatic brain injury.

Methods

Conventional MRI (T1- and T2-weighted spin echo; 5 min) was used to provide accurate localization of clear conventional brain injury and evidence of an alteration of T1. Diffusion-weighted images (ba = 20, 250 ms; bx, by, bz = 250 ms; 6 min) were also collected to give structural information on pathological processes such tissue edema. Increased brain tissue temperature should produce an increase in the ADC, but we know that other pathological processes also can profoundly alter the ADC. Ischemia has been shown to decrease the ADC in the early stages, with an increase in ADC when tissue necrosis occurs.

These data are then used to select regions of the brain for hemodynamic studies using a first-pass bolus (gadolinium DTPA; SEG-EPI). Proton spectroscopy (PRESS, TE = 130 ms; 4 min) with and without water suppression alternating the transmitter frequency [2] for brain tissue temperature (BTT) were collected from the same region. Phosphorus spectroscopy (1D CSI from a tuned 7 cm surface coil) was used to measure intracellular pHi, phosphocreatine (PCr), and adenosine triphosphate (ATP) levels.

We studied mildly, moderately, and severely head-injured patients and compared them to 20 controls of similar age.

Results

The control subjects had a mean BTT of 37.3°C (range 36.8°–37.9°C). The head-injured patients (BTT mean 37.6°C) were overall not significantly different. The BTT with mild or moderate head injury did not show a significant alteration. The severely head-injured patients [n = 3; Glasgow Coma Scale (GCS) <7; >7 days, diffuse injury] demonstrated a persistent alteration in brain tissue temperature (38.2° and 39.0°C, mean delay of study from injury 13 days (4–24 days) (Fig. 1). This increase in BTT appeared to be associated with regions near but not involved in the MRI (T2) changes. A similar voxel in the contralateral hemisphere (internal control) had a BTT within the normal range. The elevation in BTT was maintained for several days (up to 24 days) after the initial injury.

Conclusions

Magnetic resonance techniques can be applied to the noninvasive study of BTT but require further validation. Direct correlation with thermocouples and indirect correlation with core body temperature are possible approaches. These developments will allow us to follow regional BTT carefully and to modify hypothermia treatment strategies to improve patients' outcome from head injury.

These techniques will also allow us to better understand the underlying pathological mechanisms that lead to an elevated BTT. New treatment strategies can then be developed that can maximize hypothermia therapy.

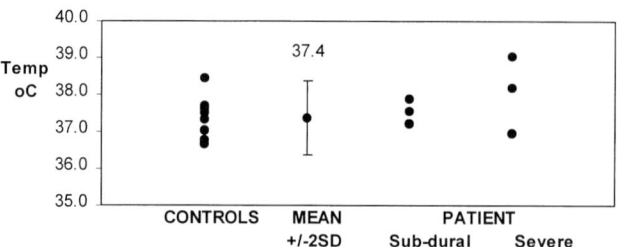

FIG. 1. Comparison of brain tissue temperatures measured by magnetic resonance spectroscopy in three patients with acute on chronic subdural hematoma and three patients with severe head injury (Glasgow Coma Scale <7) days after initial injury. There were mine controls

Magnetic resonance technologies can be applied to the difficult and complex clinical science of brain injury in acute and longitudinal studies. This technology may help us select suitable patients for specific neuroprotective strategies, such as brain hypothermia, and directly measure the acute effects and long-term outcomes.

References

1. Arus C, Chang YC, Barany M (1985) N-Acetylaspartate as an intrinsic thermometer for 1H NMR of brain slices. J Magn Reson 63:376–379
2. Cady EB, D'Souza PC, Penrice J, Lorek A (1995) The estimation of local brain temperature by in vivo 1H magnetic resonance spectroscopy. Magn Res Med 33:862–867
3. Clifton GL (1995) Systemic hypothermia in treatment of severe brain injury: a review and update. J Neurotrauma 12:923–927
4. Hindman JC (1966) Proton resonance shift of water in the gas and liquid states. J Chem Phys 44:4582–4592
5. Jiang JY, Lyeth BG, Clifton GL, Jenkins LW, Hamm RJ, Hayes RL (1991) Relationship between body and brain temperature in traumatically brain-injured rodents. J Neurosurg 74:492–496
6. Kataokà K, Yanase H (1998) Mild hypothermia: a revived countermeasure against ischaemic neuronal injury Neurosci Res 32:103–117
7. Richard D, Rivest R, Huang Q, Bouillaud F, Sanchis D, Champigny O, Ricquier D (1998) Distribution of the uncoupling protein 2 mRNA in the mouse brain. J Comp Neurol 397:549–560
8. Rosen BR, Belliveau JW, Vevea JM, Brady TJ (1990) Perfusion with NMR contrast agents. Magn Reson Med 14:249–265
9. Siminia P, van der Zee J, Wondergem J, Haveman J (1994) Effect of hyperthermia on the central nervous system: a review. Int J Hyperthermia 10:1–30
10. Young IR, Hand JW, Oatridge A, Prior MV, Forse GR (1994) Further observations on the measurement of tissue T1 to monitor temperature in vivo by MRI. Magn Reson Med 31:342–345

Bacteria Detected and the Pharmacokinetics of Antibiotics During Brain Hypothermia

Morio Kaburagi[1], Miwa Yoshida[1], Toshimitsu Nakayama[1],
Nariyuki Hayashi[2], Kosaku Kinoshita[2], Takashi Moriya[2],
and Akira Udagawa[2]

Summary. We examined the state of bacteria detected from patients during brain hypothermia and the pharmacokinetics of antibiotics administered for antibiotic prophylaxis. Samples including blood were collected from patients who underwent brain hypothermia at the Nihon University Itabashi Hospital Emergency and Critical Care Center, and the type of bacteria and interval until detection were investigated using these samples. Simultaneously, we measured concentrations of antibiotics administered for antibiotic prophylaxis [cefmetazole (CMZ), flomoxef (FMOX), cefoperazone/sulbactam (CPZ/SBT), aspoxicillin (ASPC), arbekacin (ABK), amikacin (AMK)] and compared the half-lives of these agents during the cooling stage or during the cooling and rewarming stages. Bacteria such as methicillin-resistant staphylococcus aureus (MRSA), *Pseudomonas aeruginosa*, and *Candida* were mainly detected. The mean interval until the bacterial detection was 4.4 days after rewarming was started. Of the administered antibiotics, half-lives of agents that are mainly eliminated via kidney excretion (CMZ, FMOX, SBT, ABK) did not differ during the cooling and rewarming stages. However, for two patients receiving CPZ, an agent metabolized in the liver, the half-life of CPZ was markedly prolonged during hypothermia in one patient with liver dysfunction, whereas there was no prolongation in the other patient. The results of this study suggest that the types of bacteria detected are similar to those in other patients hospitalized in the intensive care unit. With respect to the pharmacokinetics of antibiotics, the half-life of CPZ was prolonged in one patient during the cooling stage, suggesting that the drug-metabolizing capacity in the liver parenchyma may be reduced during hypothermia. Therefore, antibiotics that are metabolized in the liver should be administered cautiously.

Key words. Detected bacteria, Antibiotic prophylaxis, Hypothermia, Pharmacokinetics, Drug metabolism

Introduction

In most patients during brain hypothermia, antibiotics are administered for antibiotic prophylaxis. However, the pharmacokinetics of these agents remain unclarified. In particular, changes in physiological function may influence pharmacokinetics during hypothermia, but

---

[1]Department of Pharmacy, [2]Department of Emergency and Critical Care Medicine, Nihon University School of Medicine, 30-1 Oyaguchi Kami-machi, Itabashi-ku, Tokyo 173-8610, Japan

few studies have reported the influence of hypothermia on pharmacokinetics. In this study, we investigated the type of bacteria detected from patients during brain hypothermia and examined the time courses of the pharmacokinetics of antibiotics administered for antibiotic prophylaxis.

Subjects and Methods

The period when the patient's blood temperature was lowest was regarded as the cooling stage. The interval from the commencement of rewarming until the final administration of antibiotics was regarded as the rewarming stage.

Bacteria Detected

We retrospectively examined bacteria clinically isolated from sputum, throat, and blood in 51 patients with severe head injury who underwent brain hypothermia between January 1995 and March 1998. The time of initial detection was classified into cooling and rewarming stages with respect to the type of bacteria.

Changes in Serum Drug Concentrations

Eleven patients with severe head injury were included: nine patients who underwent brain hypothermia between January 1997 and May 1997 and were treated with cefmetazole (CMZ, $n = 4$), flomoxef (FMOX, $n = 2$), cefoperazone/sulbactam (CPZ/SBT, $n = 2$), or arbekacin (ABK, $n = 1$) and two patients in whom these agents were combined with amikacin (AMK) or aspoxicillin (ASPC) (one patient each) only during the cooling stage. In these patients, blood was collected over 6 h after the end of administration during the cooling stage or during the cooling and rewarming stages. Using blood samples, drug concentrations were measured according to the standard method by liquid chromatography or fluorescence polarization immunoassay (TDXFLXR). Changes in serum concentrations of antibiotics were applied to a one-compartment open model, and the area under the concentration time curve (AUC), volume of distribution (V_d), disappearance rate constant (kel), half-life ($t_{1/2}$), and total clearance (CL) were calculated.

Results were compared for the cooling stage and the rewarming stage. The kel value was calculated by the least squares method. AUC was calculated by the diagonal method using concentrations until the final measurement (extrapolation and approximation of the elimination curve to infinity). CL was calculated as dose/AUC. V_d was calculated as CL/kel.

Results

Bacteria Detected

For the bacteria detected from the sputum, throat, and blood of 51 patients who underwent brain hypothermia, the detection rate of gram-positive coccis was 35.9%. Of these bacteria, the detection rate of MRSA (15.9%) was the highest of all detected gram-positive cocci. The detection rate of gram-negative bacillus was 46.8%. Of these bacteria, the detection rate of P. aeruginosa (9.7%) was the highest of all detected gram-negative bacillus. The detection rate of Candida was 14.5%, demonstrating the second highest rate following that of MRSA among all detected bacteria (Fig. 1).

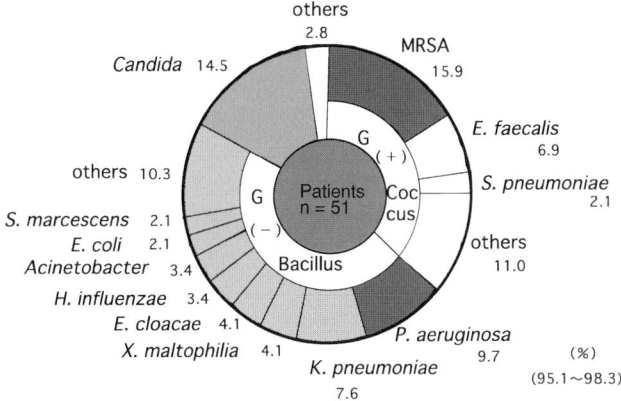

FIG. 1. Bacterial detection during brain hypothermia in all therapeutic time windows. *MRSA*, methicillin-resistant *Staphylococcus aureus*

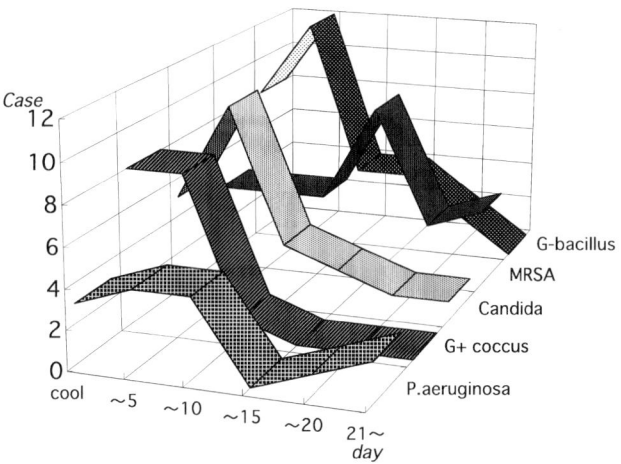

FIG. 2. Changes of phlogistic bacteria detected from patients during brain hypothermia. *G*–, gram-negative; *G*+, gram-positive

The mean interval until major bacteria were initially detected was 4.3 days after treatment was started during the cooling stage and 4.4 days after rewarming was started. During the cooling stage, gram-negative bacilli were the most frequently detected. During the rewarming stage, *Candida* was frequently detected just after rewarming was started. MRSA and *P. aeruginosa* were frequently detected 2 weeks or more after rewarming was started. The interval until MRSA and *P. aeruginosa* were detected was similar to that in other patients hospitalized in the intensive case unit (ICU) at our center (Fig. 2).

Changes in Serum Drug Concentrations

During the cooling stage, pulmonary artery temperatures ranged from 32.2° to 35.1°C. During the rewarming stage, arterial blood temperatures ranged from 34.8° to 38.4°C. Administration

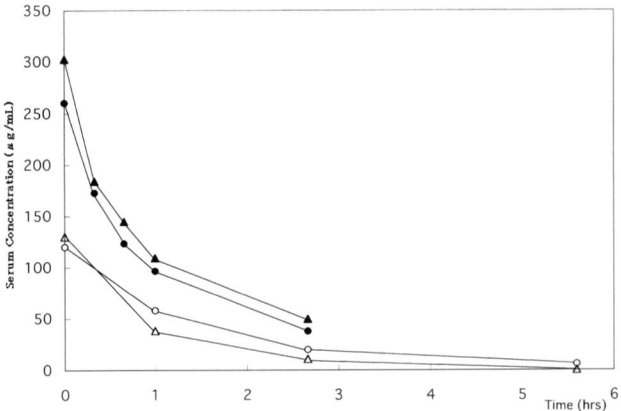

FIG. 3. Changes of serum cefmetazole (CMZ) concentration. *Filled symbols*, N.S., a 56-year-old woman with a subarachnoid hemorrhage. *Filled circles*, serum concentration at the lowest temperature of cooling stage during hypothermia. *Filled triangles*, serum concentration at the rewarming stage, almost 7 days after initiation of cooling. *Open symbols*, Y.M., a 37-year-old woman with a subarachnoid hemorrhage. *Open circles*, serum concentration at the lowest temperature of the cooling stage during hypothermia. *Open triangles*, serum concentration at the rewarming stage, almost 7 days after initiation of cooling

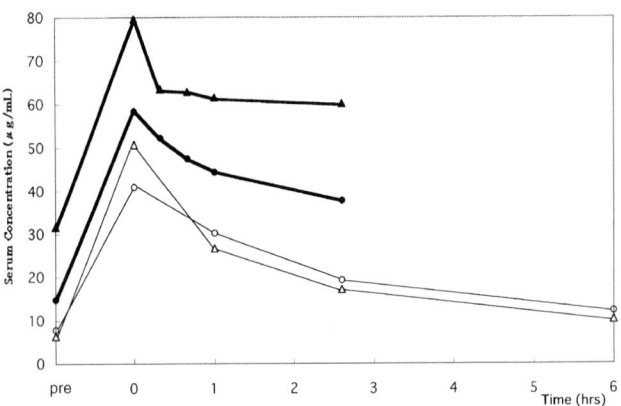

FIG. 4. Changes of serum cefoperazone (CPZ) concentration. *Filled symbols*, K.S., a 65-year-old man with cardiopulmonary arrest. *pre*, just before application of CPZ. *Filled circles*, serum concentration at the lowest temperature of the cooling stage during hypothermia. *Filled triangles*, serum concentration at the rewarming stage, almost 7 days after initiation of cooling. *Open symbols*, A.U., a 54-year-old man with an acute subdural hematoma. *Open circles*, serum concentration at the lowest temperature of the cooling stage during hypothermia. *Open triangles*, serum concentration at the rewarming stage, almost 7 days after initiation of cooling

periods for each antibiotic ranged from 2 to 7 days. As representative patients in whom blood drug concentrations were measured, the time courses of serum concentrations of antibiotics in patients treated with CMZ or CPZ are shown in Figs. 3 and 4. The pharmacokinetic parameters calculated from time courses of the serum concentration of each agent are shown in Table 1.

Half-lives of CMZ, FMOX, SBT, and ABK during the cooling stage did not differ from those during the rewarming stage. Furthermore, half-lives of ASPC and AMK, of which serum

TABLE 1. Pharmacokinetic parameters of antibiotics during brain hypothermia

Drug and patient	kel (h⁻¹)		t$_{1/2}$ (h)		AUC (μg·h/ml)		V$_d$ (L)		CL (l/h)	
	Cooling	Rewarming	Cooling	Rewarming	Cooling	Rewarming	Cooling	Rewarming	Cooling	Rewarming
CMZ										
Y.M.	0.62	0.20	1.1	3.5	222.9	—	14.5	—	9.9	—
R.K.	0.26	0.39	2.7	2.2	796.7	668.6	9.7	9.7	2.5	3.0
N.S.	0.47	0.40	1.5	1.8	500.6	535.8	8.5	9.4	4.0	3.7
Y.M.	0.52	0.63	1.3	1.1	258.5	296.1	13.8	10.7	7.2	6.8
ASPC										
A.U.	0.63	—	1.1	—	55.6	—	28.5	—	18.0	—
FMOX										
I.K.	0.40	—	1.7	—	211.9	—	23.7	—	9.4	—
A.U.	0.70	0.80	1.0	0.9	130.2	133.0	21.6	18.6	15.4	15.3
CPZ										
S.K.	0.01	0.09	60.3	8.2	3650.3	613.8	11.4	9.6	0.1	0.8
A.U.	0.19	0.18	3.6	3.8	205.1	224.1	12.7	12.3	2.4	2.2
E.U.[a]	—	0.27	—	2.5	—	150.6	—	12.1	—	3.3
SBT										
K.S.	0.62	0.48	1.1	1.4	54.3	45.5	14.8	22.9	9.2	10.9
A.U.	0.99	0.64	0.7	101.0	42.3	10.8	12.0	72.4	11.8	46.5
E.U.[a]	—	0.85	—	0.8	—	41.5	—	14.1	—	12.0
ABK										
A.U.	0.34	0.29	2.0	2.4	18.6	17.3	15.8	20.2	5.4	5.8
S.I.[a]	—	0.30	—	2.3	—	14.9	—	22.3	—	6.7
T.I.[a]	—	0.11	—	6.4	—	41.1	—	22.5	—	2.4
F.H.[a]	—	0.23	—	3.0	—	23.7	—	18.3	—	4.2

CMZ, cefmetazole; ASPC, aspoxicillin; FMOX, flomoxef; CPZ, cefoperazone; SBT, sulbactam; ABK, arbekacin; kel, elimination rate constant; t$_{1/2}$, elimination half-life; AUC, area under the concentration time curve; Vd, volume of distribution; CL, total clearance

[a] Nonhypothermic

concentrations were measured only during the cooling stage, were similar to those reported in healthy adults (ASPC 1.4h, AMK 1.8h). The $t_{1/2}$ of CPZ was prolonged, the AUC increased, and the CL decreased. In one patient (A.U.) (Fig. 4, thin line) in whom 1 g of CPZ/SBT was intravenously infused for 1 h, the serum concentration curves of CPZ/SBT during the cooling stage (34.0°–34.3°C) were similar to those during the rewarming stage (34.9°–35.1°C). However, in the patient with liver dysfunction (K.S.) (Fig. 4, thick line), the serum concentration of CPZ was higher during the cooling stage (34.5°–34.8°C), and the $t_{1/2}$ was markedly prolonged compared to that during the rewarming stage (36.0°C). In these patients treated with CPZ, the half-life of CPZ during the rewarming stage was similar to that reported in healthy adults (3.7h) in our previous studies.

Discussion

Detected Bacteria

The detection rate of bacteria during the hypothermic period was not increased compared to that in other inpatients. This may have been because brain hypothermia was started immediately after surgery, and administration of antibiotics for the prophylaxis was started immediately after admission to the ICU, inhibiting bacterial growth. A relation between hypothermia and bacterial proliferative capacity is unclear. However, when hypothermia returns to normal body temperature, the function of the patient's protective immune cells and energy reserve do not sufficiently return to the pretreatment state, and infection may easily develop [1]. This may be related to increased bacterial detection during the rewarming stage. Therefore, when administering antibiotics the tendency of bacteria detected during the rewarming stage should be carefully examined. Antibiotics must be selected and the administration method examined when the cooling stage is switched to the rewarming stage. The state of the bacteria detected after the rewarming stage was similar to that of bacteria (including MRSA and *P. aeruginosa*) in other ICU inpatients in our center, suggesting the influence of administered agents and hospital infection. Strategies for treating nosocomial infection should be further examined.

Changes in Serum Drug Concentrations

Of the five antibiotics investigated in this study, four agents (excluding CPZ) are mainly excreted in urine. There were no time courses of pharmacokinetics between the cooling stage and rewarming stage. Furthermore, the half-lives of these agents were similar to those in healthy adults. Therefore, hypothermia may not influence renal function or the rate of drug elimination. Sufficient serum concentrations of these agents were obtained. When administering this kind of agent during hypothermia, routine administration methods may be appropriate.

Cardiac output is decreased during hypothermia, and hepatic blood flow is decreased by a similar percentage [2]. The arterial blood ketone body ratio (AKBR) is decreased to approximately 0.7 during the cooling stage and returns to the normal value (1.0 or more) during the rewarming stage [3]. In CPZ-treated patients, especially those with liver dysfunction, there were time courses of pharmacokinetic parameters. This may have been because hypothermia-related liver dysfunction delayed metabolism, as CPZ is mainly metabolized in the liver. Therefore, the dose and dosing interval of agents that are metabolized in the liver must be carefully selected.

Conclusions

The state of bacterial detection during brain hypothermia and pharmacokinetic parameters of antibiotics were investigated. The following findings were obtained: (1) The state of bacterial detection was similar to that in other ICU inpatients in the emergency center. (2) Pharmacokinetic parameters of antibiotics that are mainly eliminated by kidney excretion, such as cefmetazole, flomoxef, and arbekacin, did not differ between the cooling stage and rewarming stage. Concerning the administration method: the method routinely used for other critically ill patients may be applied here. (3) Because hypothermia may decrease the drug-metabolizing capacity in the liver parenchyma, the administration schedule of an antibiotic that is metabolized in the liver, such as cefoperazone, should be carefully established.

References

1. Hayashi N (1995) The cerebral hypothermia treatment. Sougouigakusha, Tokyo, pp 53–59
2. Kawata K, Sakaguchi M, Higashizawa T (1997) The pharmacokinetics of lidocaine and its metabolite (MEGX) in hypothermic state. Jpn J Ther Drug Monit 14:311–317
3. Sirai K, Tanjyou K, Hayashi N (1998) Nutrional support on hypothermia. Intensive Crit Care Med 12:1369–1370

The Clinical Issue and Effectiveness of Brain Hypothermia Treatment for Severely Brain-Injured Patients

Nariyuki Hayashi, Hidehiko Kushi, Akira Utagawa, Kosaku Kinoshita, Toru Izumi, Katuhisa Tanjoh, Takashi Moriya, Shozo Yoshida, and Atushi Sakurai

Summary. Treatment for brain injury has focused on neuroprotection against brain edema, brain ischemia, and control of intracranial hypertension in animal studies. However, these concepts are not successful in the management of in severely brain-injured patients, because animal studies do not include information about the influence of the excess response of systemic circulatory-metabolic changes and hypothalamus–pituitary endocrine axis dysfunction caused by anesthesia. In our recent clinical studies of severe brain injury, the management of restoration therapy of dying neurons in injured brain tissue before neuroprotection therapy produced successful clinical results. Three major targets of treatment are important: Adequate administration of oxygen and metabolic substrates, control of excess release of vasopressin and growth hormone for prevention of blood–brain barrier dysfunction and cytokine encephalitis, and preclusion of selective neuronal radical damage of the dopamine A 10 nervous system for prevention of vegetation. Management of intensive care is focused on three subsequent targets: Initial care management is to maintain sufficient cerebral oxygenation and adequate brain metabolism by control of PaO_2/FiO_2 above 300, systolic blood pressure above 100 mmHg, serum glucose at 120–140 mg/dl, brain temperature at 34°–32°C, ICP below 20 mmHg, antithrombin-III (AT-III) above 100%, hemoglobin 2,3 diphosphoglycerate at 12–15 mmol/mL, serum pH above 7.3, oxygen delivery above 800 ml/min, and fluid resuscitation. The second target is control of hypothalamus–pituitary axis activation by management of brain tissue temperature at 34°C with 120–140 mg/d serum glucose, 9% saline followed by 4% saline fluid resuscitation, AT-III above 100% followed by replacement of albumin drip, and maintaining serum albumin higher than 3.5 g/dl within 2–3 h after injury. The third target is to prevent the selective neuronal damage of the dopamine A 10 nervous system by controlling brain tissue temperature at 32°–33°C with management of Hb above 11 g/dl and administration of vitamin E and C. However, in brain hypothermia treatment, there are five major pitfalls: hemoglobin dysfunction associated with masking brain hypoxia, inadequate management of brain tissue temperature with hyperglycemia, undesirable duration of brain hypothermia, inadequate care management of systemic infections, and misunderstanding of nutritional issues in the management of brain injury. These pitfalls are discussed in this chapter. A novel technique for control of these clinical issues, the success of adequate neuronal oxygenation and brain metabolism, neurohormonal control of the blood–brain barrier dysfunction, and preservation of the dopamine A 10 nervous system are explained. Preven-

Department of Emergency and Critical Care Medicine, Nihon University School of Medicine, 30-1 Oyaguchi Kami-machi, Itabashi-ku, Tokyo 173-8610, Japan

tion of brain edema, elevation of ICP, and neuroexcitaion are not mechanisms of brain hypothermia. The effectiveness of brain hypothermia treatment was studied by comparing the clinical results of brain hypothermia (99 cases) and normothermia (65 cases) of head injury with Glascow Coma Scale (GCS) less than 6. Patients with initial GCS scores of 3 did not benefit from brain hypothermia treatment, but with GCS 4, 5, and 6, clinical benefit was observed. As clinical signs, memory, intelligence, and personality were not much disturbed in the brain hypothermia-treated group.

Key words. Brain hypothermia, Brain thermopooling, Masking brain hypoxia, Dopamine nervous system, Vegetation

Introduction

As a mechanism of secondary brain damage after severe brain injury, brain edema, brain ischemia, and elevation of intracranial pressure (ICP) associated with NO radical reactions, blood–brain barrier (BBB) dysfunction, and neuroexcitation by release of excitatory amino acids have been suggested by experimental animal studies [1,43,52]. Therefore, treatment for brain-injured patients has focused on the management of brain edema, brain ischemia, and control of ICP elevation after trauma. However, these concepts are not successful in the management of human brain injury, especially in severely brain-injured patients because animal studies do not include information about the influence of excessive response of systemic circulatory and metabolic changes and hypothalamus–pituitary endocrine axis dysfunction caused by anesthesia.

In clinical treatment for severe brain injury, it is necessary to first initiate recovery therapy for dying neurons in the injured brain tissue, and then start neuroprotection therapy for prevention of brain damage by secondary mechanisms, such as brain edema, brain ischemia, and ICP elevation. For successful neuronal restoration therapy of primarily injured neurons, control of catecholamine surge with mild to moderate brain hypothermia [25,27,30], prevention of brain thermopooling [24,26,28,30], prevention of masking brain hypoxia (with normal PaO_2 and cerebral perfusion pressure) [31], and prevention of BBB dysfunction associated with vasopressin release and hyperglycemia are necessary (see also "Enhanced neuronal damage in severely brain-injured patients by hypothalamus, pituitary, and adrenal axis neurohormonal changes" by Hayashi, this volume). Without understanding the effects of these catecholamine surges [6] and hypothalamus–pituitary endocrine dysfunction on pathophysiological changes in injured brain tissue (see Hayashi, this volume), brain resuscitation is difficult in severe cases.

We have developed a brain hypothermia treatment based on a new concept of the brain injury mechanism and compared it to normothermia treatment with the previous concept of neuroprotection [24,26,28–31]. In this chapter, the clinical issues and effectiveness of brain hypothermia treatment were studied in severely brain-injured patients [Glasgow Coma Score (GCS) <6].

Methods

The clinical studies were carried out in 65 cases of normothermia treatment and 99 cases of brain hypothermia treatment as follows. For the normothermia group: GCS 3, 9 patients; GCS 4, 24; GCS 5, 14; and GCS 6; 18 cases; in total, 65 patients were treated. For the brain hypothermia group, the severity of randomized patients was recorded as GCS 3, 13; GCS 4, 21; GCS 5, 27; and GCS 6, 38 cases; in total, 99 patients were treated.

The effectiveness of brain hypothermia treatment was studied by comparing the clinical prognosis 3 months later in both groups, hypothermia and nonhypothermia treatment. The technical issues and pitfalls of brain hypothermia treatment were studied. Normothermia treatment was focused on the previous concept of neuroprotection with control of ICP elevation and brain edema, prevention of brain ischemia, and preclusion of brain hypoxia. Brain hypothermia treatment was performed using the following guideline.

Guidelines for Brain Hypothermia Treatment

Targets of Treatment in the Acute Stage

The three major targets — adequate administration of oxygen and metabolic substrates, control of excessive release of vasopressin and growth hormone for prevention of BBB dysfunction combined with cytokine encephalitis, and preclusion of selective neuronal damage of the dopamine A 10 nervous system for prevention of vegetation — were addressed in the ICU (Fig. 1).

Adequate Administration of Oxygen and Metabolic Substrates

To maintain sufficient microcirculation and cerebral oxygen metabolism, control of ICP below 20 mmHg, PaO_2/FiO_2 above 300, antithrombin-III (AT-III) above 100%, and serum glucose control between 120 and 140 mg/dl were fundamentals of management. If serum glucose is higher than 140 mg/dl, glycerol is contraindicated to avoid increasing brain tissue glucose. The body (or core) temperature is controlled at 34°C for prevention of catecholamine surge initially and after stabilization of systolic blood pressure above 100 mmHg; brain tissue temperature (BTT) is reduced to 33°–32°C with 3 to 6h of intake in cases of moderate brain hypothermia treatment.

Hemoglobin dysfunction as shown by reduced 2,3-diphosphoglycerate (DPG) [16,47] must be corrected when serum pH is lower than 7.3. Oxygen delivery is maintained at greater than 800 ml/min. Cerebral perfusion pressure (CPP) is controlled at higher than 80 mmHg with sufficient fluid resuscitation. If fluid resuscitation is not successful in maintaining systolic blood pressure above 100 mmHg, temporary block of the abdominal aorta using an abdominal

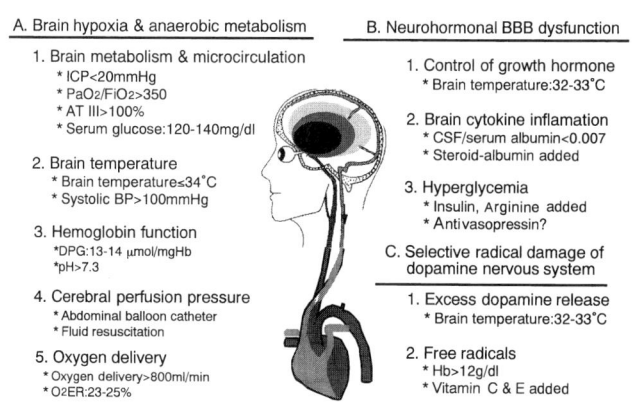

FIG. 1. Targets of brain hypothermia treatment in the acute stage

balloon catheter is available. Oxygen therapy is focused on management at greater than 800 ml/min/kg with an oxygen extraction ratio (O_2ER) of 22% to 25%.

Control of Excessive Release of Vasopressin and Growth Hormone for Prevention of BBB Dysfunction and Cytokine Encephalitis

Hypothalamus–pituitary axis activation by direct injury and stimulation of the neuropeptide Y receptor with excess release of norepinephrine and hyperglycemia produces BBB dysfunction and cytokine encephalitis-associated vasopressin release [9,40] (see also Hayashi, this volume). These pathophysiological changes should be prevented initially by control of BTT at 34°C with 120–140 mg/dl serum glucose. To avoid the progression of catecholamine surge and hyperglycemia, infuse with 7% acetic Ringer's solution and then 4% saline. If serum glucose increased above 150 mg/dl, an insulin drop should be scheduled.

Administration of AT-III alone or combined with low molecular weight heparin (LWHP) reduces vascular inflammation by activation of prostaglandin I_2 (PGI_2). Therefore, both BBB dysfunction and cytokine encephalitis could be treatable by AT-III or AT-III combined with LWHP followed by a 5% albumin drip to maintain serum albumin above 3.5 g/dl within 2 to 3 h after injury.

Preclusion of Selective Neuronal Damage of the Dopamine A 10 Nervous System for Prevention of Vegetation

BTT control between 32° and 33°C prevents dopamine release within 3 h after trauma. Control of Hb above 11 g/dl and administration of vitamin E and C are useful for scavenging of radicals.

Contraindication

Contraindication of Brain Hypothermia

For patients in shock, cases of difficult control of blood pressure even with vasoconstrictive medicines, and clinically brain dead patients, hypothermia is contraindicated [27] (see also Hayashi, this volume). In cases of unstable systolic blood pressure, mild hypothermia to 34°C of BTT could be induced by fluid resuscitation. However, moderate brain hypothermia (32°–33°C) should be induced after stabilizing cardiopulmonary functions and controlling serum glucose below 180 mg/dl. The goal of management of hyperglycemia is control of serum glucose at 120 to 140 mg/dl in moderate brain hypothermia treatment.

Decision for Mild or Moderate Brain Hypothermia Treatment

Mild Brain Hypothermia Treatment

Treatment at 34°C of BTT is indicated for patients with GCS below 8, serum glucose less than 180 mg/dl, and no clinical signs of herniation. Duration is variable at 3 to 7 days. However, brain hypothermia should be started within 3 to 6 h (Fig. 2).

Moderate Brain Hypothermia Treatment

Treatment at 32° to 33°C of BTT is indicated for patients with GCS of 6 or less 6 and serum glucose of 180 mg/dl or more. Duration is variable, 4 to 14 days. However, brain hypothermia should be started within 3 to 6 h. A flat electroencephalogram (EEG) and auditory brainstem evoked potential (ABER), arrested breathing, and dilated pupils are not signs of contraindication in the acute stage (Fig. 2). However, after 3 to 6 h, these critical clinical signs suggest contraindication of brain hypothermia treatment.

1. Mild brain hypothermia treatment (34°C)

Indication: coma, serum glucose<180mg/dl, no herniation
Duration: 3-7days

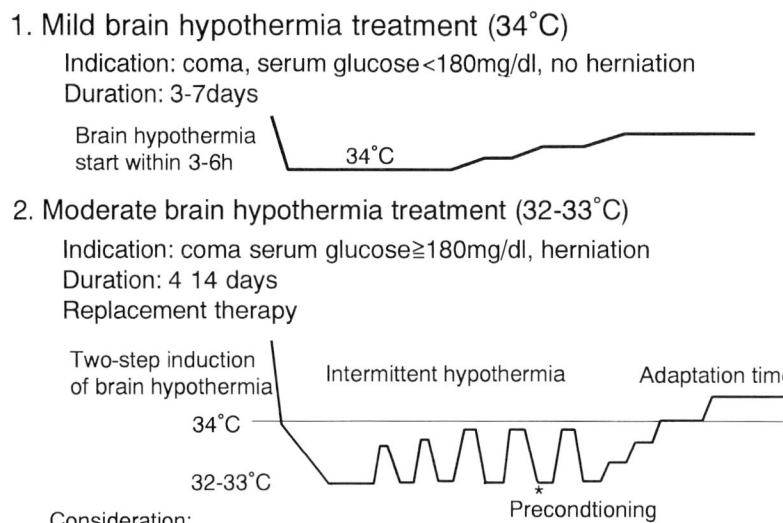

Brain hypothermia
start within 3-6h

34°C

2. Moderate brain hypothermia treatment (32-33°C)

Indication: coma serum glucose≥180mg/dl, herniation
Duration: 4 14 days
Replacement therapy

Two-step induction
of brain hypothermia

Intermittent hypothermia   Adaptation time

34°C

32-33°C

Consideration:

Precondtioning

If hyperglycemia progresses rapidly or it is difficult to control serum glucose
lower than 180mg/dl, BTT reduction should be stopped.

FIG. 2. Design of brain hypothermia treatment

Control of BTT and Schedule of Brain Hypothermia

Control of BTT using the cold water blanket technique throughout reducing the systemic blood temperature is a fundamental technique [24,25,27,31]. Selective cooling of the head and neck produce insufficient lowering of BTT and cause uncontrollable BTT elevation at the rewarming stage because the warmed core temperature is carried into the brain after stopping selective head cooling and produces a rebound elevation of BTT with vascular engorgement and activation of acute brain swelling. Figure 3 shows the design of brain cooling using the blanket technique (Modified BLANKETROL II; CSZ Cincinnati Sub-Zero, Nihon MDM, Tokyo, Japan) [27].

The patient is placed on a dry towel, which is placed on the cooling blanket, and the patient is covered with another dry towel with a cooling blanket from the chest-abdominal side, like a sandwich. Then, again wrap both the patient's body and the cooling blanket completely with another large dry towel. Communication between body temperature and room temperature should be avoided to stabilize BTT. If the heavy patient is weight >80 kg, the cooling system should be separate, using two machines for their front and back.

1. Mild brain hypothermia: Initially, the water temperature of the cooling device should be set between 28° and 30°C, and then water temperature is gradually reduced to 23° to 26°C while monitoring BTT and setting BTT at 34°C.
2. Moderate brain hypothermia: Initially, the water temperature of the cooling device is set between 16° and 18°C, and then water temperature is gradually elevated to 20° to 24°C to stabilize BTT at 33.5° to 34°C. After stabilizing systemic circulation and cardiopulmonary function, BTT is reduced to 33° to 32°C, step by step, over 5 to 6h (see Fig. 3).

1) Blanket technique.

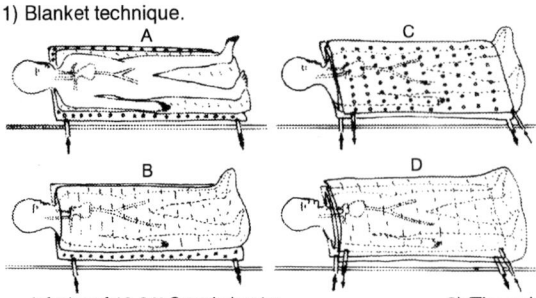

A. Patient lies on the sheet or towel,
   which is placed on the cooling blanket.
B. Patient is covered with dry towel and
   protected from skin injury by cooling blanket.
C. Cooling blanket covers the body like a
   sandwith
D. Body and cooling blanket are wrapped again
   with dry towels to shut down the
   temperature communication between body
   and room air.

Infusing of 18-24° C cooled water

2) The time schedule for management of cooling
   water temperature to control brain tissue
   temperature between 34° and 32°C.

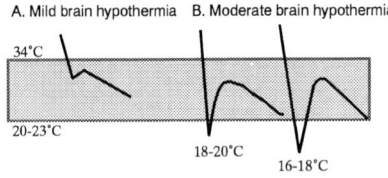

3) The schema of brain cooling by precisely controlled
   lowering of systemic circulating blood temperature.

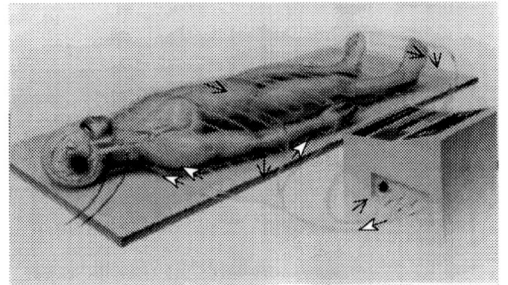

FIG. 3. Brain cooling technique using cooling water blanket and Modified BLANKETROL II machine

Cardiac arrhythmia, hypopotassemia, elongation of QT interval more than 450 mm/s on ECG, and progression of hyperglycemia to more than 180 mg/dl are warning signs.

Prolonged control of BTT at 32°C is not recommended because growth hormone (GH) will be reduced, which produces an immune crisis, lymphocytopenia, and uncontrollable hyperglycemia. Intermittent control of the moderate brain hypothermia technique, with temporary elevation of BTT around 33.5° to 34°C BTT during 1800 to 2200, is recommended to prevent an immune crisis (see Fig. 2).

At the rewarming stage, rewarming speed and time course are very important following prolonged brain hypothermia treatment. Rewarming of BTT for 0.1°C needs 1 h, fundamentally. When BTT is rewarmed to 34° to 35°C, BTT should be kept at this temperature for 1 to 2 days to provide physiological adaptation time. This technique is very successful in preventing systemic infection. The adaptation times differ depending on the level of hypothermia. Rewarming should take at least 1 day to increase 1°C. The recommended rewarming speed of BTT is 0.1°C/1 h. We prefer localized cooling of the head and neck for 3 to 5 days, even after rewarming has been completed.

Rapid elevation of blanket water temperature produces, at the same time, uncontrollable marked elevation of BTT. Blanket water temperature should not be higher than 30°C. To avoid rapid elevation of BTT, remove the cooling blanket from the body step by step without rewarming the blanket water. The reduced contact area of the cooling blanket to the patient's body also provides precise control of rewarming. This technique is much easier for rewarming after 34° to 35°. Rewarming at a slow and steady speed is less likely to cause complications.

In cases of more than 4 days of prolonged brain hypothermia, we recommend an adaptation time of 1 to 2 days for stabilizing metabolic changes. The adaptation time could be provided by control of blanket water temperature, when elevated to 28°C from 23°C and then again reduced to 26°C. This inverse control of blanket water temperature prevents progressing elevation of BTT by hypermetabolism and provides adaptation time.

Anesthesia for Surgical Operation and ICU Management

Anesthesia During Surgery

After fluid resuscitation, patients were provided ventilation with anesthesia: drip of propofol, 1–2 mg/kg (i.v.), and combination of phenteramine (i.v.), lidocaine, 1–2 mg/kg, fentanest, 0.1 mg (i.v.), succinylcholine, 1.5 mg/kg (i.v.), and vecronium, 0.02 mg/kg (i.v.). The patients received a combination of nitrous oxide, sebofulen, and fountain anesthesia.

All patients were operated on in the supine jackknife position with head position elevated to about 35°–40° to prevent brain explosion at the dural incisions. To maintain successful CPP, all patients were prepared by elastic bandage of extremities and/or insertion of an abdominal aortic balloon catheter during surgery. Removal of acute subdural hematoma, stopping of hemorrhage of contused brain tissue, evacuation of necrosed brain tissue, removal of compressive pressure to the upper brainstem, and external decompression for accidental brain swelling at the rewarming stage were the major purposes of neurological surgery. The injured brain was cooled directly by application of cooled saline throughout surgery. Body temperature was controlled between 34° and 36°C.

Anesthesia in ICU Management

All patients were cared for by ventilation with continuous drip of midazolam, 0.15–0.25 mg/kg/h; pancuronium, 0.05 mg/kg/h; and buprenorphine, 1.0–2.0 mg/kg/h after surgery. While undergoing treatment, patients were monitored for ICP, SjO_2, SvO_2, SaO_2, CPP, cardiac output (CO), oxygen delivery (DO_2), oxygen extraction ratio (O_2ER), BTT or jugular venous blood temperature (JvT), tympanic membrane temperature (TMT), bladder temperature, pulmonary arterial pressure, and end-tidal CO_2. Brain hypoxia was evaluated by changes of changes of PaO_2, SaO_2, DPG, BTT (or JvT), and DO_2. The CBF–metabolic imbalance was evaluated by interactive changes in SjO_2 and cerebral thermal index (CTI = BTT/TMT) [27]. All patients were cared for in the ICU with direct participation of doctors using the EMTEK computer management care system [24]. Nitric oxide-induced free radical reactions were evaluated from the changes of serum NO_2 and serum NO_2/urinary NO_3 ratio in the patients [32].

Intensive Care During Brain Hypothermia Treatment

BTT control at 32° to 34°C for 1 to 2 weeks depends on the severity of brain injury. There are six major stages in the ICU management (Table 1) of cooling.

1. Stabilization of vital signs: sBP > 100 mmHg and PaO_2/FiO_2 > 300.
2. Brain hypoxia: oxygen delivery (DO_2) > 800 ml/min; pH > 7.3; 6 L/min tidal volume, with 6–12 cmH$_2$O PEEP; O_2ER, 23%–25%.
3. Management of CBF and metabolism: CPP > 80 mmHg; SjO_2, 65%–70%; serum glucose, 120–160 mg/dl (BTT $\geqq$ 34°C) and 120–140 mg/dl (BTT < 34°C).
4. Care of microcirculation: AT-III > 100%; gastric pH_i > 7.3; BTT/TMT ratio, 1.01–1.03.
5. Prevention of cytokine encephalitis: AT-III > 100%; serum albumin > 3.0 g/dl; CSF/serum albumin ratio < 0.02.
6. Prevention of infections: washing of stomach, gastric juice pH < 3.5, gastric pH_i > 7.35; prevention of abdominal hypertension using a long intestinal decompression catheter; nutritional considerations; digestive decontamination (intestinal administration of VCM + AMPH-

TABLE 1. ICU management during cooling stage

1. Stabilization of vital signs
    Systolic BP > 100 mmHg
    $PaO_2/FiO_2 > 300$
2. Brain oxygenation
    $DO_2 > 800$ ml/min
    O_2ER, 23%–25%
    DPG, 10–14 μmol/ml Hb
    pH > 7.3
    6 l/min tidal volume with 6–12 cm H_2O PEEP
3. Managment of CBF and metabolism
    CPP > 80 mmHg
    SjO_2, 65%–70%
    Serum glucose:
        120–160 mg/dl (BTT $\geqq$ 34°C)
        120–140 mg/dl (BTT < 34°C)
4. Care of microcirculation
    AT-III > 100%
    Gastric pH_i > 7.3
    BTT/TMT ratio, 1.01–1.03
5. Prevention of cytokine encephalitis
    AT-III > 100%
    Serum albumin > 3.0 g/dl
    CSF/serum albumin ratio < 0.02
6. Prevention of infection
    Washing of stomach
    Gastric juice pH < 3.5
    Gastric pH_i > 7.35
    Prevent abdominal hypertension using long intestinal
        decompression catheter
    Nutritional considerations
    Digestive decontamination: VCM·AMPH-B·albekasin
    Vitamin A > 50 μg/dl
    AT-III + LWHP → S. albumin > 3.0 g/dl
    Cleaning of oral cavity and airway
    Intermittent culture study of airway secretions
    Early rehabilitation

B + albekasin); vitamin A > 50 μg/dl; AT-III + LWHP → serum albumin > 3.0 g/dl; cleaning of oral cavity and airway and intermittent culture study of airway secretions are important.

Prevention of Infections During Brain Hypothermia Treatment

The management points of care at each stage are described in Table 2. The control of catecholamine surge by 34° to 35°C of mild hypothermia, control of hyperglycemia by insulin drip, prevention of pulmonary vascular engorgement by administration of AT-III, followed by albumin replacement throughout the activation of PGI_2, preclusion of intestinal edema by replacement of albumin, nutritional support, maintaining oxygen delivery above 800 ml/min, and activation of immune function after 3 to 4 days by administration of L-arginine are important ICU management steps for prevention of systemic infection during brain hypothermia treatment. Especially, preconditioning of serum glucose (<150 mg/dl), vitamin A (>50 mg/dl), lymphocytes (>1500 mm^3), serum albumin (>3.5 g/dl; prealbumin, >20 mg/dl), Hb (>12 g/dl),

TABLE 2. Management care point at each stage

Induction stage
    1. Clean nasooral cavity
    2. Gastric lavage
    3. Digestive decontamination
    4. $DO_2I > 600$ ml/min; $DO_2 > 800$ ml/min

Cooling stage
    1. Nasooral cavity managment
    2. Gastric juice pH < 3.5
    3. Prevent abdominal hypertension < 10 mmHg
    4. Gastric decontamination antibiotics (GDC)
    5. AT-III > 80%–100%; gastric $pH_i > 7.3$
    6. Gastric immune nutrition replacement > nutritional care
    7. Ventilator care and urinary care
    8. Breathing rehabilitation (alveolar dysfunction, atelectasis)
    9. Intermittent elevation of BT from 32°C to 34°C at evening
   10. Replacement of ZnCl, arginine with Hb > 11 g/dl (if lymphocytopenia occurs keep BT at 34°C + GH + γ-globulin added)
   11. Serum albumin > 3.5 g/dl
   12. Low dosage of antibiotics
   13. O_2ER, 23%–25%; 2.3-DPG, 15–10 μmol/g Hb

Precooling stage
    1. Preconditioning:
       no severe infection, SG < 150 mg/dl, vitamin A < 50 μg/dl, lymphocyte > 1500 mm³, S. albumin > 3.5 g/dl (prealbumin > 20 mg/dl), Hb > 12 g/dl, DPG > 10 μmol/g Hb, AT-III > 100%, platelet, 50 000–80 000, digastric decontamination, muscle massage, abdominal pressure < 10 mmHg
    2. antibiotics + γ-globulin
    3. $DO_2 > 800$ ml/min, O_2ER, 23%–25%

Rewarming stage
    1. Very slow step-up rewarming (0.1°C/h, stop at 34°–35°C)
    2. Prevent rapid shift from lipid to glucose metabolism
    3. Control of SG at 150–170 mg/dl
    4. O_2ER, 23%–25%
    5. Managment of neuromuscular junction
    6. 34°–35°C BT for 2–3 days and BT > 36°C, then stop muscle relaxant > anesthesia
    7. Nutritional management

DD, antibiotics-associated colitis (diarrhea); treatment is stop the antibiotics, metronidazole 250 mg pr qi, (severe case IV) > oral vancomycine 125 mg qid

DPG (>10 mmol/g Hb), AT-III (>100%), platelets 50 000–80 000), digastric decontamination, muscle massage, and abdominal pressure (<10 mmHg) are very useful for preventing the worsening of rewarming stage infections. As causes of hypothermia-specific infection, GH-reduced immune crisis, metabolic changes from lipid to glucose at the rewarming stage, pulmonary atelectasis with unsuccessful ventilator care, and misunderstanding of nutritional support must be considered.

    Early nutritional support is recommended in critically ill patients. However, early enteral and parenteral nutrition produces an increase of serum glutamate, about twofold. If the BBB dysfunctions, such as the CSF/serum albumin ratio increasing above 0.02, serum glutamate and serum cytokines can easily pass through the BBB and activate secondary neuronal damage [35,36]. The mechanism of BBB dysfunction is not simple, with multiple factors being associated with release of vasopressin and activation of cytokines (see Hayashi, this volume).

The peak time of BBB dysfunction is concentrated at 3 to 4 days after brain injury. From these results, nutritional support that includes amino acids and glucose is recommended, starting after 3 to 4 days after severe brain injury (see Hayashi, this volume).

We prefer two categories of nutritional consideration. When BBB function is not severely damaged, with the CSF/serum albumin ratio less than 0.02, we schedule early enteral administration of ZnCl and glutamine until 3 days after trauma and follow with enteral-parenteral amino acid nutrition. In cases of severely damaged BBB function (CSF/serum albumin $\geq$ 0.02), enteral-parenteral administration of ZnCl with replacement therapy of AT-III and albumin until 3 to 4 days is followed by enteral nutritional therapy through the long intestinal abdominal decompression catheter.

Rewarming Time

Timing of rewarming is one of the key points for successful brain hypothermia treatment. Because recovery of intracerebral pathophysiological changes is not obtained during the cooling stage, that is, the stop (or delay) of progression of pathophysiological changes by brain cooling, in these patients the stopped or delayed secondary brain injury mechanism starts again with rewarming. The shift of the secondary brain mechanism at the rewarming stage is made much worse by the imperative metabolic shift from lipid to glucose, cytokine activation, and neurohormonal changes [31].

For these reasons, the decision as to rewarming time must be made with an exact diagnosis of the way of recovery. The recording of θ waves on the background of δ waves on EEG, no ICP elevation, SjO$_2$ control between 60% and 75%, and no brain swelling on CT scan are indirect evaluation parameters for the decision to start rewarming.

Cerebral Dopamine Replacement Therapy

After brain hypothermia treatment, cases with no recovery of consciousness should be programmed for replacement therapy with cerebral dopamine [29–31]. As a method of replacement of cerebral dopamine, the combination of pharmacological treatment such as amantadine (300 mg/kg/day) or parodel (2.5–20 mg/day), increasing uptake of cerebral dopamine by administration of estrogen (Estraderm TTS, 1 set/day), and intermittent electrical stimulation of the median nerve (20 s on, 50 s off, 10–20 mA, 30 pulses/s, duration 300 ms) is effective [30,31]. Reduced CSF dopamine after brain hypothermia is suggested as a good indicator of cerebral dopamine replacement therapy. In most cases of vegetative state after brain hypothermia treatment, more than 3 weeks of replacement therapy are appropriate.

Clinical Study of Neuroprotection by Brain Hypothermia

As mechanisms of neuroprotection by preliminary hypothermia, prevention of free radicals, brain edema, ICP elevation, gene damage, and BBB dysfunction have been shown in animal studies [3,4,7,14,33,34,37,39,45,52]. However, in all clinical cases, application of brain hypothermia treatment includes differences in meaning compared to animal studies [30,31]. Detailed data concerning neuroprotection by brain hypothermia treatment after trauma are not made clear. As negative factors for neuronal restoration after severe brain injury, brain tissue glutamate, BBB dysfunction, increased brain tissue glucose and lactate, excess release of dopamine in the CSF, release of vasopressin, and release of norepinephrine were studied to understand needed changes during brain hypothermia treatment. Changes of neurotransmitters and metabolic substrate in the brain tissue and CSF were studied using CMA/Micro-dialysis AB System (CMA/MICRODIALYSIS, Solna, Sweden) and the Neurotome Colloquium Electrode Array System (MC MEDICAL, Tokyo, Japan).

Analysis of Causes of Lack of Success and of Pitfalls of Brain Hypothermia Treatment

Brain hypothermia treatment based on a new concept of brain injury mechanism and target of treatment may include many different pathophysiological changes [25,27,29,30,31]. The imbalance of brain tissue glucose and neurohormonal release of vasopressin throughout feed-back mechanism of macronutrients, changes of immune function-associated GH release, car-diopulmonary dysfunction caused by reduced serum catecholamine, reactivity of cytokine inflammations, and medication function. Therefore, useful brain hypothermia treatment requires not only understanding a new concept of brain injury mechanism but also under-standing protective pathophysiological reactions under hypothermia conditions and the special care management technique during brain hypothermia treatment. We carefully studied the reasons for unsuccessful clinical results and the pitfalls of brain hypothermia treatment throughout all our experiences with brain hypothermia treatment in severely brain-injured patients.

Clinical Results of Brain Hypothermia and Normothermia Treatment

Eligible patients were randomly assigned in our two medical centers of emergency and crit-ical care medicine, Nihon University of Itabashi Hospital and Surgadai Hospital. Brain hypothermia treatment was executed mainly at Itabashi Hospital and normothermia treat-ment was performed at Surugai Hospital.

The severity of brain-injured patients was evaluated by the Glasgow Coma Scale (GCS) score, and the clinical outcome for all patients was evaluated by Glasgow Outcome Scale (GOS) scores, 3 months later.

Results

Neuronal Protection by Brain Hypothermia Treatment

Changes of Brain Energy Metabolism and Neuroexcitatory Amino Acids

The concentration of brain tissue glucose is maintained at lower levels than that of serum glucose (about one-third). However, the sequential dynamic changes are very tightly corre-lated to the changes of serum glucose (Fig. 4). The effects of BTT on brain tissue glucose metabolism are not clear in clinical brain-injured patients. In this study, a specific pattern of metabolic changes of glucose and glutamate under 33°C BTT for 4 days is demonstrated.

Neurotoxic amino acid neurotransmitters, glutamate release, is successfully prevented at lower than 100 μmol/l by control of BTT at 33°C. When BTT was reduced to 33°C for a couple of days, glutamate release was suppressed for a more prolonged period than brain hypother-mia. At the rewarming stage, a small rebound of glutamate release is recorded in many cases. This small rebounding of glutamate is, however, associated with many factors, not only intracranial pathophysiological changes, but also systemic activation of cytokines and nutri-tional supply, which includes immune function-activating glutamine and glutamate. BTT control at 34°C produced reduction of brain tissue glutamate release to about 400 μmol/l, which is four times higher than at BTT of 33°C.

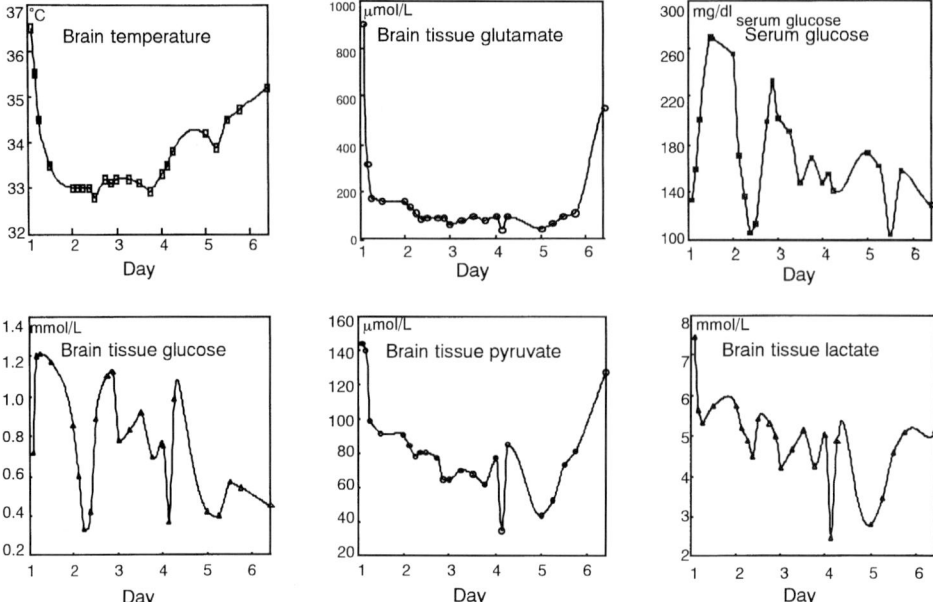

FIG. 4. Sequential changes of brain tissue glutamate and glucose metabolism during brain hypothermia treatment

Following brain hypothermia treatment, the specific metabolic changes of brain tissue glucose are impressive. The changes of brain tissue glucose, pyruvate, and lactate are not similar in pattern to the reduction in BTT (see Fig. 4). Dynamic changes of brain tissue glucose and lactate, which related to the changes of serum glucose, were recorded. Otherwise, brain tissue pyruvate was not changed dynamically. The effect of brain hypothermia on the metabolism of brain tissue glucose suggested a step-by-step downgrade reduction pattern (see Fig. 4). No recording of immediate suppression of glucose metabolism was evident.

Changes of Vasoactive Hormones, Metabolic Substrate, and BBB Function

The intercerebral excess releases of dopamine produce OH^- radicals, which react to oxygen [1,50]. Clinically, prevention of dopamine release is very important for prevention of selective radical attacks to the dopamine nervous system, which includes the A10 nervous system [29,31]. In this study, the release of dopamine was very similar in pattern to the changes in BTT (Fig. 5). In the acute stage, control of BTT below 33°C is very useful for prevention of free radical reactions, which are associated with dopamine.

In contrast to the immediate successful prevention of dopamine release, other vasoconstrictive metabolic substrates, glucose, and vasoactive neurohormones such as epinephrine and vasopressin are reduced step by step. Especially, serum vasopressin and brain tissue glucose are not reduced until 4 to 5 days after trauma (Fig. 5).

Dysfunction of the BBB, evaluated by CSF/serum ratio, suggested a pattern very similar to that of the release of vasoactive hormones. The very high correlation between changes of brain tissue glucose, BBB function, and vasopressin was very impressive (Fig. 6). Therefore, during brain hypothermia treatment, the management of hyperglycemia is very important for prevention of brain edema and cytokine encephalitis.

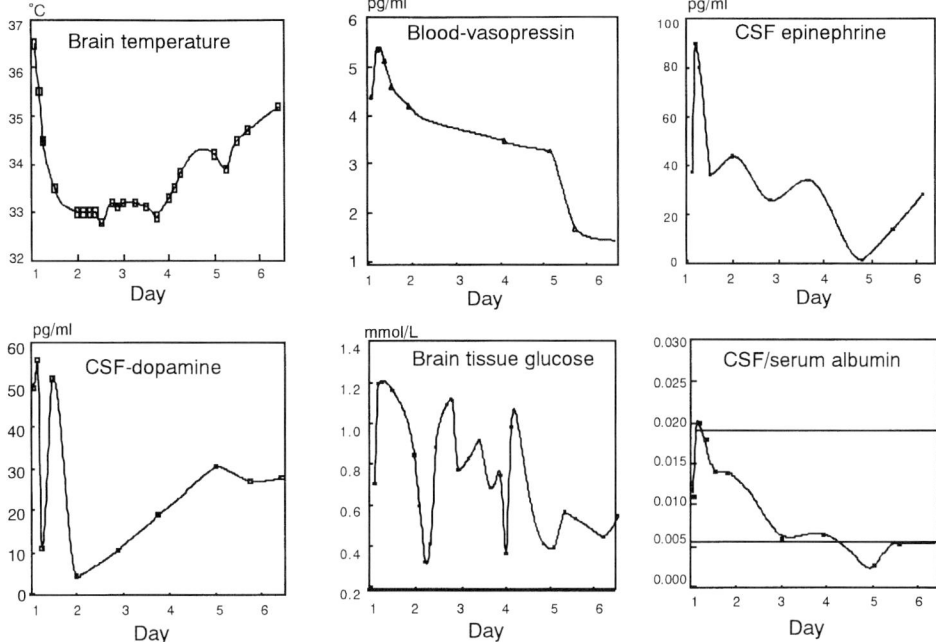

FIG. 5. Sequential changes of vasoactive neurohormones, metabolic substrate, and BBB function (evaluated with changes of CSF/serum albumin) following brain hypothermia treatment in traumatic brain injury

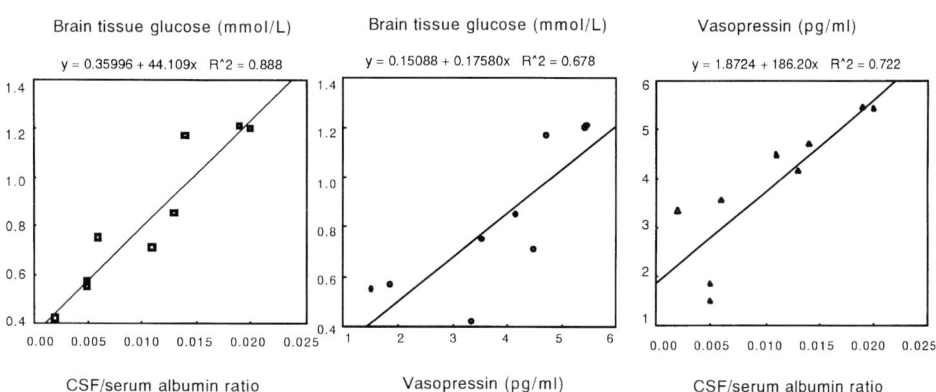

FIG. 6. Relationships between changes of brain tissue glucose, release of vasopressin, and BBB function, evaluated by changes in the CSF/serum albumin ratio. Normal values of CSF/serum albumin are less than 0.007; the recorded interrelation was highly significant

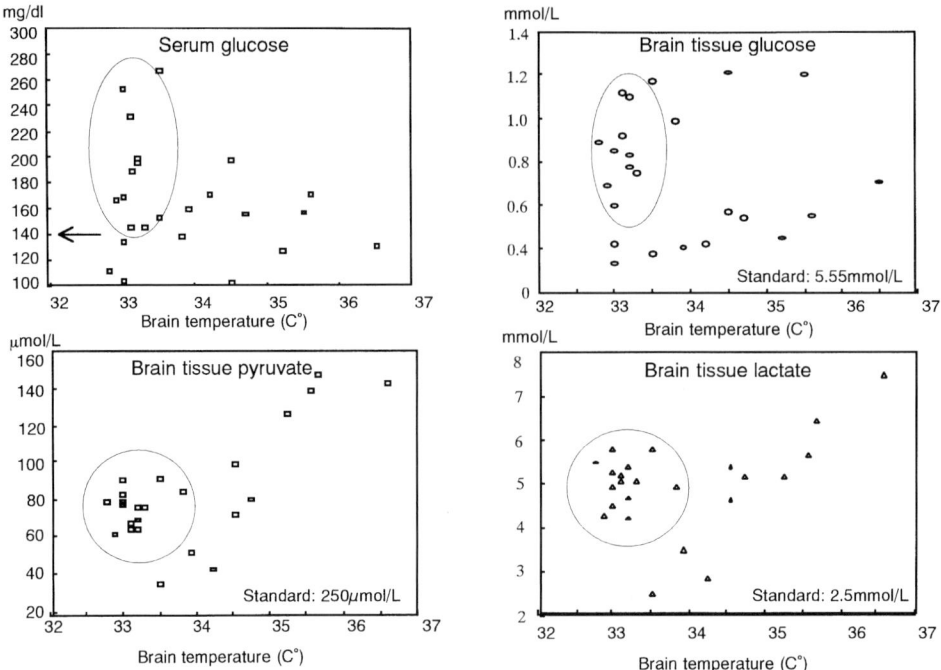

FIG. 7. Brain tissue pyruvate and lactate increased more severely at 33°C than at 34°C of brain hypothermia because of inadequate control of hyperglycemia

Causes of Unsuccessful Brain Hypothermia Treatment

Adequate Brain Temperature and Hyperglycemia

In severely brain-injured patients, catecholamine surge-associated hyperglycemia is unavoidable (see Hayashi, this volume). This catecholamine surge could be prevented by brain hypothermia and the easy control of hyperglycemia. However, brain hypothermia at lower than 33°C some times produces increasing serum glucose by systemic reduction of glucose consumption. This inadequate control of serum glucose causes an increase of brain tissue lactate and pyruvate with increasing brain tissue glucose (Fig. 7). The critical level of hyperglycemia to cause an increase in lactate is higher than 140 mg/dl under the condition of BTT at 33°C. Increased brain tissue glucose enables activation of cytokines and BBB permeability. Therefore, in the management of moderate brain hypothermia treatment, we must control serum glucose at 120 to 140 mg/dl, exactly. At the induction stage, if difficult control of hyperglycemia is experienced, further hypothermia is not indicated (see Fig. 2).

Inappropriate Duration of Brain Hypothermia

Brain hypothermia of short duration cannot produce recovery and is limited for stopping pathophysiology or delaying its progression in the injured brain. Without recovery from brain injury during the cooling stage, in these cases, rewarming promotes the progression of stopped pathophysiological changes and makes them much worse [31]. Therefore, before starting rewarming, we must make sure whether the injured brain is on the way to recovery. Two days of brain hypothermia treatment are too short, especially for severely brain-injured patient.

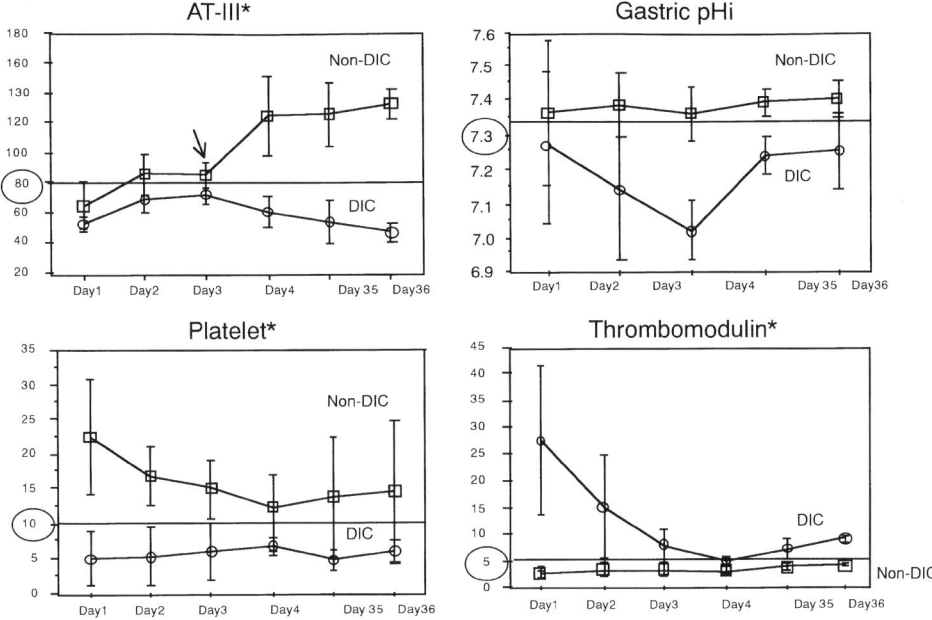

FIG. 8. Changes of DIC-promoting factors* and gastric pH$_i$ during brain hypothermia treatment ($n = 8$)

Adequate duration of brain hypothermia is theoretically variable. However, with prolonged brain hypothermia treatment, it is easy to cause an immune crisis with reduced GH and severe systemic infections. To provide adequate duration of brain hypothermia, we need skillful care technique for control of immune crisis and infections.

Activation of Brain Damage by Systemic Infections

Severe damage of the BBB function, such as an elevated CSF/serum albumin ratio greater than 0.02, is a serious complication of pulmonary infection because increased cytokines in systemic circulation caused by pulmonary infections can easily permeate the BBB and make a cytokines encephalitis (see Hayashi, this volume). The systemic infection itself is a direct cause of the worsening of the brain injury. Therefore, management of infection during brain hypothermia treatment includes not only the prevention of infections but also caring for vascular inflammations, vascular permeability, and BBB dysfunctions. To control these pathophysiological changes, management of AT-III at higher than 100% to prevent vascular inflammations and microemboli, which was derived from disseminated intravascular coagulability (DIC) complication studies (Fig. 8), management of hyperglycemia to prevent increasing vascular permeability, and then control of serum albumin above 3.5 g/dl to maintain BBB function are required. Replacement therapy using albumin is very successful to prevent intestinal mucosa edema, obstructive pancreatic dysfunction, free bacteria, and free pharmacology. Recent brain hypothermia treatment has dramatically reduced the incidence of infections (Table 3) and improved neuronal recovery.

Inadequate Nutrition

In the ICU management of critically ill patients, early administration of parenteral and enteral nutrition is recommended. The recent parenteral and enteral nutritive solutions are rich

TABLE 3. Alteration of incidence of severe systemic infections with cerebral hypothermia treatment during 8 years

Time period	Treatment	Cases	Percent
1991–1993	Antibiotics γ-Globulin Physiological rehabilitation Prevention of hypoproteinemia	9/14	64.2
1994–1995	GI washing O$_2$ER control at 23%–25% Kinetic therapy Early intestinal nutrition Electrical muscle stimulation	16/50	32.0

1996–1998	Replacement of growth hormone
	L-arginine, glutamin, Zn immune-
	  enhancing early nutrition
	Hemoglobin > 12 g/dl
	Vitamin A and lipid nutrition at
	  rewarming stage
		5/44	11.3

TABLE 4. Changes of serum amino acids after parenteral nutrition of AMIZET and combination of AMIZET + glutamine AMIZET XB ($n = 4$) and AMIZET XB + glutamine ($n = 6$)

Serum amino acid (standard values, mmol/ml)	Nutrition	Brain tissue temperature (34°C)	Brain tissue temperature (36°C)
Arginine (54–130)	AMIZET + glutamin AMIZET ® XB	86 ± 21.8 71 ± 10.1 — N.S.	126 ± 23.6 62 ± 13.8 — $P = 0.0105$
Ornithine (30–100)	AMIZET + glutamin AMIZET ® XB	62 ± 14.6 72 ± 27.3 — N.S.	95 ± 25.0 57 ± 12.2 — $P = 0.0190$
Citrulline (17–43)	AMIZET + glutamin AMIZET ® XB	18 ± 10.0 18 ± 6.4 — N.S.	25 ± 10.7 12 ± 1.10 — $P = 0.0105$
Glutamine (420–700)	AMIZET + glutamin AMIZET ® XB	407 ± 50.0 372 ± 48.1 — N.S.	503 ± 91.7 421 ± 66.8 — N.S.
Glutamate (12–63)	AMIZET + glutamin AMIZET ® XB	105 ± 23.7 136 ± 65.3 — N.S.	125 ± 23.6 137 ± 40.2 — N.S.

in glucose and glutamate. We wondered if excess glucose and glutamate could activate BBB dysfunction and produce neuroexcitation neuronal death. Parenteral amino acid nutrition increased neurotoxic glutamate in the serum about twofold (Table 4). In cases with a CSF/serum albumin ratio higher than 0.02, meaning cases of severe BBB dysfunction, early nutrition after trauma within 3 to 4 days and active amino acid nutrition at the rewarming stage produced an uncontrollable increase of brain tissue glutamate.

Clinical Results

At 3 months after severe brain injury (GCS < 6) in the normothermia group, 41 of 65 (63%) had died, 6 of 65 (9%) were in a vegetative state, 7 of 65 (11%) had severe disability, 8 of 65 (12%) had mild disability, and 3 of 65 (5%) had mild or no disability. In the brain hypothermia group, 45 of 99 (45%) had died, 5 of 99 (5%) were in vegetative state, 8 of 99 (8%) had severe disability, 14 of 99 (14%) had mild disability, and 27 of 99 (28%) had mild or no disability (Table 5).

TABLE 5. Clinical prognosis of traumatic severe brain injury 3 months later with moderate brain hypothermia and normothermia treatment

Glasgow Outcome Score	3 Hypothermia	3 Normothermia	4 Hypothermia	4 Normothermia	5 Hypothermia	5 Normothermia	6 Hypothermia	6 Normothermia
1. Death	11 (84%)	9 (100%)	11 (52%)	17 (71%)	7 (26%)	9 (64%)	16 (42%)	6 (33%)
2. Vegetative state	—	—	1 (5%)	4 (17%)	2 (7%)	1 (7%)	2 (5%)	1 (6%)
3. Severe disability	—	—	—	1 (4%)	5 (19%)	2 (15%)	3 (9%)	4 (22%)
4. Moderate disability	1 (8%)	—	3 (14%)	1 (4%)	6 (22%)	1 (7%)	4 (11%)	6 (33%)
5. Mild or no disability	1 (8%)	—	6 (29%)	1 (4%)	7 (26%)	1 (7%)	13 (34%)	1 (6%)
Total	13	9	21	24	27	14	38	18

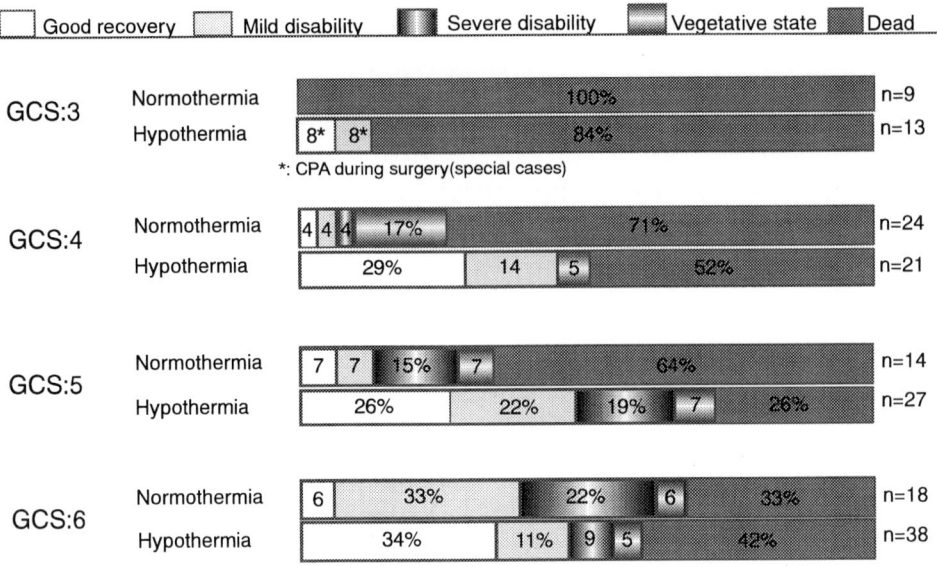

FIG. 9. Difference in clinical prognosis at 3 months after normothermia treatment (65 cases) and moderate brain hypothermia treatment (99 cases)

The efficacy of brain hypothermia was related to the severity of the injury as indicated by the Glasgow Coma Score on admission. The patients with initial coma scores of 3 did not benefit from brain hypothermia treatment, except for 2 cases of cardiac arrest that occurred during surgery. Of these 2 cases, 1 was GCS 5 with bilateral acute subdural hematoma with diffuse brain injury. The 15-min cardiac arrest occurred because of uncontrollable bleeding from the base of the skull. Consciousness returned 56 days after surgery; however, 3 months later, mild disability of mental retardation was recorded. Now, 3 years later, his mental retardation has completely disappeared and the patient has made a good recovery in lifestyle. The other case was a 26-year-old man with acute subdural hematoma (GCS 6) on admission, because of a cardiac arrest incident for 9 min during surgery after cardiac arrhythmia, ventricular fibrillation with lower body temperature, and hypopotassemia. Three months later, no neurological deficits were observed. In both cases, oxygen was inhaled at the time of cardiac arrest. These 2 special cases probably should be excluded from the GCS 3 category.

In GCS 4 to 6, in contrast, clinical benefit is observed (Fig. 9; see Table 5). Among these patients with higher scores, 29% at GCS 4, 26% at GCS 5, and 34% at GCS 6 in the brain hypothermia group had a good outcome. However, good outcome was limited in the normothermia group with high scores; 4% in GCS4, 7% in GCS 5, and 6% in GCS6, respectively. As clinical signs, memory, intelligence, and personality specifically are maintained better in the brain hypothermia-treated group than in the normothermia group. The effectiveness of cerebral dopamine replacement therapy was limited in cases of lower CSF dopamine, except 1 case. The 11 of 28 (40%) cases in vegetative state suggested the clinical effect. In this series of brain hypothermia treatment with cerebral dopamine replacement therapy, 5 of 28 (18%) of those experiencing vegetation recovered to a useful lifestyle with good memory, good personality, and good intelligence results.

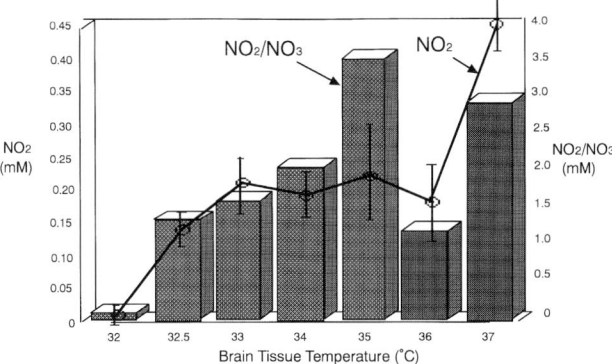

FIG. 10. Effects of brain hypothermia on changes in NO_2 and NO_3 in the severe brain injury patient ($n = 8$). (From [29] with permission)

Discussion

History of Clinical Approach of Hypothermia

In 1943, Fay reported the effectiveness of hypothermia for brain trauma. In 1954, Rosomoff and Holaday measured the changes in CBF during hypothermia treatment and initiated clinical trials of the procedure. Subsequently, many clinicals trial of hypothermia have been undertaken over a period of decades, and deep global hypothermia has been established as a principal cerebral protective technique for circulatory arrest procedures. The classical mechanism proposed for the neuronal protection afforded by hypothermia is a reduction of oxygen and glucose consumption by lowering the rates of enzymatic reactions subserving metabolism. Brain hypothermia has thus been recommended to effect neuronal protection during anesthesia [10,15,52]. However, the use of hypothermia in neurosurgical procedures has been restricted by postoperative complications such as severe pulmonary infections, cardiac dysfunction, and thrombocytopenia-induced intravascular microcirculatory disturbances. Numerous hazards of hypothermia have compromised its clinical application to the management of brain injury patients.

In 1989, Busto et al. demonstrated that mild and moderate degrees of hypothermia (2°–4°C temperature reduction) are also associated with substantial effects, involving histological damage by reducing excitatory neurotransmitters [11]. Several other animal studies have shown that mild hypothermia can stabilize ion homeostasis [45], membrane permeability [52], protein synthesis [52], acid–base balance, downregulation of protein kinase [4], the arachidonic acid cascade [14], membrane lipid peroxidation [45], free radical reactions, and permeability of the blood–brain barrier [37]. However, intraischemic rather than postischemic brain hypothermia can protect chronically after global forebrain ischemia in rats [15].

Based on clinical studies, Hayashi et al. [27] reported that the threshold of disappearance of cortical loop responses is at 33°C of BTT and that of NO-induced free radicals is 32°C of BTT. However, prevention of NO-induced free radicals is limited to about 50% at 34°–35°C BTT (Fig. 10) [31,32]. The effects of hypothermia for neurological protection could thus differ according to the actual BTT.

Mild to moderate hypothermia may be expected to offer safer treatment when compared to the deep hypothermia treatment previously used [43]. Recently, details of two controlled, randomized clinical studies on the use of therapeutic moderate hypothermia for severe closed head injuries have been published [8,44]. Marion et al. [44] randomly assigned 40 patients with severe closed head injury (Glasgow Coma Scores 3–7) to either a hypothermia group or a normothermia group. The hypothermia patients were cooled to 32°–33°C (as BTT) within 10 h after injury, maintained at that temperature for 24 h, and rewarmed to 37°C over a period of 12 h. Hypothermia significantly reduced the ICP (40%) and CBF (26%) during the cooling period, and neither parameter exhibited a significant rebound increase after rewarming of the patients. At 3 months after injury, 12 patients in the hypothermia group had moderate, mild, or no disabilities, as opposed to 8 patients in the normothermia group. Systemic complications were similar in both groups. The authors concluded that therapeutic hypothermia (32°C) following severe closed head injury represents a safe procedure, and that the tendency toward a better outcome with hypothermia indicates a limitation of secondary brain injury [44]. Clifton et al. [8] randomized 46 patients with severe nonpenetrating brain injury (Glasgow Coma Scores 4–7) into groups undergoing either standard management at 37°C ($n = 22$) or standard management with systemic hypothermia at 32°–33°C ($n = 24$). Surface cooling was initiated within 6 h of injury and maintained for 48 h. There were no cardiac or coagulopathy-related complications, and the incidence of seizures was significantly lower in the hypothermia group. The mean Glasgow Outcome Score at 3 months after injury showed an absolute increase of 16% in terms of the number of patients in the good recovery/moderate disability category as compared with those in the severe disability/vegetative/dead categories. The evidence of an improved neurological outcome suggested that phase III testing of moderate systemic hypothermia in patients with severe head injury is warranted [8]. Although the effectiveness of neuroprotection by prolonged cerebral hypothermia has been clearly demonstrated in animal studies and clinical trials, such hypothermia treatment is still limited to within a 48-h period of cooling to avoid severe pulmonary infections and sepsis.

The Concept of Brain Hypothermia Treatment

The Clinical Issues in Previous Hypothermia Treatment

On the management of severe brain injury, it has been considered that recovery of the primary injured tissue was difficult. Therefore, the target of treatment was focused on the prevention of secondary brain injury such as brain edema, ICP elevation, neuroexcitation, and tolerance to CBF disturbances [42,46]. However, many neurons in injured tissue do not die immediately; they are only on the way to dying. Therefore, as an initial treatment for severe brain injury, the management is restoration therapy of dying neurons in injured brain tissue, and then follows neuroprotection therapy for prevention of secondary brain injury mechanisms such as brain edema, ischemia, and ICP elevation. For successful neuronal restoration therapy of primary injured neurons, control of catecholamine surge with mild to moderate brain hypothermia, prevention of brain thermopooling, prevention of masking brain hypoxia, even with normal PaO_2 and CPP, and of hyperglycemia-vasopressin release-associated BBB dysfunction are necessary [31] (see also Hayashi, this volume).

Recent animal studies have revealed that mild hypothermia is very successful to prevent secondary pathophysiological changes, such as delayed neuronal injury, release of glutamate, excessive excitation of nerve synapses, free radical reactions, and ICP elevation [14,38,45,52]. Also, it has been demonstrated that mild hypothermia is very successful to prevent catecholamine surge, reduce excess release of GH, and prevent cytokine encephalitis. For successful neuronal restoration in severely injured patients, enough administration of oxygen, adequate administration of metabolic substrate to the injured neurons, prevention of catecholamine surge with brain thermopooling, and management of cytokine encephalitis are necessary. Brain hypothermia without intensive management of oxygen delivery, hemoglobin function, hyperglycemia, vasopressin, GH, BBB function, and prevention of systemic infections in severely injured cases of BBB function that cause activation of cytokine encephalitis cannot provide clinical success.

However, hypothermia-induced severe infections have become a major issue in clinical trials such that this therapy remains limited to a 48-h duration even with mild to moderate hypothermia treatment [8,44]. In severely injured patients, especially in cases of GCS less than 5, 48 h of brain hypothermia is too short to provide recovery of pathophysiological changes during the cooling stage and will cause a shift of secondary brain injury mechanisms at the rewarming stage. Secondary brain injury mechanism will be much worse in these cases because of combined cytokine activation, glucose metabolism imbalance, increased oxygen demand, and vascular engorgement at the rewarming stage.

Hypothermia treatment with the goal of effective prevention of brain edema, ICP elevation, free radicals, and BBB dysfunction is not enough to result in the survival of severely injured patients. Brain hypothermia treatment that includes the novel technique of ICU management as described in the guideline in this chapter has a much more precise treatment target, which is based on the new concept of brain injury mechanism as described in our previous paper, and must be developed. The previous concept of hypothermia, which was based on animal experimental studies, is too simple to allow survival of severely injured patients.

Initial Care Management of Brain Hypothermia Treatment

The mechanism of neuronal recovery by the first trial of mild to moderate brain hypothermia treatment is summarized as stabilization of oxygen delivery, neuroprotection, and preservation of the dopamine nervous system.

Treatment for Brain Hypoxia Associated with Catecholamine Surge in the Acute Stage

Most neurons in primary injured brain tissue do not die immediately and otherwise can be sustained on the way to death. To recover these neurons in primary injured brain tissue, maintaining adequate oxygen and glucose metabolism is basically necessary. However, our recent clinical studies recorded a very high incidence of brain hypoxia even with normal PaO_2 and CPP within 6 h of the acute stage (see Hayashi, this volume). As reasons for such a discrepancy between brain hypoxia and normal PaO_2 and BP in the acute state, catecholamine surge-induced masking brain hypoxia, such as blood shift to the intestine by excess release of dopamine, brain thermalpooling by lower systolic BP (at <90–100 mmHg), hemoglobin dysfunction causing release oxygen from combined hemoglobin, and undesirable oxygen delivery by lower CO or hemoglobin were recorded (see Hayashi, this volume). Mild to moderate hypothermia was very successful to control this catecholamine surge (Fig. 11) and masking brain hypoxia. Therefore, in the acute stage, the most important beneficial mechanism of brain hypothermia is prevention of masking brain hypoxia by control of catecholamine surge (see Fig. 1).

The desirable brain temperature to control catecholamine surge is about 34°C of BTT. Moderate brain hypothermia, 32°–33°C of BTT, some times reduces serum catecholamines (dopamine > epinephrine > norepinephrine) extensively and brings about an unstable systemic circulatory disturbance without appropriate fluid resuscitation (see Fig. 11). Therefore, adequate fluid resuscitation and oxygenation are important for care management throughout brain hypothermia treatment. Dehydration therapy for prevention of brain edema is not suitable for management, especially in the acute stage.

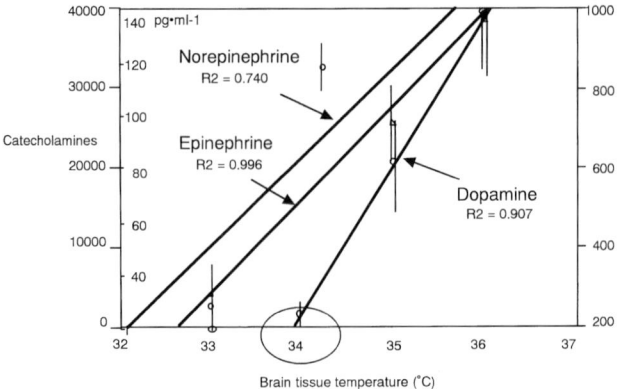

FIG. 11. Effects of brain hypothermia on catecholamine surge

Neuronal recovery requires a desirable oxygen–glucose metabolism. However, for a long time it has been believed that suppression of brain metabolism causes tolerance to ischemia by reducing oxygen and glucose demand. This idea might be beneficial for protection from coming insults or neurons not as severely injured after trauma and stroke. However, severely injured neurons need enough ATP to maintain cellular homeostasis. Our clinical studies of systemic metabolic changes during moderate hypothermia suggested that a systemic energy metabolism shift from glucose to lipid occurs after BTT lower than 34°C [28,30,31]. Some metabolic changes could be considered in the brain metabolism during brain hypothermia. Our clinical studies of brain metabolism during brain hypothermia treatment using a microdialysis monitor suggested that precise control of serum glucose is important to maintain brain metabolism and also prevent BBB dysfunction (Hayashi, this volume). Hyperglycemia occurs initially depending on the severity of catecholamine surge (indirect parameter of harmful stress and severity of brain damage) and secondarily with reduced systemic glucose utilization by brain hypothermia. In most cases below BTT of 33°C it is easy to manage hyperglycemia with increasing brain tissue pyruvate and lactate (see Fig. 7). The critical level of serum glucose for prevention of brain tissue lactate accumulation is above about 140 mg/dl. From these results, we can say that brain hypothermia treatment is necessary for enough neuronal oxygenation and adequate control of serum glucose for maintaining balanced metabolism, as shown in Fig. 1. This fundamental care management only could be provide a chance for recovery for brain-injured patients with a GCS of less than 6.

Prevention of Excess Release of Vasopressin and GH

The excessive release of vasopressin causes BBB dysfunction with activation of cytokines (Hayashi, this volume). Activation of cytokines stimulates GH release [2]. Our clinical studies about immune dysfunction during prolonged brain hypothermia management suggested that GH is one of the regulators of immune function [27,28] by activating CD4 with increase of IL-1 and IL-6 and suppressing CD8 with reduced antiinflammatory cytokine, IL-10 [13]. If BBB function is severely damaged, as monitored at a CSF/serum albumin ratio greater than 0.02, increased serum cytokines easily permeate the BBB [35,36] and cause activation of cytokine inflammation in the injured brain tissue. Therefore, too much release of GH causes greatly complicated severe secondary brain damage by cytokine encephalitis and diminishes the anti-inflammatory mechanism. Recent clinical studies in ICU care management of critically ill patients have also suggested the poor prognosis of GH [9]. The peak time of release of GH is between 3 and 4 days. The release of GH could be prevented by brain hypothermia with correlation to the level of lower BTT.

The precise mechanism of vasopressin release in severely brain-injured patients is not clarified. The hypothalamus neuropeptide Y network stimulates the release of vasopressin for control of macronutrient intake by a feedback mechanism and cerebral vascular reactions [12,21,40,41]. The hypothalamus neuropeptide Y network is stimulated by norepinephrine and increased brain tissue glucose (see Fig. 6). Therefore, excess release of vasopressin and GH is also associated with catecholamine surge, which is observed as a neuroendocrinological hormonal reaction following harmful stress such as severe brain injury, stroke, and subarachnoid hemorrhage.

The management of excess release of vasopressin and GH is very important for survival of severely brain-injured patients. Reduction of catecholamine surge by mild to moderate brain hypothermia, control of hyperglycemia, suppression of inflammatory reactions by activating prostaglandin I (PGI) 2 with AT-III, and maintenance of BBB function by replacement of hypoalbuminemia are summarized for the initial treatment of neurohormonal excess released by pathophysiological changes.

Prevention of Excess Release of Cerebral Dopamine

Excitatory amino acids, such as glutamate, released in response to neuronal injury, have been interesting [1]. Hypothermia is one of the successful methods to prevent injury by these mechanisms (see Fig. 4). As another neuronal injury mechanism, dopamine has been reported to make free radicals, which is associated with H_2O_2 formation [1,50], this means the occurrence of selective radical damage of the dopamine nervous system, which includes the dopamine A10 nervous system. In our preliminary clinical studies, CSF levels of dopamine were recorded at much lower levels during brain hypothermia treatment [30,31]. Which means that excess release of dopamine from the injured brain is prevented, protecting the dopamine nervous system from selective radical damage in the acute stage, by brain hypothermia. We experienced good clinical recovery as to awaking, thinking, memory, volition, and emotional expression, which is associated with the neuronal functions of dopamine A10 nervous system, when patients were treated by brain hypothermia [30,31]. The clinical effectiveness of the vegetative state, in all these patients, was related to reduced CSF NO_2/NO_3 in the acute stage and increasing CSF dopamine in chronic stages [29–31]. Therefore, we have hypothesized that excess release of dopamine causes selective radical damage of the dopaminergic central nervous system, which includes the A10 nervous system, and results in difficulty in using the mind, prolonged memory disturbances, reduced activity, and disturbed volition. Dr. Marion's cooperative studies on the effectiveness of hypothermia treatment for severe head injury patients (GCS < 7) have recorded that the hypothermia group had a lower incidence of vegetation [44] than the nonhypothermia-treated group even without cerebral dopamine replacement therapy. Our combination therapy of brain hypothermia and replacement of cerebral dopamine was very useful for the prevention of the vegetative state for severe brain injury patients (GCS < 6). Prevention of excess release of neurotransmitters in the acute stage and the replacement of these neurotransmitters in the chronic stage are very important for neuronal recovery after severe brain injury. This concept supports the reasons that dopamine-related management is effective for vegetation, memory disturbances, and aphasia [5,11,18,22,23].

Regulation of Mechanism of BTT and Advanced Technique for Control of BTT

The BTT is influenced by cerebral blood flow. However, the precise mechanism of regulation of BTT has not yet been clarified. We found recently that changes of BTT can be determined by four factors, including (1) the core temperature, (2) the BP that carries the core temperature to the brain tissue, and (3) brain metabolism. Thus, BTT is highest at physiological conditions, at $37.0° \pm 0.29°C$, compared to the core temperature of $36.3° \pm 0.23°C$, tympanic membrane temperature of $36.7° \pm 0.27°C$, and bladder temperature of $36.6° \pm 0.25°C$. The BTT value is controlled ultimately by the fourth factor, the CBF. An elevated BTT can be reduced through washout by the CBF [31] (see also this volume). Therefore, the BTT was measured at values similar to the jugular venous blood temperature rather than the tympanic membrane temperature, which may reflect carotid blood temperature. Under physiological conditions, the BTT is maintained at a level very close to that of the systemic circulating blood temperature. To control the BTT precisely, when lowering or elevating its value, the best way is to effect changes through reducing or increasing the systemic circulating blood temperature. Localized cooling of the neck and head can lead to difficulty in control of BTT at the rewarming stage, because the warmed blood temperature is carried into the brain abruptly after the cessation of head cooling. Three-compartment cooler blanket techniques have been developed to control BTT at 32°–36°C in our ICU [24–30]. We understand the mechanism of alteration of BTT, and began another brain cooling technique, the direct blood cooling method using an external circulating system. This technique is very useful for management of brain resuscitation after cardiac arrest.

Prevention of Infections during Brain Hypothermia Treatment

A major issue in hypothermia treatment is the high incidence of severe systemic infections associated with prolonged hypothermia. Pneumonia is extremely common, because of the loss of protective cough reflexes, and the occurrence of aspiration pneumonia, which is accelerated by H_2-blocker therapy, cold-induced bronchorrhea, and bacterial translocation from the intestine. These complications are strongly activated by an increase of free radicals, intravascular coagulability, deficiency of the energy source to the T cells and B cells, intestinal mucosa edema associated with hypoalbuminemia, reduced antiinflammatory protection by lower AT-III, activation of cytokines by hyperglycemia, and an imbalance of oxygen delivery versus consumption at the rewarming stage [28–30]. Even with appropriate prophylactic treatment, a high incidence of infections still tends to occur at the rewarming stage.

The mechanism of the impaired immune function was studied by means of the interactions between changes of BTT, lymphocytes, pituitary hormones (ACTH, LH, and GH), and catecholamines and indirect parameters of immune function such as CD3, CD4, CD4/CD8, PHA, and IGF-1 of the internal jugular vein [25,30,31]. Decrease of jugular venous pituitary hormone and catecholamine levels was recorded depending on the level of hypothermia. The sensitivities of reducing pituitary hormones and serum catecholamines to hypothermia were ACTH > LH > GH and dopamine > NE > E, respectively. The immune function was also modified and activated by IGF-1 with activation of GH. Statistical studies on GH in relation to the effects on the immune system demonstrated activation of CD4 and T helper cells and suppression of CD8 and suppressor T cells (Fig. 13) [27]. Severe immune dysfunction through pituitary dysfunction following brain hypothermia was a major cause of the high incidence of severe infections during hypothermia treatment. Based on the detailed findings, a novel technique for prolonged cerebral hypothermia treatment has been developed in our ICU (see Tables 1, 2, Fig. 2).

Intestinal cleaning after surgery, control of gastric juice pH below 3.5, intermittent control of BTT during brain hypothermia (see Fig. 2), an adequate schedule of nutritional support with monitoring of serum glutamate as described in our guideline, careful management of serum glucose between 120 and 140 mg/dl, oxygen delivery maintained at higher than 800 ml/min., control of AT-III higher than 100%, and careful management of hypoalbuminemia are major points of care management for prevention of infection during brain hypothermia treatment. Unfortunately, if severe infections occur during brain hypothermia treatment, the inflammatory reaction is initially suppressed by replacement of AT-III with low molecular weight heparin and then followed by replacement of albumin, activating the immune function with replacement of L-arginine, and administration of antibiotics and a combination of albekasine (IV) and digestive decontamination as described are useful. The most useful care management for prevention of infection is maintaining preconditioning as described before starting rewarming. Management of hypoalbuminemia is especially important in preconditioning care because severe hypoalbuminemia (<2.5 g/dl) produces various negative factors for severe infections such as intestinal mucosa edema with difficulty in enteral nutrition, increase in free bacteria, unstable antibiotic function, easy cytokine penetration of the BBB, no mannitol for control of brain edema, and the uncontrollable increase of brain tissue glutamate by moderate brain hypothermia.

A careful rewarming schedule, keeping an adaptation time as described in the guideline, will be very effective to maintain not only immune activity but also cerebral glucose metabolism in the injured brain tissue. This management care technique will be successful for brain hypothermia treatment prolonged for more than 1 week.

Pitfalls of Brain Hypothermia Treatment

Five major pitfalls were experienced in this treatment: masking brain hypoxia, inadequate management of BTT and hyperglycemia, undesirable duration of brain hypothermia, inadequate care management of systemic infections, and nutritional misunderstanding in the management of brain injury.

Masking Brain Hypoxia

The normal PaO_2 and ICP management is not enough for recovery of injured neurons in severe head trauma patients. As a result of this masking brain hypoxia could be produced by subsequent pathophysiological changes such as circulating blood shifts to the intestinal organs caused by excess release of dopamine, difficulty in release of oxygen from hemoglobin by reduced hemoglobin enzymes, oxygen delivery below 800 ml/min, and the increased demand of oxygen in the injured brain by brain thermopooling. These specific maskings of brain hypoxia in the acute stage of severe brain injury produce uncoupling of brain metabolism and CBF (see Hayashi, this volume).

To avoid this masking brain hypoxia, control of the BTT at 34°C to prevent excess release of dopamine, systolic blood pressure above 100 mmHg to avoid brain thermopooling, serum pH > 7.3 to prevent hemoglobin enzyme/DPG reduction, and management of oxygen delivery at greater than 800 ml/min are important.

Intestinal blood shift by excess release of dopamine is sometimes very difficult to monitor because of increasing cardiac contraction; however, intestinal vasodilatations produce normal blood pressure and normal CPP. Only the changes of BTT at lower than bladder temperature by continuous monitoring of these parameters can diagnose this blood shift.

The most common pitfall is lower cardiac output and 90–100 mmHg of systolic blood pressure by reduced fluid resuscitation or cardiac dysfunction by catecholamine surge. This lower systolic blood pressure is not sufficient to prevent brain thermopooling without brain hypothermia [27]. Too rapid induction of brain hypothermia causes unstable cardiac function serum catecholamine release is too greatly suppressed (see Fig. 10).

For the management of brain hypothermia, maintaining sufficient cerebral oxygenation and adequate delivery of glucose are very important.

Inadequate Brain Temperature and Hyperglycemia

In severely brain-injured patients, catecholamine surge associated with hyperglycemia is unavoidable (see Hayashi, this volume) because glycogen and ATP in the major organs metabolizes to glucose by activation of epinephrine. This catecholamine surge could be prevented by brain hypothermia, and hyperglycemia is easy to control at the induction stage. However, in the cooling stage of brain hypothermia, reduced BTT below 33°C sometimes produces increased serum glucose by systemic reduction of glucose consumption. This inadequate control of hyperglycemia causes an increase of brain tissue lactate and pyruvate with increased brain tissue glucose (see Fig. 7). The critical level to increase brain tissue lactate is greater than 140 mg/dl serum glucose at BTT of 33°C.

Increased brain tissue glucose allows activation of cytokines and increases the permeability of BBB, as described elsewhere. Therefore, in the management of moderate brain hypothermia treatment, we must control serum glucose at 120 to 140 mg/dl, exactly. At the induction stage, if control of hyperglycemia is difficult, BTT should be elevated at 0.5°C of BTT and maintained as mild brain hypothermia treatment until stabilize systemic circulation and hyperglycemia have stabilized (see Fig. 2).

Inappropriate Duration of Brain Hypothermia

A short duration of brain hypothermia cannot allow recovery and is limited in halting pathophysiological changes during the cooling stage, especially in severely injured patients. Unless recovery from brain injury occurs during the cooling stage, in these cases rewarming promotes the progression of delayed pathophysiological changes and makes these much worse. Therefore, before starting rewarming, we must make sure whether the injured brain is on the way to recovery. The 2-day brain hypothermia treatment is too short to allow recovery, especially in severely brain-injured patients. Adequate duration of brain hypothermia is theoretically variable. However, prolonged brain hypothermia treatment facilitates an immune crisis with reduced GH and severe systemic infections [28–30].

To maintain adequate duration of brain hypothermia, we need skillful care management for control of immune crisis-associated infections and criteria for starting rewarming.

Activation of Brain Damage by Systemic Infections

Severe infections during brain hypothermia decide the prognosis and success of the treatment for two reasons: additional brain damage can be caused by cytokine encephalitis, and prolonged brain hypothermia treatment makes it difficult for critically ill patients with brain injury to survive.

The severe damage to BBB function such caused by as CSF/serum albumin ratio elevated above 0.02 is a serious condition when systemic and/or severe pulmonary infections are complications because increased cytokines in the systemic circulation, caused by pulmonary infections, easily penetrate the BBB and worsen the brain injury by cytokine encephalitis (see

Hayashi, this volume). The systemic infection itself also a negative factor to the brain injury by causing brain hypoxia and venous congestion with increased mediastinal pressure. Therefore, in the management of brain hypothermia treatment, severe pulmonary infections not only disturb the pulmonary functions but also worsen cerebral vascular inflammation, vascular permeability, brain edema, and cytokine encephalitis with BBB dysfunction. To control these pathophysiological changes, management of AT-III above 100% for prevention of vascular inflammation and microembolus, which was derived from disseminated intravascular coagulability (DIC) complication studies (see Fig. 8), management of hyperglycemia to prevent increasing vascular permeability, and then control of serum albumin above 3.5 g/dl to maintain BBB function are necessary. Serum albumin replacement therapy is very successful to prevent fundamental promoting factors of infections such as intestinal mucosa edema, obstructive pancreatic dysfunction, free bacteria, and free pharmacology. Our recent brain hypothermia treatment dramatically reduced the incidence of infections (see Table 3) and improved neuronal recovery.

Inadequate Nutrition

In the ICU management of critical ill patients, early administration of parenteral and enteral nutrition is recommended. Recent parenteral and enteral nutrition solutions are rich in glucose, lipid, and amino acid glutamate for support of immune functions. We wonder whether excessive glucose and glutamate could activate BBB dysfunction and produce neuroexcitational neuronal death in cases of severe BBB dysfunction. Parenteral amino acid nutrition increased of neurotoxic glutamate in the serum about twofold (see Table 4). In cases of a CSF/serum albumin ratio higher than 0.02, that means early nutrition in severe BBB dysfunction increases neurotoxic glutamate in the injured brain tissue. The peak time of BBB dysfunction by vasopressin is 24 h; however, GH-related BBB dysfunction is 3 to 4 days after the trauma (see Hayashi, this volume). Therefore, we prefer the following criteria of nutritional management during brain hypothermia treatment. In cases of BBB dysfunction that is not severely damaged, as shown by a CSF/serum albumin ratio less than 0.02, early nutrition that includes ZnCl, glutamine, and arginine for activation of the immune function is started 2 days after trauma. However, in cases of CSF/serum albumin ratio higher than 0.02, initial enteral nutrition is limited to saline with ZnCl and, 3 to 4 days later, amino acid nutrition is started with monitoring of serum glutamate. We have experienced an uncontrollable increase of brain tissue glutamate even with 32°C of moderate brain hypothermia management with pulmonary infection, BBB dysfunction, and erroneous administration time for amino acid nutrition.

Replacement Therapy for Prevention of Vegetative State Following Brain Hypothermia Treatment

For the recovery of neurons in the primarily injured tissue, prolonged brain hypothermia lasting more than 48 h is considered indispensable. The clinical results of these treatments in severely brain-injured patients (GCS < 6) revealed a good recovery and an extremely low incidence of the vegetative state (see Table 2). The initial purpose of brain hypothermia treatment is to provide sufficient cerebral oxygen supply within 3 to 6 h after insults through stabilization of systemic circulation. Oxygen delivery that is greater than 800 ml/min is most important to follow the mild or moderate brain hypothermia treatment to allow recovery from serious neuronal conditions in primarily injured brain tissue. After 6 h, brain hypothermia is very effective to prevent secondary pathophysiological changes in injured neurons. However, brain hypothermia has another, third, beneficial mechanism to prevent vegetation by reducing excess release of cerebral dopamine from the injured brain tissue. In previous studies, some cases of the vegetative state, the effectiveness of pharmacological activation of dopamine [11,19,22] and electrical stimulation of the central nervous system [20] to increase the CSF dopamine have been reported [29–31]. Low values of dopamine and luteinizing hormone (LH) in the jugular venous blood were also recorded in prolonged vegetation [25]. Following brain hypothermia, jugular venous blood dopamine decrease was strictly correlated to lowering of the BTT (see Fig. 5), and we speculated prevention of dissipation of dopamine in the injured brain tissue had occurred. From these results, we hypothesized that the dopamine nervous system may play an important role in vegetation, and that excitatory neuronal death within the dopamine nervous system can be prevented by a lower BTT.

The reason for the low incidence of vegetation in brain hypothermia-treated patients is not only prevention of intracellular secondary injury but also reduction of excess leak of dopamine from injured brain tissue. We have experienced 5 of 28 cases (18%) who returned to an ordinary lifestyle from the vegetative state, while others retained neuronal deficits caused by the original brain disease. However, in all these patients, intelligence and personality were maintained 3 months later. Therefore, as a late treatment after brain hypothermia, replacement of dopamine is necessary in severely brain-injured patients.

Our clinical trials of pharmacological activation of dopamine synapses with the combination of amantadine, Estraderm patching, and increasing CSF dopamine by intermittent stimulation of the median nerve have revealed very useful effects for neuronal recovery and the prevention of vegetation [29–31]. We must focus on the protection of specific parts of the nervous system to prevent vegetation, not only on the general management of neuronal recovery in the primarily injured brain tissue.

Clinical Results

In this series, we have focused on the effect of brain hypothermia treatment for critically ill patients with GCS less than 6. The efficacy of brain hypothermia was related to the severity of the injury, as indicated by the Glasgow Coma Score on admission. The patients with initial coma scores of 3 did not benefit from brain hypothermia treatment; however, in GCS 4, 5, and 6, clinical benefit was observed (see Fig. 9, Table 5). Among these patients with higher scores, 29% with GCS 4, 26% with GCS 5, and 34% with GCS 6 in the brain hypothermia group had a good outcome. However, in the normothermia group with previous concept treatment, a good outcome was limited, to 4% with GCS4, 7% with GCS 5, and 6% with GCS6, respectively.

As clinical signs, memory, intelligence, and personality are not much disturbed specifically in the brain hypothermia-treated group. As for the reasons, in the acute stage, the dopamine A10 nervous system is protected by the combination of 20 managements (Fig. 1). However, many patients cannot make a recovery soon after brain hypothermia treatment. In these cases, replacement therapy of cerebral dopamine with the combination therapy of amantadine administration, estrogen patching, and intermittent electrical stimulation of the peripheral median nerve for 3 to 4 weeks is successful if low levels of CSF dopamine are observed. The 40% of vegetations suggested a clinical effect from the combination of cerebral dopamine replacement therapy. We have found very good recovery of 18% of vegetation cases with useful lifestyle, good memory, good personality, and intelligence. The quality of neuronal recovery was not stopped at 3 month after the trauma, and continued over a few years. Therefore, even after brain hypothermia treatment, clinical recovery could be expected to continue for 2 to 4 years with rehabilitation.

Conclusion

The initial purpose of brain hypothermia treatment is to provide sufficient cerebral oxygen supply by protecting masking brain hypoxia in the severely injured brain. Brain hypothermia is very successful to prevent other secondary pathophysiological changes in injured neurons, such as delayed neuronal death, release of glutamate, radical damage by dopamine leak, synaptic excitation by potassium, calcium free radical reactions, and ICP elevation. However, hypothermia-induced severe infections have become a major issue in the clinical setting.

The mechanism of the brain hypothermia treatment is to provide sufficient cerebral oxygen supply with adequate control of glucose metabolism in the brain, prevention of BBB dysfunction and cytokine encephalitis by control of hypothalamus–pituitary axis hormonal abnormality, and protection of selective radical attack on the dopamine A10 nervous system.

In brain hypothermia treatment, five major pitfalls such as hemoglobin dysfunction associated with masking brain hypoxia, inadequate management of BTT and serum glucose, undesirable duration of brain hypothermia, inadequate care management of systemic infections, and nutritional misunderstanding in the management of brain injury have been demonstrated in this study. A novel technique for control of these clinical issues, success of adequate neuronal oxygenation and brain metabolism, neurohormonal control of BBB dysfunction, and preservation of dopamine A10 nervous system have been developed. The effectiveness of brain hypothermia treatment was studied by comparing the clinical results of brain hypothermia (99 cases) and normothermia (65 cases) of head injury with a GCS less than 6. The patients with initial coma scores of 3 did not benefit from brain hypothermia treatment; however, in those with GCS 4, 5, or 6, clinical benefit was observed. As clinical signs, memory, intelligence, and personality are not much disturbed, specifically in the brain hypothermia-treated group.

References

1. Baker AJ, Zornow MH, Scheller MS, Yaksh TL, Skilling SR, Smullin DH, Larson AA, Kuczenski R (1991) Changes in extracellular concentrations of glutamate, asparate, glycine, dopamine, serotonin, and dopamine metabolites after transient global ischemia in the rat. J Neurochem 57:1370–1379
2. Billiau A, Vankelecom H (1992) Interferon-γ: general biological properties and effects on the neuro-endocrine axis. In: Bartfai T, Ottoson D (eds) Neuro-immunology of fever. Pergamon Press, Oxford, pp 65–77
3. Busto R, Dietolich WD, Globus MY-T, Martinez E, Valdes I, Ginsberg MD (1989) Effect of mild hypothermia on ischemia-induced release of neurotransmitters and free fatty acids in rat brain. Stroke 20:904–910
4. Cardell M, Boris MF, Wieloch T (1991) Hypothermia prevents the ischemia-induced translocation and inhibition of protein kinase C in the rat striatum. J Neurochem 57:1814–1817
5. Chandra B (1978) Treatment of disturbances of consciousness caused by measles encephalitis with levodopa. Eur Neurol 17:265–270
6. Clifton G, Robertson C, Kyper K, Taylor AA, Duncan RD, Grossman R (1983) Cardiovascular response to severe head injury. J Neurosurg 59:447–457
7. Clifton GL, Jiang JY, Lyeth BG, Jenkins LW, Hamm RJ, Hayes RL (1991) Marked protection by moderate hypothermia after experimental traumatic brain injury. J Cereb Blood Flow Metab 11:114–121
8. Clifton GL, Allen S, Barrodale P, Plenger P, Berry J, Koch S, Fletcher J, Hayes R, Choi SC (1993) A phase II study of moderate hypothermia in severe brain injury. J Neurotrauma 10:263–271

9. Corte FD, Mancini A, Valle D, Gallizzi F, Carducci P, Mignani V, De Marinis L (1998) Provocative hypothalamopituitary axis tests in severe head injury: correlations with severity and prognosis. Crit Care Med 26(8):1419–1426

10. Crawford ES, Saleh SA (1981) Transverse aortic arch aneurysm: improved result of treatment employing new modifications of aortic reconstruction and hypothermic cerebral circulatory arrest. Ann Surg 194:180–188

11. Crisman LM, Childs A, Wilcox RE, Barrow N (1988) The effect of bromocriptine on speech dysfunction in patients with diffuse brain injury (akinetic mutism). Clin Neuropharmacol 11:462–466

12. Chronwall BM, Di Maggio DA, Massari VJ, Pickel VN, Ruggiero DA, O'Donohue TL (1985) The anatomy of neuropeptide Y-containing neurons in rat brain. Neuroscience 15:1159

13. Davila DR, Breif S, Simon J, et al. (1987) Role of growth hormone in regulating T-dependent immune events in aged, nude, and transgenic rodents. J Neurosci Res 18:108–116

14. Dempsey IRJ, Combs DJ, Maley ME, Cowen DE, Roy MW, Donaldson DL (1987) Moderate hypothermia reduces postischemic edema development and leukotriene production. Neurosurgery (Baltim) 21:177–181

15. Dietrich WD, Busto R, Valdes I, Loor Y (1990) Effects of normothermic versus mild hyperthermic forebrain ischemia in rats. Stroke 21:1318–1325

16. Dudariev VP, Lanovenko II (1999) Changes in the oxygen-binding properties of the blood in white rats under the influence of hypoxia and its pharmacological correction. Fiziol Zh 45(1–2):97–103

17. Fay T (1943) Observations on generalized refrigeration in cases of severe cerebral trauma. Assoc Res Nerv Ment Dis Proc 24:611–619

18. Feeney DM, Hovda DA (1985) Reinstatement of binocular depth perception by amphetamine and visual experience after visual cortex ablation. Brain Res 342:352–356

19. Galski T, Krotenberg R (1989) The usefulness of Hydergine on cognition in patients with traumatic head injury. Arch Phys Med Rehabil 70:A-12

20. Glenn MB (1986) CNS stimulants: applications for traumatic brain injury. J Head Trauma Rehabil 1:74–76

21. Goadsby PJ, Edvinsson L (1997) Extrinsic innavation: transmitters, receptors, and functions — the sympathetic nerve system. In: Welch KMA, Caplan LR, Reis DJ, Siesjø Bo K, Weir B (eds) Primer on cerebrovascular diseases. Academic Press, San Diego, pp 60–63

22. Gualtieri CT, Chandler M, Coons TB, Brown LT (1989) Review. Amantadine: a new clinical profile for traumatic brain injury. Clin Neuropharmacol 12:258–270

23. Haig AJ, Ruess LM (1990) Recovery from vegetative state of six months duration associated with Sinemet (levodopa/carbidopa). Arch Phys Med Rehabil 71:1081–1083

24. Hayashi N, Hirayama T, Ohata M (1993) The computed cerebral hypothermia management technique to the critical head injury patients. Adv Neurotrauma Res 5:61–64

25. Hayashi N, Hirayama T, Utagawa A, Daimon W, Ohata M (1994) Systemic management of cerebral edema based on a new concept in severe head injury patients. Acta Neurochir 60:541–543

26. Hayashi N, Hirayama T, Utagawa A (1994) The cerebral thermo-pooling and hypothermia treatment of critical head injury patients. In: Nagai H (ed) Intracranial pressure, vol IX. Springer, Tokyo, pp 589–599

27. Hayashi N (1995) Cerebral hypothermia treatment. In: Hayashi N (ed) Cerebral hypothermia treatment. Sogo Igaku, Tokyo, pp 1–105

28. Hayashi N (1996) Advance of cerebral hypothermia treatment. J Crit Med 8:295–300

29. Hayashi N, Kinoshita K, Shibuya T (1997) The prevention of cerebral thermo-pooling, damage of A10 nervous system, and free radical reactions by control of brain tissue temperature in severely brain injured patients. In: Teelken AW (ed) Neurochemistry. Plenum, New York, pp 97–103

30. Hayashi N (1997) Combination therapy of cerebral hypothermia, pharmacological activation of the dopamine system, and hormonal replacement in severely brain damaged patients. J Jpn Intensive Care Med 4:191–197

31. Hayashi N (1997) Prevention of vegetation after severe head trauma and stroke by combination therapy of cerebral hypothermia and activation of immune-dopaminergic nervous system. Proc Annu Meet Soc Treat Coma 6:133–145
32. Hayashi N, Utagawa A, Kinosita K, Izumi T (1999) Application of a novel technique for clinical evaluation of nitric oxide-induced free radiacal reactions in ICU patients. Cell Mol Neurobiol 19:3–17
33. Jiang JY, Lyeth BG, Kapasi MZ, Jenkins LW, Povlishock JT (1992) Moderate hypothermia reduces blood-brain barrier disruption following traumatic brain injury in the rat. Acta Neuropathol (Berl) 84:495–500
34. Katsura K, Minamisawa H, Ekholm A, Folbergrova J, Siesjo BK (1992) Changes of labile metabolites during anoxia in moderately hypo- and hyperthermic rats: correlation to membrane fluxes of K^+. Brain Res 590:6–12
35. Kossmann T, Hans V, Imhof HG, Stocker R, Grob P, Trentz O, Morgani-Kossmann MC (1995) Intrathecal and serum interleukin-6 and acute-phase response in patients with severe traumatic brain injuries. Shock 4:311–317
36. Kossmann T, Hans V, Lenzlinger PM, Csuka E, Stsahel PF, Trentz O, Morgani-Kossmann MC (1996) Analysis of immune mediator production following traumatic brain injury. In: Schlag G, Redel H, Traber D (eds) Shock, sepsis and organ failure. Springer, Berlin, pp 263–297
37. Kristian T, Katsura K, Siesjo BK (1992) The influence of moderate hypothermia on cellular calcium uptake in complete ischaemia: implications for the excitotoxic hypothesis. Acta Physiol Scand 146:531–532
38. Lau S, Merbitz CP, Grip JC (1988) Modification of function in head-injured patients with Sinemet. Brain Inj 2:225–233
39. Lel B, Tan X, Cai H, Xu Q, Guo Q (1994) Effect of moderate hypothermia on lipid peroxidation in canine brain tissue after cardiac arrest and resuscitation. Stroke 25:147–152
40. Leibowiz SF, Sladek C, Spencer L, Temple D (1988) Neuropeptide Y, epinephrine and norepinephrine in the paraventricular nucleus: stimulation of feeding and the release of corticosterone, vasopressin and glucose. Brain Res Bull 21:905
41. Leibowitz SF (1999) Macronutrients and brain peptides: what they do and how they respond. In: Berthoud HR, Seeley RJ (eds) Neural and metabolic control of macronutrient intake. CRC Press, Boca Raton, pp 389–406
42. MacIntosh TK (1994) Neurological sequelae of traumatic brain injury: therapeutic implications. Cerebrovasc Brain Metab Rev 6:109–162
43. Marion DW, Obrist WD, Carlier PM, Penrod LE, Darby JM (1993) The uses of moderate therapeutic hypothermia for patients with severe head injuries: a preliminary report. J Neurosurg 79:354–362
44. Marion DW, Penrod LE, Kelsey SF, et al. (1997) Treatment of traumatic brain injury with moderate hypothermia. N Engl J Med 336:540–546
45. Mitani A, Kadoya F, Kataoka K (1991) Temperature dependence of hypoxia-induced calcium accumulation in gerbil hippocampal slices. Brain Res 562:159–163
46. Mysiw WJ, Jackson RD (1982) Tricyclic antidepressant therapy after traumatic brain injury. J Head Trauma Rehabil 2:34–42
47. Pas'ko SA, Volosheniuk TG (1990) Disordered phosphorus metabolism and its correction in the acute period of severe craniocerebral trauma. Zh Vopr Neirokhir Im N N Burdenko 3:14–16
48. Rosomoff HL, Holaday DA (1954) Cerebral blood flow and cerebral oxygen consumption during hypothermia. Am J Physiol 179:85–88
49. Sahgal A (1984) A critique of the vasopressin-memory hypothesis. Psychopharmacology 83:215–228
50. Silvka A, Coben G (1985) Hydroxyl radical attack on dopamine. J Biol Chem 260:15466–15472
51. Spuler A, Tan WKM, Meyer FB (1996) Molecular events in cerebral ischemia. In: Raffel C, Harsh GR (eds) The molecular basis of neurosurgical disease. Williams & Wilkins, Baltimore, pp 248–269
52. Widmann R, Miyazawa T, Hossmann KA (1993) Protective effect of hypothermia on hippocampal injury after 30 minutes of forebrain ischemia in rats is mediated by postischemic recovery of protein synthesis. J Neurochem 61:200–206

Development and Status of Hypothermia for Brain Injury: National Acute Brain Injury Study: Hypothermia

Guy L. Clifton

Summary. After laboratory studies of moderate hypothermia (30°–33°C) in rodent models, clinical studies were organized to investigate the potential application of moderate systemic hypothermia in patients after severe brain injury. These preliminary clinical studies indicated improved neurologic outcome and low toxicity in patients. Accordingly, the multicenter, randomized trial, National Acute Brain Injury Study: Hypothermia (NABIS:H) was funded by the National Institutes of Health. This study is designed to test the hypothesis that systemic hypothermia to 32°–33°C, if rendered within 6 h of injury, improves the Glasgow Outcome Score (GOS) at 6 months after injury in patients with severe brain injury in the range of Glasgow Coma Scale (GCS) 3–8. Five hundred patients are to be tested in an intent-to-treat protocol with randomization stratified by GCS. Power is 80% and is set to detect a 10%–12% absolute shift in the percentage of patients in the good outcome category using dichotomized GOS (good results/moderate disability vs. severe disability/vegetative/dead). This chapter presents a summary of the trial as of April 1998.

Key words. Hypothermia, Brain injury, Glasgow Coma Scale (GCS), Moderate, Systemic

Introduction

The National Acute Brain Injury Study: Hypothermia (NABIS:H) was approved and funded by National Institutes of Health (NIH) in 1994, with patient enrollment beginning in October 1994. The specific aim of this randomized, prospective, multicenter trial is to determine whether surface-induced moderate hypothermia (32°–33°C), begun rapidly after severe traumatic brain injury (TBI) and maintained for 48 h, improves outcome with low toxicity. The rationale for this study is based on earlier laboratory and clinical studies. Moderate hypothermia (30°–33°C) was shown to diminish neurononal loss in rodent models of global ischemia when administered during and after ischemia [5]. Improved behavioral outcome and reduced mortality were shown in rodent brain injury models with moderate systemic hypothermia administered after injury [4]. Concurrent clinical studies of series of patients with severe brain injury [2,3,6,7] indicated improved neurologic outcome in the hypothermia group.

Department of Neurosurgery, Vivian L. Smith Center for Neurologic Research, University of Texas-Houston Health Science Center, 6431 Fannin, Suite 7.148, Houston, TX 77030, USA

In accordance with preestablished stopping rules, enrollment in the trial was terminated by the NABIS:H Performance and Safety Monitoring Board on May 5, 1998. On the date of termination, 392 patients had been enrolled in the study. Because data specific to each treatment group may not be analyzed by the investigators until data entry is complete at the time of the last patient's 6-month outcome evaluation, data specific to centers but not to treatment groups are presented here. At the time of this presentation, completed data were not available for all enrolled patients. The material presented here is based on data available on 344 patients as of April 2, 1998.

Patient Eligibility

The NABIS:H has been using the following inclusion and exclusion criteria since the initiation of patient enrollment in October 1994.

Inclusion Criteria

1. Patients not following commands: Glascow Coma Scale (GCS) motor score 1–5, total GCS 8
2. Age 16–65 years
3. Available to initiate cooling within 6 h of injury
4. Nonpenetrating brain injury

Exclusion Criteria

1. GCS 7–8 with normal computed tomography (CT) scan, only mild subarachnoid hemorrhage, or a skull fracture
2. Hypotension (systolic blood pressure 90 mmHg) for 30 min postresuscitation
3. Hypoxia (saturation 94%) for 30 min postresuscitation
4. Estimated Abbreviated Injury Severity Score (AIS) of 4 for any organ system except head
5. Follow-up unlikely to be possible
6. Patients not available for cooling within 6 h of injury
7. GCS of 3 with unreactive pupils
8. Pregnancy

Sample Size Calculation

The estimate of the sample size required for the NABIS:H two-arm trial was calculated using a simple asymptotic method for the binary outcome. The sample size was determined so as to detect an absolute difference of 10% or more with power of at least 85%. A 10% difference in dichotomized Glasgow Outcome Scale (GOS) is considered to be clinically important. The approximate sample size for the trial is presented in Table 1. It is assumed that the variance is reduced by the use of the well-known prognostic factors as co-variables and that the expected attrition rate is 5%. Table 1 also shows the approximate sample size needed for detecting 4- and 5-point differences in the mean Disability Rating Scale (DRS).

Center Enrollment Data

The seven active centers in the trial and the inactive centers with the numbers of patients enrolled as of May 5, 1998, by each center are shown in Table 2. Patients eligible for enrollment but meeting one or more exclusion criteria are shown in Table 3. The percentages of

TABLE 1. Sample size estimates for NABIS:H

Power	Glasgow Outcome Scale: % Difference (no. of patient[a])			Disability Rating Scale: mean difference (no. of patients[a])	
	10%	11%	12%	4	5
85	482	399	335	370	236
90	563	465	391	432	275
95	696	575	484	533	341

Number of patients needed for statistical analysis
NABIS:H, National Acute Brain Injury Study: Hypothermia

TABLE 2. Randomizing centers in NABIS:H

Center	Enrollment (as of 5/5/98)
Houston	96
St. Louis	77
Sacramento	73
Pittsburgh	69
Indianapolis[a]	30
Portland[a]	9
Toronto[a]	5
Inactive centers	33
Total enrolled patients	392

[a] Active small centers

TABLE 3. Reasons for exclusion of 450 screened NABIS:H patients[a]

Reason for exclusion	No.[b]	% Excluded
GCS = 3, *and* unreactive pupils	101	22
GCS 7–8, normal CT scan	93	21
AIS >4, except head	84	19
Unavailable for cooling within 6h	83	18
BP <90 for 30 min after resuscitation	44	10
No consent	38	8
Medical condition	35	8
Hypoxic >30 min after resuscitation	31	7
Rewarming required for bleeding	18	4
Follow-up unlikely	9	2
Pregnant	0	0

GCS, Glasgow Coma Scale; CT, computed tomography; AIS, Abbreviated Injury Security Score; BP, blood pressure
[a] Data available on April 2, 1998
[b] Patients may fail more than one exclusion

excluded patients were evenly distributed between those with GCS 3, GCS 7–8 with normal scan, admission after 6h, severe multiple trauma. Patient characteristics on admission are shown by center in Table 4. There were center differences in terms of the severity of injury. Admission temperatures are shown in Table 5. Hypothermia upon admission was common.

TABLE 4. Patient characteristics on admission to NABIS:H: age, pupil reaction, and initial Glasgow Coma Score[a]

Active center	No.	Mean age (years)	Pupils (%)			Initial GCS (%)	
			Bilateral reactive	Unilateral reactive	non-reactive	3–5	6–8
Houston	88	31	62	14	24	34	67
St. Louis	75	30	56	9	35	53	47
Sacramento	72	32	71	13	17	42	58
Pittsburgh	63	32	51	17	32	41	59
Small centers	38	33	63	13	24	31	69
All patients	336	31	61	13	26	41	59

All data given as percents are mean values
[a] Data available on April 2, 1998

TABLE 5. NABIS:H patient temperature on admission[a]

Active center	No. of patients randomized	Admission temperature		
		Mean ± SD	Minimum	Maximum
Houston	88	33.1 ± 2.41	29.9	38.8
St. Louis	75	35.9 ± 1.81	30.3	39.1
Sacramento	72	34.6 ± 2.52	28.5	38.6
Pittsburgh	62	35.6 ± 1.69	30.0	39.3
Small centers	37	33.8 ± 2.40	27.0	37.5
All patients	334	34.8 ± 2.33	27.0	39.3

All temperatures are expressed as degrees celsius (°C)
[a] Data available on April 2, 1998

TABLE 6. NABIS:H cooling times for enrolled patients: target 8 hours[a]

Active center	Year 1		Year 2		Year 3		Year 4		Active centers	
	No.	Hours	No.	Hours	No.	Hours	No.	Hours	No.	Hours
Houston	5	9.81	20	6.65	17	5.28	3	7.26	45	6.52
St. Louis	7	8.10	17	9.13	11	5.00	2	5.00	37	7.57
Sacramento	7	11.40	12	5.75	14	6.86	6	6.21	39	7.24
Pittsburgh	7	10.55	8	6.92	12	7.81	4	6.52	31	8.03
Small centers		n/a	6	8.21	8	7.05	7	8.01	21	7.70
All patients	26	9.98	63	7.33	62	6.31	22	7.02	173	7.32

[a] Data available on April 2, 1998

Cooling times by year of the study and by center are shown in Table 6. The mean time from injury to target temperature was 7.32 h. Mean cooling times diminished by the second year as centers improved their logistics of randomization.

Alerting Rules

The mortality and complication rates are monitored and reported to the Performance Safety Monitoring Board monthly. This board is composed of three MDs and three PhDs from various U.S. universities and from the NIH. If mortality rates or total critical complication rates in two of seven body systems examined are significantly different between the two treatment arms at $P < 0.05$, the chairman of the Monitoring Board is notified immediately by the Biostatistics Center.

The revised stopping rule for NABIS:H is based on two interim analyses used in the trial. The Lan-Demets approach based on the O'Brien-Fleming form of critical boundary was used when 6-month outcomes were observed from 160 and 320 patients. There are two conditions under which the Patient Safety and Monitoring Board must decide whether to advise the NIH to terminate the trial. They are that (1) the differences at either interim analysis are significant or (2) the likelihood of a positive outcome in favor of the hypothermia group (if the trial were to continue to completion) is less than 10%.

Consent Procedures and Use of Waiver

For patients eligible for the study, efforts are made to contact next of kin/legal guardian to obtain consent. If next of kin/legal guardian cannot be reached or the patient cannot be identified, efforts to document these attempts are noted on the consent procedures form. In this situation, waiver of consent should be invoked. In the event that waiver is used, next of kin/legal guardian is apprised of the patient's participation in the study as soon as possible and additional pertinent information provided to next of kin/legal guardian.

Randomization Procedures

The study nurse assesses the patient in the emergency department as soon as possible after injury. To randomize the patient to normothermia or hypothermia, the study nurse calls a toll-free phone number for the Touch Tone Randomization Service, enters the answers to required questions, and receives a randomization number and treatment arm assignment. Randomization assignments are stratified by GCS 3–5 and 6–8 for each center.

Initial Patient Management

Initial patient management includes standard resuscitation and trauma management procedures. Early intubation, preferably at the scene of the injury, is desirable. Prompt treatment or, preferably, avoidance of hypoxia, hypotension, and other secondary insults to the injured brain are key principles in early patient management. In addition, treatment of other injuries is initiated.

Standard Management for Normothermia Patients

The principles of standard management for normothermia patients are in accordance with the Guidelines for the Management of Severe Head Injury developed as a joint initiative of the American Association of Neurological Surgeons and the Brain Trauma Foundation in 1995 [1]. Standard management used in this trial includes the following.

1. No active rewarming of patients who are hypothermic on arrival.
2. Early removal of hematomas, replacing the bone flap.
3. Routine sedation for 72 h with morphine 5–10 mg intravenously every hour regardless of the intracranial pressure (ICP).

4. Use of vecuronium 5–10 mg every hour only as needed for ventilatory control (if ICP is 20 mmHg).
5. Management of ICP (used in sequence).
    a. Optimal head position for ICP is first found.
    b. Morphine (5–10 mg/h) is used for sedation.
    c. Ventricular drainage of cerebral spinal fluid (CSF) if a ventriculostomy is in place.
    d. Vecuronium (5–10 mg/h) is administered for agitation or resistance to the ventilator. (Hypothermia patients receive vecuronium automatically, normothermia patients if needed.)
    e. Mannitol (0.5–1.0 g/kg) is given in repeated doses until serum osmolality is 315.
    f. Hyperventilation is to a $PaCO_2$ no lower than 30 mmHg.
    g. If the ICP fails to respond, based on the criteria below pentobarbital coma is started.
        (i)   ICP > 25 mmHg for 30 min
        (ii) ICP > 30 for 15 min
        (iii) ICP > 40 at all
6. Cerebral perfusion pressure is kept at 70 mmHg, with use of vasopressors if necessary.
7. Dehydration is avoided by replacement of urine volume. Adequate hydration is monitored by pulmonary artery catheter, daily weight, and intake and ouput (I&O).
8. Hyperthermia of 38.5°C or more is treated with Tylenol and a cooling blanket.
9. Phenytoin is administered with an initial loading dose on admission (18 mg/kg) and for 1 week after injury. It should be discontinued in the absence of seizures during this time.
10. Nutrition is begun enterally or parenterally within 48 h of admission.
11. All patients are placed on Roto-Rest beds (Kinetic Comcepts, San Antonio, TX, USA). Two beds are always on standby in the hospital for this study. Patients should be kept in rotation on a bed for a minimum of 18 h.

Standard Management for Hypothermia Patients

Patients randomized to hypothermia are managed exactly as the normothermia patients with the following modifications.

1. Hypothermia is established with goal of reaching 33°C within 8 h of injury or less.
    a. Hypothermia is established as soon as possible using ice packs and gastric lavage.
    b. Patient is placed on a Roto-Rest bed with plumbing. Cooling pads are wrapped securely around the patient to ensure maximum contact. The cooling unit (Cincinnati Sub-Zero, Cincinnati, OH, USA) is set at 33.2°C.
    c. Setting is adjusted on the cooling machine to maintain patient temperature between 32.5° and 34°C for 48 h.
    d. Ice saline gastric lavage is used to speed core cooling.
    e. Temperature of ventilator air is adjusted to 90°–94°F.
2. Administration of morphine (5–10 mg hourly) begins as soon as surface cooling is initiated and continues until patient is rewarmed and bladder temperature is 37°C.
3. Administration of vecuronium (5–10 mg hourly) begins as soon as surface cooling is initiated. It is maintained until the patient is rewarmed and the bladder temperature is 37°C.
4. Hypokalemia is managed.
    a. Hypokalemia is treated with intravenous potassium administered to maintain normokalemia.
    b. Potassium replacement is stopped 3 h before rewarming is begun to allow for the return of intracellular potassium.

TABLE 7. Most frequently occurring complications: "top 10 list" for all patients and study centers[a]

Active center	All patients (n = 340)	Houston (n = 89)	St. Louis (n = 74)	Sacramento (n = 72)	Pittsburgh (n = 64)	Small centers (n = 41)
Decreased CPP	81	80	82	81	78	83
Increased ICP	69	73	72	65	80	46
Pneumonia	65	67	70	78	42	64
Hypotension	26	26	12	39	22	39
UTI	26	30	35	22	25	5
Bradycardia	24	19	23	29	25	26
Decubitus	20	29	20	10	25	10
Pneumothorax	19	29	19	13	13	18
Catheter +	19	25	31	4	20	5
Sinusitis	14	27	18	7	8	5

All data are percents
CPP, cerebral perfusion pressure; ICP, intracranial pressure; UTI, urinary tract infection
[a] Data available on April 2, 1998

5. Rewarming is induced gradually by increasing the setting of the cooling unit to warm the patient at a rate of 0.5°C every 2 h (4 h to rise 1°C).

Complications

On average, NABIS:H patients experienced 5.23 complications (range 6.07–4.81 complications) per patient. Twenty-one percent of all complications were coded as critical. The most frequent complications included decreased cerebral perfusion pressure (CPP), intracranial hypertension, pneumonia, urinary tract infection, hypotension, pneumothorax, catheter positive culture, bradycardia, decubitus, and sinusitis. The percentage of patients experiencing each of these complications is shown in Table 7. Decreased CPP is defined as CPP < 70 mmHg for two or more consecutive hours. Increased ICP is defined as ICP > 20 mmHg for two or more consecutive hours. Pneumonia is defined as the presence of three of the following: (1) elevated temperature; (2) presence of polymorphonuclear leukocytes (PMNs) (>15 000/min^3); (3) treatment with antibiotics for purulent sputum; and (4) infiltrate on chest radiograph. Hypotension is defined as mean arterial pressure (MAP) <70 mmHg or significantly less than baseline, requiring intervention.

Outcome Evaluation and Assessment

The following outcome measures are assessed by blinded neuropsychology technicians at 3 and 6 months after injury. The results of the outcome studies are forwarded directly to the Biostatistics Center.

3 Months: GOS, neurological examination, Neurobehavioral Rating Scale
6 Months: GOS, Disability Rating Scale (DRS), symbol digit modality, controlled oral word association, grooved pegboard, trailmaking B, Rey complex figure, neurological examination, Neurobehavioral Rating Scale

Of 392 patients, 5 have been lost to follow-up. All other patients had 6-month outcome assessment. Table 8 shows results of the 6-month assessments. Mortality rates by center for

TABLE 8. Six-month assessments: primary outcome measure aggregate data

Category	No.	%
Good recovery	59	20
Moderate disability	70	23
Severe disability	74	25
Vegetative state	11	4
Dead	83	28
Total	214	

Categories of recovery are based on the Glasgow Outcome Score

TABLE 9. NABIS:H: mortality by center

Center	Mortality (%)	
	3 Months	6 Months
Houston ($n = 93$)	29.03	33.70
St. Louis ($n = 70$)	22.86	23.94
Pittsburgh ($n = 69$)	18.84	20.00
Sacramento ($n = 65$)	29.23	27.94
Inactive centers ($n = 29$)	37.93	33.33
Small centers ($n = 35$)	31.43	31.84
Total ($n = 361$)	26.87	28.02

the study are shown in Table 9. The results of the study relative to treatment effect will be available by early 1999.

References

1. Bullock R, Chesnut RM, Clifton GL, Shajar J, Marion DW, Narayan RK, Newell DW, Pitts LH, Rosner NJ, Wilberger JW (1996) Guidelines for the management of severe head injury. Eur J Emerg Med 2:109–127
2. Clifton GL, Allen S, Barrodale P, Plenger P, Berry J, Koch S, Fletcher J, Hayes RL, Choi SC (1993) A phase II study of moderate hypothermia in severe brain injury. J Neurotrauma 10:263–271
3. Clifton GL, Allen S, Berry J, Koch SM (1992) Systemic hypothermia in treatment of brain injury. J Nuerotrauma 9:S487–S495
4. Clifton GL, Jiang JY, Lyeth BG, Jenkens LW, Homm RJ, Hayes RL (1991) Marked protection by moderate hypothermia after experimental traumatic brain injury. J Cereb Blood Flow Metab 11:114–121
5. Clifton GL, Taft WC, Blair RE, Choi SC, De Lorenza RJ (1989) Conditions for pharmacologic evaluation in the gerbil model of forebrain ischemia. Stroke 20:1545–1552
6. Marion DW, Obrist WD, Carlier PM, Penrod LE, Darby JM (1993) The use of therapeutic moderate hypothermia for patients with severe head injuries: a preliminary report. J Neurosurg 79:354–362
7. Shiozaki T, Sugimoto H, Taneda AM, Yoshida H, Iwai A, Yoshioka T, Sugimoto T (1993) Effect of mild hypothermia on uncontrollable intracranial hypertension after severe head injury. J Neurosurg 79:363–368

Intravascular Volume Expansion During Therapeutic Moderate Hypothermia for Brain-Injured Patients: Preliminary Report

Mayuki Aibiki[1], Shuji Kawaguchi[1], Osamu Umegaki[2], Shinji Ogura[2], Nobuyuki Kawai[3], Yoshihiro Kinoshita[2], and Satoshi Yokono[2]

Summary. Hemodynamic depressions during moderate hypothermia may worsen cerebral ischemia after brain injury. In this preliminary report, we examined retrospectively the effects of intravascular volume expansion on hemodynamic changes, intracranial pressure (ICP), and internal jugular oxygen saturation (SJO_2) in seven brain-injured patients, who were selected because of their elevated ICPs even after induction of hypothermia. All patients were ventilated, and hypothermia was induced by surface cooling using midazolam, buprenorphine, and vecuronium. After the hypothermic period (divided into the initial, middle, and late phases), patients were gradually rewarmed at a rate of approximately 1°C per day. Mean blood pressure (MBP), central venous pressure (CVP), cerebral perfusion pressure (CPP), cardiac output (CO), ICP, and SJO_2 were measured. Despite a large amount of infusion ranging from approximately 4000 to 5000 ml/day, ICP decreased from the middle phase compared to the initial phase of the therapy. After such volume expansion, higher levels of CVP (ranging from 9.7 ± 0.8 to 10.7 ± 1.5 mmHg) were found during the hypothermic period in association with CO levels (5.2 ± 0.1 to 5.3 ± 0.2 l/min) similar to those of normothermia. Sustained CPP was accompanied by reduced ICP, increased SJO_2, and augmented CO. These results suggest that even a large amount of infusion to the brain-injured patients decreases ICP and improves CO during moderate hypothermia, which may be beneficial to the cerebral circulation and metabolism in the patients. The current study warrants further future studies to test such a hypothesis.

Key words. Cardiac output, Cerebral perfusion pressure, Internal jugular oxygen saturation, Moderate hypothermia, Volume expansion

Introduction

Therapeutic moderate hypothermia of 32°–33°C appears to be neuroprotective in patients with brain injury [1,10]. However, hypothermia produces circulatory depressions resulting from decreases both in blood volume and heart rate [4,19], which are the major affecting

---

[1] Intensive Care Unit, [2] Department of Anesthesiology and Emergency Medicine, [3] Department of Neurosurgery, Kagawa Medical University, 1750-1 Ikenobe, Miki, Kita, Kagawa 761-0793, Japan

factors for cardiac output [17]. Hemodynamic depressions may worsen ischemic conditions in the area surrounding contusion or intracerebral hematoma after traumatic brain injury (TBI) [14]. Such derangements would be a crucial determinant for subsequent neuronal damages in brain-injured victims [18]. If adequate circulatory management is not applied, even moderate hypothermia would fail to produce neurological improvements in brain-injured patients. We therefore have undertaken intravascular expansion to obtain adequate cerebral perfusion pressure during hypothermia for brain-injured patients, but such expansion may raise concerns regarding exacerbation of intracranial hypertension even during hypothermia. To the best of our knowledge, there are no reports examining whether such volume replacement during hypothermia is deleterious or beneficial for cerebral circulation or metabolism. In this preliminary report, we present the effects of intravascular volume expansion on hemodynamic changes, intracranial pressure, and internal jugular oxygen saturation during moderate hypothermia for brain-injured patients.

Subjects and Methods

This study was approved by the Ethics Committee of Kagawa Medical University, and informed consent from families or relatives was obtained before including the patients in this study. Thirteen brain-injured patients underwent moderate hypothermia of 32°–33°C. Body temperatures were monitored at a tympanic membrane, an internal jugular vein, or both. Inclusion criteria included a Glasgow Coma Scale (GCS) assessment of ≤ 8 on admission to the emergency room and evidence of injury on computed tomography (CT) scanning of the brain. The background of the patients in the present study is shown in Table 1. The GCS score of the patients ranged from 3 to 8 on admission. Moderate hypothermia was induced and maintained by surface cooling after administration of midazolam at a dose of 3–7 μg/kg/min, vecuronium at a dose of 2–4 mg/h, and buprenorphine at a dose of 0.4–0.6 mg/day. These agents were infused continuously until the end of the study. All patients were artificially ventilated to adjust their $PaCO_2$ levels to a level of 30–33 mmHg. After the hypothermic period, patients were gradually rewarmed at a rate of approximately 1°C per day. The rewarming process was started if there were no signs of brain swelling on CT findings. Thus, the duration of hypothermia was anticipated to last 4 days; but depending on the CT findings and intracranial pressure, the duration of hypothermia could be prolonged beyond the predetermined period. Consequently, the duration of hypothermic period ranged from 4 to 12 days.

Parameters Measured

Mean blood pressure (MBP), central venous pressure (CVP), and cardiac output (CO) using the Swan-Ganz CCOmbo (Baxter Healthcare Corp., CA, USA) were measured. As cerebral circulatory variables, the intracranial pressure (ICP) using Codman ICP sensors (Johnson & Johnson, MA, USA) and the internal jugular venous oxygen tension (SJO_2) using the Oximetrix SO_2 System (Abbott, IL, USA) were monitored.

Treatment Protocol

A subdural, epidural hematoma or intracerebral hematoma producing brain compression was evacuated as soon as possible. Using mainly colloid infusion, the mean arterial pressure was maintained between 90 and 100 mmHg so cerebral perfusion pressure would be ≥ 70 mmHg. The daily water balance during the hypothermic phase was aimed at approximately 1000–

TABLE 1. Background of patients

Pt. no.	Age (years)	Gender	Diagnosis	GCS	ST	GOS Outcome	CT class[b]	Pupil abnormalities on admission[c]
1	17	M	EH	7	+	GR	5	+
2	16	M	SH	8	+	GR	5	−
3	9	M	CC ICH	5	+	GR	5	−
4	52	M	ICH	6	+	MD	5	+
5	69[a]	F	CPA	3	ND	V	1	+
6	48	M	CC ICH	7	+	GR	5	−
7	18	M	DAI TSAH	7	ND	GR	2	−
8	22[a]	M	SH CC	6	+	MD	5	+
9	72[a]	F	CPA	4	ND	V	1	+
10	17[a]	F	TSAH	8	ND	GR	2	+
11	30[a]	M	EH	5	+	MD	5	−
12	20[a]	F	ICH AVM	4	+	MD	5	+
13	24[a]	M	ICH AVM	5	+	MD	5	+

GCS, Glasgow Coma Scale on admission; ST, surgical treatment; GOS, Glasgow Outcome Scale at 6 months after injury; GR, good recovery (score 5); MD, moderate disability (score 4); SD, severe disability (score 3); V, vegetative (score 2); D, death (score 1); CT class, CT classification; ND, not done; CC, cerebral contusion; EH, epidural hematoma; SH, subdural hematoma; TSAH, traumatic subarachnoid hemorrhage; CPA, cardiopulmonary arrest; ICH, intracerebral hematoma; DAI, diffuse axonal injury; AVM, arteriovenous malformation; NS, not significant
[a] Included in this study
[b] CT classification was done according to the following criteria: 1, no visible evidence of injury; 2, cisterns present with a midline shift of less than 5 mm and no lesion of less than 25 ml; 3, cisterns compressed or absent; 4, midline shift of more than 5 mm; 5, a lesion requiring surgical evacuation
[c] Pupillary abnormalities were defined as abnormalities in size or light response in one or both pupils

1500 ml. Dobutamine at a dose of 2–4 μg/kg/min was given to improve cardiac depression if bradycardia below 50 beats per min (bpm) occurred. If the temperature difference between the internal jugular blood and the palmer skin surface, which may be an indicator of reflecting the condition of peripheral circulations [15], increased beyond 4°C, hydralazine (a vasodilator) in a dose of 1–3 μg/kg/min was administered after further volume expansion. In all patients, 800 ml of 10% glycerol was administered daily for the purpose of reducing ICP. Daily dexamethasone 6–8 mg was given to all patients for 4 days.

Patient Selection

Among 13 brain-injured victims, 7 underwent surface cooling shortly after admission because of a low GCS, obvious anisocoria, or CT findings suggesting elevated ICP. An ICP sensor was inserted in such patients, and they showed ICPs of more than 15–20 mmHg even after induction of moderate hypothermia. The effects of a large intravenous infusion on ICP and the other parameters were evaluated in these patients.

Assessment of Neurologic Outcome

Independent neurosurgeons who were not aware of the study presented here determined the neurologic outcome approximately 6 months after the injury. The neurologic outcome was graded according to the Glasgow Outcome Scale [9]: 1, death; 2, vegetative state; 3, severe disability (unable to live independently but able to follow commands); 4, moderate disability (ability to live independently but unable to return to work or school); and 5, good recovery (able to return to work or school).

Statistical Analysis

Data were expressed as the mean ± SE. To standardized the period of hypothermia therapy, which differed for each patient, the time course of the therapy was divided into four periods: the hypothermic period (initial, middle, and late phases) and the rewarming period. Data for each parameter were taken from values obtained at 0 and 12 o'clock of each ICU day. Statistical analyses were done with ANOVA followed by Scheffe's F-tests for comparisons within a group and among means at different phases during hypothermic therapy. A P value of <0.05 was considered significant.

Results

As shown in Fig. 1, despite of a large positive water balance (2700 ± 600 at the initial phase and 3031 ± 260 at the middle phase), the ICP decreased significantly from the middle phase of the hypothermic period to the initial phase. This change was sustained until the end of the study. Oxygen saturation of internal jugular blood increased both in the middle (from 61 ± 3% to 73 ± 2%) and late phases (72 ± 3%) of the therapy, in association with decreases in the ICP during the hypothermic period.

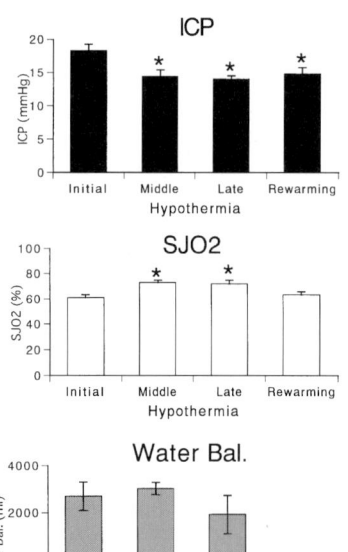

FIG. 1. From top to bottom: Time course of intracranial pressure (*ICP*), internal jugular oxygen saturation (*SJO₂*), and water balance (*Water Bal.*) at each phase. *Asterisks* show significant differences between the initial phase ($p < 0.05$). Data are shown in mean ± SE ($n = 7$). From among 13 victims, 7 patients were selected for this study for their elevated ICPs even after inducing hypothermia

FIG. 2. From top to bottom: time course of ICP, SJO$_2$, and cerebral perfusion pressure (*CPP*) at each phase. *Asterisks* show significant differences between the initial phase ($p < 0.05$). Data are shown as mean ± SE ($n = 7$)

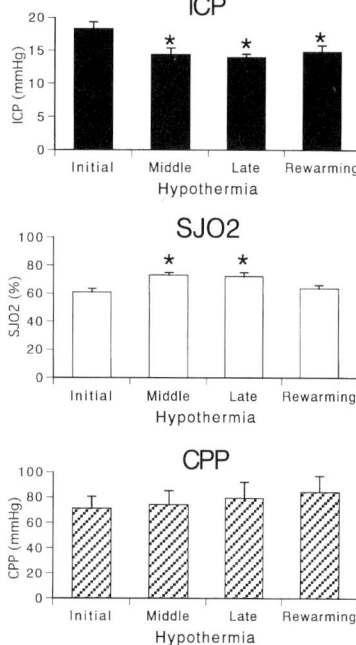

As demonstrated in Fig. 2, CPP was sustained at 71 ± 9 mmHg even from the initial phase of the therapy and was maintained throughout the course. These CPP changes were associated with reduced ICP and increased oxygen tension of internal jugular blood.

As shown in Fig. 3, the CVP during the hypothermic period ranged from 9.7 ± 0.8 at the initial phase to 10.7 ± 1.5 mmHg at the middle phase. These relatively high levels of CVP were accompanied by normal levels of CO (ranging from 5.2 ± 0.1 to 5.3 ± 0.2 l/min). Although the CVP level during the rewarming period decreased to 7.9 ± 1.8 mmHg, compared to that of the middle phase, the CO at rewarming increased from 5.2 ± 0.3 l/min at the late phase to 6.0 ± 0.5 l/min. SJO$_2$ levels both at the middle and late phase were significantly higher than that at the rewarming period, but this response was not associated with significant changes in COs.

Discussion

Effects of Volume Expansion

We demonstrated herein that blood volume expansion diminished hemodynamic deterioration during moderate hypothermia, which may favor the maintenance of cerebral perfusion pressure. Hemodynamic depressions during hypothermia, if not adequately treated, may worsen ischemic conditions at sites near the contusion or intracerebral hematoma after sustaining brain injury. Such derangements could be a determinant for neurological outcome [18]. Thus, we have undertaken intravascular expansion to obtain adequate cerebral perfusion pressure during hypothermia for brain-injured patients, but such expansion may aggravate intracranial hypertension during hypothermia. However, as demonstrated in this study, even a large infusion to brain-injured patients who exhibited intracranial hypertension did

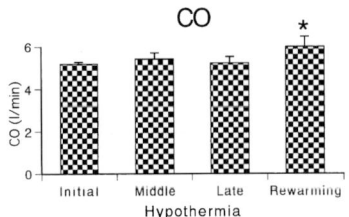

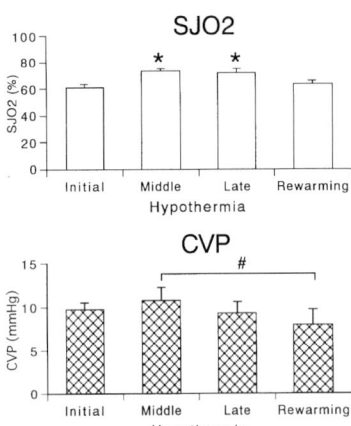

Fig. 3. From top to bottom: time course of cardiac output (*CO*), SJO$_2$, and CPP at each phase. Asterisks show significant differences between the initial phase. #, differences between the middle phase and the rewarming period ($p < 0.05$). Data are shown as mean ± SE ($n = 7$)

not further increase their ICP but, rather, served to decrease it significantly during hypothermia therapy of 32°–33°C.

In a previous paper, CPP was shown to improve after volume expansion for traumatic brain-injured patients whose body temperatures were not controlled [13]. In that paper, vasopressors such as phenylephrine or norepinephrine were also used to maintain systemic blood pressure to ensure the CPP. However, it is well known that prolonged usage of catecholamine causes low perfusion to organs such as kidneys, resulting in renal insufficiency [11]. More importantly, it is possible that an increase in systemic blood pressure induced mainly by vasopressor, and not by adequate volume expansion, causes low perfusion of injured brain tissue, in which blood supply is required. In this study, we applied a small amount of dobutamine (a β-stimulant) to reverse bradycardia during hypothermia. It may also contribute to an increase in cardiac output. Thus, it is likely that this course of treatment itself does not cause organ dysfunction.

Major mechanisms for hemodynamic impairment during induced hypothermia have been indicated to be (1) cardiac output depletion caused by a decreased heart rate [19]; and (2) reduction in the intravascular blood volume [4,8]. During hypothermia a body fluid shift to the interstitial space due to an increase in vascular permeability occurs, resulting in a decrease in intravascular plasma volume [12]. This change in vascular permeability seems to be due to sympathetic activation during hypothermia [20]. Thus, we need to replenish the intravascular volume to overcome such hemodynamic derangements during hypothermia. In this study, CVPs during the hypothermic period were at relatively high levels and did not change significantly, which may reflect intravascular volume expansion. This treatment may contribute to the maintainance of cardiac output during therapeutic moderate hypothermia.

Why Did ICP Not Increase after Significant Intravascular Expansion during Hypothermia?

The blood–brain barrier (BBB) can be disrupted, even from the early phase of traumatic brain injury [3,7]. The alterations are associated with leukocyte accumulation, suggesting the importance of the role of leukocytes in the development of the barrier impairment [5]. These changes appear to be an important cause of acute brain swelling. Recently, we reported that hypothermia may exert neuroprotective effects mediating through interleukin-6 depletion, which means that it may have antiinflamatory effects [1]. Hypothermia attenuates an increase in BBB permeability after brain trauma [16], resulting in a reduction of ICP. Therefore, we need to test the hypothesis as to whether mechanisms that reduce ICP even after massive infusion in brain-injured patients with elevated ICP are attributable to a rapid improvement of the BBB function due to moderate hypothermia.

Is Maintaining Cardiac Output at Normothermia Beneficial in Brain-injured Patients during Moderate Hypothermia?

It is well known that brain injury causes a hyperdynamic state characterized by increased cardiac output, moderate hypertension, and decreased systemic and pulmonary vascular resistance [6]. These cardiovascular responses may be adaptive in brain-injured patients, possibly to improve cerebral circulation [6]. Hypovolemia associated with low cardiac output may impair oxygen delivery to systemic tissues including injured brain tissue. In animals, hypovolemia may decrease cardiac output without a drop in arterial blood pressure by increasing systemic vascular resistance mediated through sympathetic activation [17]. Thus, monitoring only the CPP in brain-injured patients may lead us to overlook cerebral low perfusion, which would occur after hypovolemia in brain-injured patients, in whom the relation between systemic blood pressure and cerebral blood flow might have been deprived.

Hypothermia itself causes hypovolemia and bradycardia, leading to low cardiac output [4,19]. These declines in hemodynamics have been thought to parallel the depressed oxygen demand [2,19]. If so, even when bradycardia occurs during hypothermia, intact heart rate responses to blood pressure changes evoked pharmacologically would develop. However, we have reported recently that in hypothermic rabbits the heart rate did not increase in response to nitroglycerine-induced hypotension, although sympathetic nerve activity did increase [20]. These discrepant data indicate that hemodynamic depression during hypothermia may not be due to reduced oxygen metabolism (metabolic–hemodynamic coupling), but to direct cardiac effects induced by hypothermia [20]. It remains uncertain whether the coupling in the injured brain occurs in brain-injured patients who have undergone moderate hypothermia. Therefore, if hemodynamic depression during hypothermia is not adequately treated, it is possible that even hypothermia could not improve subsequent brain ischemia after brain injury. Further studies are required to define the effects of intravascular expansion on cerebral perfusion and metabolism in brain-injured patients who have undergone moderate hypothermia.

References

1. Aibiki M, Maekawa S, Ogura S, Kinoshita Y, Kawai N, Yokono S (1999) Effect of moderate hypothermia on systemic and internal jugular plasma IL-6 levels after traumatic brain injury in humans. J Neurotrauma 16:225–232

2. Baraka A (1994) Influence of surface cooling and rewarming on whole-body oxygen supply-demand balance. Br J Anaesth 73:418–420
3. Barzo P, Marmarou A, Fatouros P, Corwin F, Dunbar J (1996) Magnetic resonance imaging-monitored acute blood-brain barrier changes in experimental traumatic brain injury. J Neurosurg 85:1113–1121
4. Chen RYZ, Chien S (1978) Hemodynamic functions and blood viscosity in surface hypothermia. Am J Physiol 235:H136–H143
5. Clark RSB, Carlos TM, Schding JK, Bree M, Fireman LA, Dekosky ST, Kochanek PM (1996) Antibodies against Mac-1 attenuate neutrophil accumulation after traumatic brain injury in rats. J Neurotrauma 13:333–341
6. Clifton GL, Robertson CS, Kyper K, Taylor AA, Dhenken RD, Grossman RG (1983) Cardiovascular response to severe head injury. J Neurosurg 59:447–454
7. Fukuda K, Tanno H, Okimura Y, Nakamura M, Yamamura A (1995) The blood-brain-barrier disruption to circulating proteins in the early period after fluid percussion brain injury in rats. J Neurotrauma 12:315–324
8. Green JF, Jackman AP (1979) Mechanism of the increased vascular capacity produced by mild perfusion hypothermia in the dog. Circ Res 44:411–419
9. Jannet B, Snoek J, Bond MR, Brooks N (1981) Disability after severe head injury: observation on the use of the Glasgow Outcome Scale. J Neurol Neurosurg Psychiatry 44:285–293
10. Marion DW, Penrod LE, Kelsey SF, Obeist WD, Kochanek PM, Palmer AM, Wisniewski SR, DeKosky ST (1997) Treatment of traumatic brain injury with moderate hypothermia. N Engl J Med 336:540–546
11. Mazze RI (1990) Renal physiology. In: Miller RD (ed) Anesthesia, 3rd edn, vol l. Churchill Livingstone, New York, pp 601–619
12. Nose H (1982) Transvascular fluid shift and redistribution of blood in hypothermia. Jpn J Physiol 32:831–842
13. Rosner MJ, Rosner SD, Johnson AH (1995) Cerebral perfusion pressure: management protocol and clinical results. J Neurosurg 83:949–962
14. Schroder ML, Muizelaar JP, Bullock MR, Salvant JB, Povlishock JT (1995) Focal ischemia due to traumatic contusion documented by stable xenon CT and ultrastructural studies. J Neurosurg 82:966–971
15. Sessler DI (1990) Temperature monitoring. In: Miller RD (ed) Anesthesia, 3rd edn, vol 2. Churchill Livingstone, New York, pp 1227–1242
16. Smith S, Hall ED (1996) Mild pre- and posttraumatic hypothermia attenuates blood-brain barrier damage following controlled cortical impact injury in the rat. J Neurotrauma 13:1–9
17. Spyer KM (1988) Central nervous system control of the cardiovascular system. In: Bannister SR (ed) Autonomic failure: A text book of clinical disorders of the autonomic nervous system, 2nd edn. Oxford University Press, New York, pp 56–78
18. Teasdale GM, Graham DI (1998) Craniocerebral trauma: protection and retrieval of the neuronal population after injury. Neurosurgery 43:723–738
19. Wong KC (1983) Physiology and pharmacology of hypothermia (medical progress). West J Med 138:227–232
20. Xu H, Aibiki M, Ogura S, Seki K, Yokono S, Ogli K (2000) Effects of induced hypothermia on renal sympathetic nerve activity, baroreceptor reflex and catecholamine changes in urethane-anesthetized rabbits. Crit Care Med (in press)

Treatment of Hyperacute Embolic Stroke with Major Cerebral Artery Occlusion by Mild Hypothermia

Hiroaki Naritomi, Kazuyuki Nagatsuka, Takemori Yamawaki, Kotaro Miyashita, Hiroshi Moriwaki, and Yoshimasa Watanabe

Summary. Mild hypothermia was utilized for the treatment of hyperacute embolic stroke with major cerebral artery occlusion. The subjects were 12 stroke patients, 61 ± 13 years of age, who had occlusions of internal carotid artery (ICA), 7; middle cerebral artery (MCA) trunk, 4; or basilar artery (BA), 1. All patients were admitted within 4 h after stroke. The initial NIH Stroke Scale classification at admission was 21.8 ± 9.3. Hypothermia was induced within 6 h after stroke, and the brain temperature was maintained at 33°C for 3–6 days. Two of seven patients with ICA occlusion, one with recurrent multiple emboli and the other with massive hemorrhagic infarction, died during the acute phase. The remainder had a considerably good functional outcome showing Rankin Scale 2.8 ± 1.5 and Barthel Index 69 ± 35 at 3 months after stroke. Computed tomography (CT) findings in those patients were similar in the following two respects: (1) the development of cerebral edema was unremarkable in both the hypothermic and post-hypothermic periods, and (2) ischemic areas were rarely enhanced by contrast agents. It should also be noted that in two patients with delayed recanalization, ischemic lesions on CT developed gradually and were completed at 3–5 days after stroke. Mild hypothermia may have protective effects on stroke preventing the development of blood–brain barrier (BBB) disruption and cerebral edema, provided the hypothermia is induced in the hyperacute phase. Our CT findings suggest that hypothermia prolongs the time window of stroke therapy.

Key words. Mild hypothermia, Cerebral infarction, Blood–brain barrier, Cerebral edema, Therapeutic time window

Introduction

It has been well established by experimental studies that even a moderate increase or decrease in brain temperature causes significant aggravation or amelioration of cerebral ischemic injury [1,9]. Stroke patients often show increased body temperature in the acute phase, and the increased body temperature appears to be closely connected with poor clinical outcome [2,8]. Therefore, it is reasonable to assume that the prevention of hyperthermia or the induction of

Cerebrovascular Division, Department of Medicine, National Cardiovascular Center, 5-7-1 Fujishiro-dai, Suita, Osaka 565-8565, Japan

mild hypothermia may be therapeutic for acute ischemic stroke. Recently, a number of institutes in Japan have been using mild hypothermia for the treatment of severe head injury [6], and the safety of mild hypothermia has been confirmed through such experiences. However, mild hypothermia has not been used extensively for the treatment of ischemic stroke. We reported our experience of hypothermic treatment of hyperacute embolic stroke in 1996 [7]. So far we have treated 12 embolic stroke patients with major cerebral artery occlusion using mild hypothermia in the hyperacute phase of stroke. Although our experience to date has been small, computed tomography (CT) findings obtained in those patients suggest the usefulness of mild hypothermia for the treatment of hyperacute stroke. The methods and results of hypothermia therapy in these 12 patients including CT findings are described as follows.

Case Materials and Methods

During the interval from 1994 to 1999, a total of 12 patients with acute cardiogenic embolism underwent mild hypothermia therapy in our department according to the following criteria: (1) ages below 70 years; (2) admission within 4h after stroke; (3) hemiparesis in association with consciousness disturbance more than 2 on the Japan Coma Scale; (4) no hemorrhagic change on computed tomography (CT); (5) ultrasonographic findings suggestive of embolic occlusion of major cerebral artery, such as internal carotid artery (ICA), middle cerebral artery (MCA), or basilar artery (BA); (6) no improvement of neurologic symptoms for more than 30min following administration of recombinant tissue plasminogen activator (rt-PA), alteplase 2000 units; and (7) no association of severe cardiac, hepatic, or renal dysfunction. The patients were eight men and four women with ages ranging from 35 to 69 years (61 ± 13 years). All of them were admitted within 4h after stroke, and ICA occlusion ($n = 7$), MCA trunk occlusion ($n = 4$), or BA occlusion was diagnosed at first by ultrasonography and was later confirmed by conventional angiography.

Mild hypothermia therapy was undertaken in the stroke care unit of our institute. Conventional angiography was performed prior to the induction of mild hypothermia in three patients and following mild hypothermia in the other nine patients. Prior to the induction of hypothermia, rt-PA was administered intravenously in seven patients and intraarterially in one patient within 4h after stroke. None of them exhibited noticeable neurologic recovery, so they underwent hypothermia therapy. Another patient with occlusion of BA top received urokinase administration in a superselective manner following the induction of hypothermia at 7h after stroke. The remaining three patients received no thrombolytic therapy.

The hypothermia therapy was induced under general anesthesia with fentanyl and midazolum. Prior to the induction of general anesthesia, 1000ml of plasma expander was rapidly infused through the venous route in order to prevent excessive reduction of blood pressure accompanied by anesthesia. Following the anesthesia, the body temperature was lowered rapidly using a hypothermic blanket combined with an alcohol compress to reach a brain temperature of 33°C. The brain temperature was monitored at the internal jugular bulb, and the core temperature was monitored at the bladder. Approximately 1.5h was required to reach the target brain temperature. Hypothermia at 33°C brain temperature was maintained for 3–6 days followed subsequently by rewarming. At the time of rewarming, the brain temperature was increased by 1–2°C/day.

Following the hypothermia therapy, CT scanning was performed repeatedly to evaluate effects of hypothermia, to determinate the time of rewarming, and to estimate the development of cerebral edema following the rewarming. Functional recovery was evaluated at 3 months after stroke using the Rankin Scale and the Barthel Index.

TABLE 1. Hypothermia therapy and clinical outcome in 12 patients

Total cases	$n = 12$
Ages	61 ± 13 years
Initial NIHSS	21.8 ± 9.3
Occluded artery	
ICA	$n = 7$
MCA	$n = 4$
BA	$n = 1$
Start of body cooling	4.0 ± 1.0 h
Time to reach 33°C	5.9 ± 1.4 h
Hypothermic duration	3–6 days
Mortality	2/12 (16.7%)
Rankin Scale at 3 months	2.8 ± 1.5
Barthel Index at 3 months	69 ± 35

NIHSS, National Institutes of Health Stroke Scale;
ICA, internal carotid artery; MCA, middle cerebral
artery; BA, basilar artery

Results

Table 1 summarizes the initial severity of stroke, the site of occlusion as confimred by conventional angiography, the times of hypothermia therapy, and the clinical outcome in the 12
patients. On admission, the grade of consciousness disturbance ranged from 3 to 100 on the
Japan Coma Scale, and the severity of stroke was 21.8 ± 9.3 on the National Institutes of Health
(NIH) Stroke Scale. Body cooling started at 4.0 ± 1.0 h, and reached 33°C brain temperature
at 5.9 ± 1.4 h. The hypothermia at 33°C in brain temperature was maintained for 3–6 days.
The hypothermic duration in each case was determined on the basis of CT findings obtained
at 2–3 days after stroke according to the following protocol: 3 days in cases of small
or medium-sized ischemic lesion without mass effects, 5 days in cases of large ischemic
lesion without mass effects, and more than 5 days in cases of large ischemic lesion with mass
effects.

Of the 12 patients, two patients with ICA occlusion died during the acute phase. Both had
received rt-PA administration prior to the hypothermia therapy. One patient had massive
hemorrhagic changes at 2 days after stroke, which expanded further at 3 days after stroke
leading to the fatal outcome. The other patient had recurrent multiple emboli resulting in
bilateral ICA occlusion with unilateral vertebral artery occlusion, which caused the fatal
outcome. Except for these two patients, none died in the acute or chronic phase. Those 10
surviving patients showed a considerably good functional recovery. At 3 months after stroke,
they showed a Rankin Scale of 2.8 ± 1.5 and a Barthel Index of 69 ± 35.

CT findings obtained in the 10 surviving patients were similar in the following two respects.
First, all the 10 patients showed no appreciable mass effects on CT. As shown in Figure 1, no
appreciable mass effect was observed even in patients with large ischemic lesions. This was
true whether CT was obtained in the hypothermic period or post-hypothermic period. Thus,
cerebral edema was unremarkable both in the hypothermic and post-hypothermic periods in
all the 10 patients. Second, little parenchymal enhancement of ischemic lesions was observed
on contrast-enhanced CT (Fig. 1) in all the eight patients undergoing contrast enhancement.
Apart from these two characteristic CT findings, which were commonly observed in the
surviving patients, an interesting CT change, i.e., a gradual development of ischemic lesions,

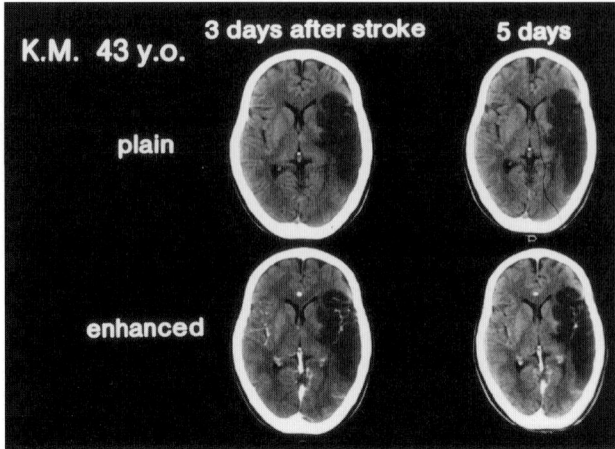

Fɪɢ. 1. Computed tomography (CT) findings during hypothermia in a case of left internal carotid artery (ICA) occlusion. *Plain* CT demonstrates a large ischemic lesion without noticeable mass effect. *Enhanced* CT exhibits no parenchymal enhancement in ischemic lesions

was observed in two of three patients without thrombolytic therapy. In these two patients, the size of low-density areas did not reach the maximum within 24 h after stroke and expanded gradually over 3–5 days (Fig. 2).

Comments

Embolic occlusion of the major cerebral artery usually causes large cerebral infarction in association with massive cerebral edema. The mortality in such large infarctions with massive edema was reported to exceed 70% [5]. Recently, Schwab et al. reported effects of mild hypothermia therapy on such malignant types of cerebral infarction [10]. They induced hypothermia (33°C brain temperature) at the average of 14 h after stroke and maintained the hypothermia for 2–3 days. The hypothermia successfully suppressed cerebral edema and decreased the intracranial pressure significantly. However, cerebral edema again developed after rewarming, resulting in increased intracranial pressure. As a consequence, 44% of patients died in their hypothermic study. Schwab et al. commented that the hypothermia therapy was useful for suppressing intracranial pressure and decreasing the mortality of malignant cerebral infarction. However, it seems that the induction of hypothermia at 14 h after stroke is too late to utilize the cerebral protective effects of hypothermia. At 14 h after stroke, the neuronal viability is likely lost in the majority areas of ischemic lesions; therefore, the hypothermia may be unable to exert its neuroprotective actions. Experimental studies indicated that hypothermia may suppress cerebral edema [3]. Such an action probably reduced the intracranial pressure during the hypothermia in the study of Schwab et al. [10]. However, the edema-suppressive action probably occurs only during the hypothermia. In the study of Schwab et al., the edema-suppressive action disappeared after rewarming, thus, resulting in the redevelopment of cerebral edema.

In this study, the hypothermia was induced at the average of 4 h after stroke, and the 33°C target brain temperature was obtained at the average of 5.9 h after stroke. At such a hyperacute phase of ischemia, many neurons in ischemic lesions may maintain their viability. The

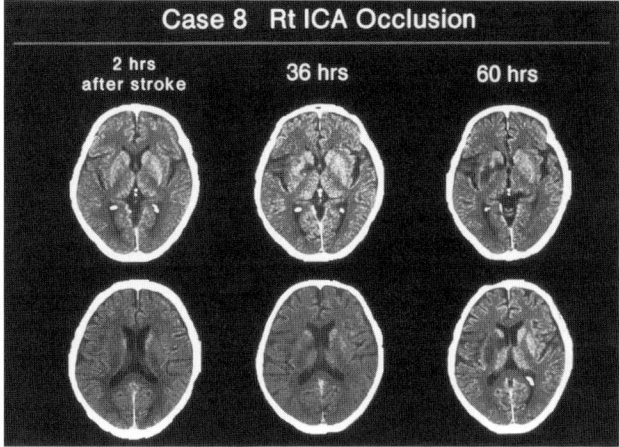

FIG. 2. Serial CT findings during hypothermia in a case of right ICA occlusion. Low-density area is unremarkable at *2h* after stroke. A small low-density area is observed in the basal ganglia areas at *36h* after stroke. A low-density area expanded further at *60h* after stroke

hypothermia induced at the hyperacute phase may exert neuroprotective action and may preserve the viability of many neurons. As a consequence, none of our patients, except for the two fatal cases, developed severe cerebral edema as confirmed by CT during the hypothermia. Furthermore, none of these patients showed the deterioration of cerebral edema after rewarming. No deterioration of cerebral edema in the post-hypothermic period is probably related with the neuroprotection of ischemic regions.

In our CT studies performed during the hypothermia therapy, the ischemic parenchyma was rarely enhanced by contrast agents. This CT observation strongly suggests that the hypothermia protects the blood–brain barrier (BBB) in ischemic lesions. Dietrich et al. in their experimental study documented that mild hypothermia protected the BBB, thereby contributing to the protection of ischemic neurons [4]. Our CT findings agree with the experimental findings of Dietrich et al. and suggest that the BBB protection is one of actions of hypothermia and may contribute to the protection of ischemic neurons.

In the present study, interesting CT findings were obtained in two patients without rt-PA administration, in whom the occluded arteries were not recanalized for a long duration. Serial CT studies in these two patients demonstrated a gradual development of ischemic areas over 3–5 days. These CT findings suggest that neurons in some areas of ischemic lesions maintained their viability for more than 2 days under hypothermic condition. Thus, hypothermia appears to prolong the viability of ischemic neurons and prolong a therapeutic time window of stroke.

In this study, the patients undergoing hypothermia therapy all had embolic occlusion of ICA, BA, or MCA trunk, and their NIH Stroke Scale on admission was 21.8 on average. The severity of stroke in these patients is comparable with that in patients undergoing hypothermia therapy in the study of Schwab et al. [10]. Nevertheless, the mortality in our patients (17%) was considerably lower as compared with that in patients in Schwab's study (44%). The difference in the mortality between the two studies is probably attributable to the time difference in the induction of hypothermia. The results of the present preliminary study suggest that the hypothermia therapy may be useful for the treatment of malignant embolic stroke, provided it is induced in the hyperacute stage. However, a randomized large-sample study is needed to ensure the effect of mild hypothermia therapy on acute stroke.

References

1. Busto R, Dietrich WD, Globus MYT, Valdes J, Schein berg P, Ginsberg MD (1987) Small differences in intraischemic brain temperature critically determine the extent of ischemic neuronal injury. J Cereb Blood Flow Metab 7:729–738
2. Castillo J, Davalos A, Marrugat J, Noya M (1998) Timing for fever-related brain damage in acute ischemic stroke. Stroke 29:2455–2460
3. Dempsy RJ, Combs DJ, Maley ME, Cowen DE, Roy MW, Donaldson DL (1987) Moderate hypothermia reduces postischemic edema development and leukotriene production. Neurosurgery 21:177–181
4. Dietrich WD, Halley M, Valdes I, Busto R (1991) Interrelationships between increased vascular permeability and acute neuronal damage following temperature-controlled brain ischemia in rats. Acta Neuropathol 81:615–625
5. Hacke W, Schwab S, Horn M, Spranger M, De Georgia M, van Kummer R (1984) Malignant middle cerebral artery territory infarction: clinical course and prognostic signs. Arch Neurol 53:309–315
6. Hayashi N, Hirayama T, Ohhata M (1993) The computed cerebral hypothermia management technique to the critical head injury patients. Adv Neurotrauma Res 5:61–64
7. Naritomi H, Shimizu T, Oe H, Kinugawa H, Sawada T, Hirata T (1996) Mild hypothermia therapy in acute embolic stroke: a pilot study. J Stroke Cerebrovasc Dis 6 (Suppl 1):193–196
8. Reith J, Jorgensen HS, Pedersen PM, Nakayama H, Raaschou HO, Jeppesen LL, Olsen TS (1996) Body temperature in acute stroke: relations to stroke severity, infarct size, mortality, and outcome. Lancet 347:422–425
9. Ridenour TR, Warner DS, Todd M, McAllister AC (1992) Mild hypothermia reduces infarct size resulting from temporary but not permanent focal ischemia in rats. Stroke 23:733–738
10. Schwab S, Schwarz S, Spranger M, Keller E, Bertram M, Hacke W (1998) Moderate hypothermia in the treatment of patients with severe middle cerebral artery infarction. Stroke 29:2461–2466

Mild Hypothermia Therapy for Severe Acute Brain Insults in Clinical Practice

Tsuyoshi Maekawa, Daikai Sadamitsu, Ryosuke Tsuruta, Takeshi Inoue, Akio Tateishi, and Fujio Murakami

Summary. Animal experiments have provided persuasive evidence that mild hypothermia confers significant protection against ischemic or traumatic brain insults. Therefore, it is very important to establish a safe and secure procedure for mild hypothermia therapy in clinical practice.

In this chapter, we describe the indications, procedures, beneficial and adverse effects, and clinical experiences of mild hypothermia in our institute. Severe head injury (GCS $\leq$ 8), cerebral embolic stroke, postoperative subarachnoid hemorrhage (aneurysm clipping, Hunt and Kosnick grade 3 or 4, Fisher CT classification 3 or 4), and post-cardiopulmonary resuscitated encephalopathy (arrest time, 5–10 min) would be good indications. In these procedures, brain-oriented intensive care is essential, and the maintenance of microcirculation is the cornerstone of success in this therapy. We demonstrate that elevation of excitotoxic glutamate was normalized, while glycine (a potent activator of glutamate neurotoxicity) and NO_2 plus NO_3, (NO metabolites and a source of free radicals) were persistently high in the cerebrospinal fluid. The latter evidence gives us key factors for future treatment in addition to mild hypothermia therapy.

Recent data from our work and that of other investigators suggest that mild hypothermia will be a promising measure against severe acute brain insults in the very near future.

Key words. Hypothermia, Nomenclature, Indication, Procedure, Glutamate, Nitric oxide

Introduction

The aim of brain protection and resuscitation in severe acute brain insults is to minimize the primary brain insult and to suppress or facilitate recovery from adverse secondary brain insults. Figure 1 shows the possible process of neuronal damage in brain hypoxia and/or ischemia. At present, excitotoxicity by glutamate and intracellular Ca^{2+} accumulation are the main causes in neuronal cell death [22]. But glutamate receptor antagonists and Ca^{2+} entry blockers are not adequate in clinical practice.

Advanced Medical Emergency and Critical Care Center, Yamaguchi University Hospital, 1-1-1 Minami Kogushi, Ube, Yamaguchi 755-8505, Japan

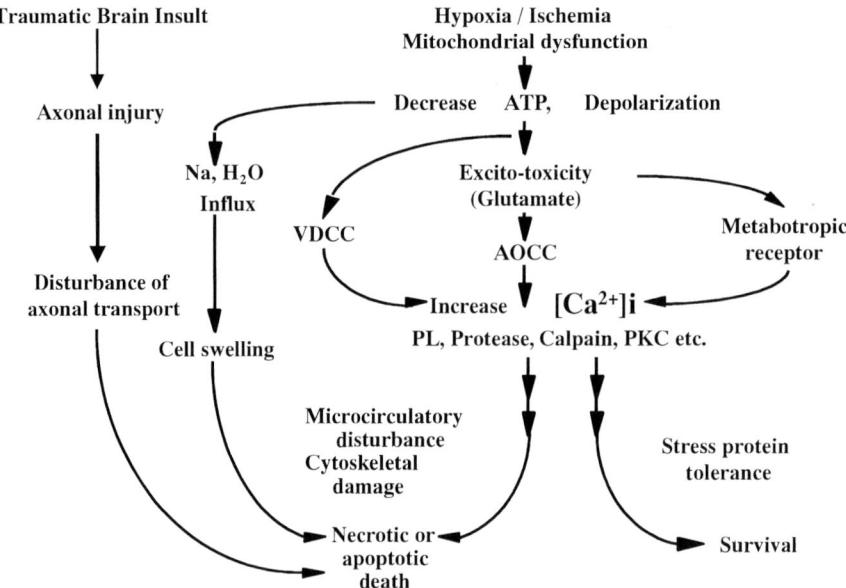

FIG. 1. Possible process of neuronal damage. At present, excitotoxicity by glutamate and intracellular Ca^{2+} accumulation are the main causes of neuronal cell death in brain hypoxia and ischemia. *ATP*, adenosine triphosphate; *VDCC*, voltage-dependent Ca^{2+} channel; *AOCC*, agonist-operated Ca^{2+} channel; *PL*, phospholipase; *PKC*, protein kinase C

Recently, animal experiments have provided persuasive evidence that mild hypothermia confers significant protection against ischemic or traumatic brain injuries [2,3,10]. In contrast to hypothermia, slight elevation of brain temperature (39°C) worsened neuronal cell death [15]. Therefore, it is very important to establish a safe and secure procedure for mild hypothermia therapy in clinical practice.

Nomenclature of Hypothermia

There has been no standardized hypothermic nomenclature, graded by the degree of core body temperature. Figure 2 compares systems of nomenclature found in the literature [14a,19] with the one used by our group since 1994 [9].

Mild Hypothermia in Clinical Practice

Indications

Mild hypothermia therapy has been and will be applied to head injury [4,14a,25], cerebral infarction [16], postoperative subarachnoid hemorrhage [12], and cardiopulmonary-resuscitated patients [7]. However, definitive indications must be determined in the near future with evidence-based studies.

The indications are shown in Table 1, which is a summary from the literature and from personal communication. These are subject to change when sufficient clinical data have been

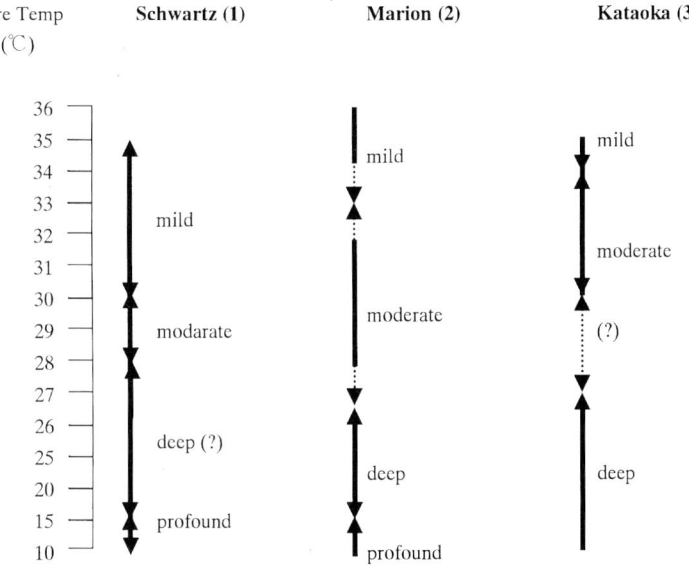

FIG. 2. Hypothermia nomenclature graded by the degree of core body temperature on Schwartz [19], Marion [14b], and Kataoka [9] Scales

TABLE 1. Indication, degree, and duration for mild hypothermia therapy[a]

Condition	Indication window	Degree (°C)	Duration (days)	Note [Reference]
Head injury	GCS ≦ 8, Large mass lesion (operation), start ≦ 6h, ICP ≦ 40 mmHg	32–34	2–5	Tateishi et al. [25]
	GCS ≦ 8, ICP < 20 mmHg	34	2 or more	Shiozaki et al. [21]
	4 ≦ GCS ≦ 7, start within 6 hr	32–33	2	Clifton [4]
	GCS ≦ 7, start within 6 hr	32–33	24 (hr)	Marion et al. [14a]
Cerebral infarction	Either reperfused or nonreperfused case by tPA (2400 × 10⁴ U iv or ia), start ≦ 6 hr	33	3–7	Naritomi et al. [16]
Postoperative subarachnoid hemorrhage	Hunt and Kosnik, 3 or 4; Fisher, 3 or 4, postoperative vasospasm period	34	3–12	Maekawa et al. [12]
	Ineffective cases of barbiturate and/or hypertensive therapies	33 ± 0.5	4–7	Nozaki et al. [personal communication]
Cardiopulmonary resuscitation	5 min < arrest time ≦ 10 min, BPs ≧ 80 mmHg, 45% ≦ SjvO₂ ≦ 80%	32–34	2–5	Maekawa et al. [unpublished data]

[a] Indication window, target core body temperature, and duration of mild hypothermia therapy may be adjusted when sufficient clinical data are accumulated
GCS, Glasgow Coma Scale; ICP, intracranial pressure; BPs, systolic blood pressure; SjvO₂, superior jugular bulb venous blood oxygen saturation

collected. The upper age limit has not been decided, but 65 years may be appropriate because of frequently coexisting complications. The time window for this therapy is 3–6 h, based on animal experiments [5,6]. However, the effectiveness of the therapy would be much greater the earlier it is started. Neurological evaluation, brain computed tomography (CT), intracranial pressure (ICP), and superior jugular bulb venous blood oxygen saturation ($SjvO_2$) are good indicators to use to select a patient for mild hypothermia therapy. The exclusion criteria are penetrated brain injury, multiple trauma, hypoxemia ($SaO_2 < 94\%$, >30 min), persistent hypotension (systolic blood pressure < 90 mmHg, >120 min), normal brain CT with Glasgow Coma Scale (GCS) more than 8, preexisting organ failure, persistent high ICP (>50 mmHg), and high $SjvO_2$ (>80%) on admission.

Procedures

Monitoring

Ordinary monitoring such as by electrocardiogram, direct arterial pressure, cardiac output and central venous pressure measured by a pulmonary arterial catheter, and core body (pulmonary artery, bladder) and peripheral (foot or palm) temperatures are essential. Blood gases and electrolytes, peripheral blood cell counts, bleeding tendency, and immune testing are also important.

Special monitoring is also needed. Superior venous blood temperature, $SjvO_2$, mean blood flow velocity of the middle cerebral artery by transcranial Doppler sonography, electroencephalogram, brain stem evoked potentials, and ICP (if possible) are included.

Anesthesia

Our sedative protocol, as shown in Table 2, is basically neurolept analgesia. We use a higher dose of droperidol (butyrophenone derivative) and a lower dose of fentanyl (a synthesized narcotic). Microcirculation should be maintained by the α-blocking effect of droperidol and intravenous infusion of plasma expander without glucose, which is effective to reduce body temperature. Fentanyl suppresses the shivering center in the brain, and pancuronium or vecuronium suppresses shivering at peripheral sites, i.e., skeletal muscles. Midazolam, which is a benzodiazepine derivative and a γ-amino butylic acid agonist, is also usable. Muscle relaxants, such as pancuronium or vecuronium, are used at earlier stages, when mechanical venti-

TABLE 2. Protocol for sedation and muscle paralysis during mild hypothermia[a]

	Initial dose	Maintenance dose
Midazolam	$0.10\,mg{\cdot}kg^{-1}$	
Droperidol	$0.50\,mg{\cdot}kg^{-1}$	$0.025\,mg{\cdot}kg^{-1}{\cdot}h^{-1}$
Fentanyl	$0.01\,mg{\cdot}kg^{-1}$	$0.020\,mg{\cdot}kg^{-1}{\cdot}day^{-1}$
Pancuronium	$0.10\,mg{\cdot}kg^{-1}$	$0.050\,mg{\cdot}kg^{-1}{\cdot}h^{-1}$

[a] Peripheral microcirculation should be maintained by the α-blocking effect of droperidol and intravenous infusion of plasma expander, which is also effective for lowering body temperature. Shivering is prevented by the opiate and the muscle relaxant. Dosage of each drug is changed in each patient. Fentanyl is used with droperidol and/or midazolam

lation is performed, but are not used at later stages. Our sedative protocol for mild hypothermia therapy is adjusted to manage postoperative SAII patients, for which hyperdynamic and hypervolemic therapies are essential. This sedative protocol is applicable to manage other brain insults, because cardiac output, oxygen-carrying capacity, and tissue perfusion are much higher than those with ordinary sedative protocols. Morphine 10–20 mg·h^{-1} with methocrine 10–20 mg·h^{-1} is used by Clifton's group and fentanyl 50–100 μg·h^{-1} and vecuronium 10 mg·h^{-1} is used for 36 h by Marion's group [4,14a]. These preparations must be performed and completed before the start of cooling, because peripheral vasoconstriction caused by surface cooling is harmful for microcirculation and organ perfusion. We must recognize that drug metabolism is suppressed; hence, the duration of the drug effects will be prolonged by mild hypothermia.

Induction

Volume loading (500–1000 ml in adults) with plasma expanders, such as hydrooxyethyl starch, low-molecular-weight dextrane, or albumin, is essential to prevent hypotension and to dilate vessels made resistant by sedatives (droperidol) or analgesics (fentanyl) used in our protocol. Centralization of blood in lower extremities by elastic bandages and with positioning (jack-knife position) are also useful. Maintenance or elevation of cardiac output, reduction of systemic vascular resistance, and maintenance of microcirculation with higher oxygen delivery are able to accomplish this therapy with or without small amounts of β-agonistic catecholamine support.

When adequate sedation, analgesia, and vasodilatation are prepared with mechanical ventilation, mild hypothermia is initiated by surface cooling with a pair of cold-water-circulating mats, gastric irrigation with cold half-saline using a double balloon nasogastroduodenal tube (Ileus tube; Y-C, Fuji System, Tokyo, Japan). Additionally, venous infusion lines are cooled. If adequate vasodilatation (with appropriate volume load) is achieved by the α-blocking effect of droperidol and by reduction of endogenous catecholamines with fentanyl, heat exchange is adequately smooth and core body temperature is reduced to 32°C within 2 h. Because core body temperature usually decreases 2°C more after stoppage of the cooling, the cooling must stop at 34°C when the target core body temperature is 32°C.

Maintenance and Brain-oriented Intensive Care

Patients are treated with brain-oriented intensive care [18], as shown in Table 3. Adequate vasodilatation during the maintenance phase of mild hypothermia therapy is very important not only for heat exchange, but also for the maintenance of organ function. When vasodilatation is achieved, the temperature difference between the core and peripheral tissues will be less than 2°–3°C. The degree and duration of mild hypothermia in each brain insult are shown in Table 1, but they may be adjusted after accumulation of sufficient clinical data.

Mechanical ventilation must continue with controlled or synchronized intermittent mandatory mode. Hypoxemia caused by neurogenic pulmonary edema and/or aspiration pneumonia is prevented by increasing inspired oxygen concentration and low-level positive end-expiratory pressure ($\leqq 5$ cmH$_2$O) with head-up tilt position, if necessary. PaCO$_2$ is kept to a near normal value (35–40 mmHg) if ICP is controllable. A minute volume of ventilation is modulated, according to SjvO$_2$, which is a good and very sensitive index of the balance between cerebral metabolic rate for oxygen and cerebral blood flow. Nondepolarizing muscle relaxant may not be needed during the maintenance phase of mild hypothermia (32°–34°C) therapy if the patient is not resisting a ventilator or shivering. Because fentanyl suppresses the brainstem respiratory center and shivering, which occurs only at the beginning of cooling, the effect

TABLE 3. Brain-oriented intensive care

Respiration
$PaO_2 > 150$ torr, or around 100 torr (long term)
$PaCO_2 = 35$–40 torr, 30–35 torr (head-injured child)
   Change by internal jugular venous oxygen saturation or by intracranial pressure
Sedation: Prevent fighting against a ventilator and excessive body movements
   diazepam: 0.2 mg·kg^{-1}, pancuronium: 0.1 mg·kg^{-1}
   thiopental: 2–5 mg·kg^{-1} (use for intracranial hypertension), narcotics

Circulation
Cerebral perfusion pressure = 60–100 mmHg
   (relatively low in children and high in hypertensive patients)
Antiarrhythmia
   lidocaine: 1–2 mg·kg^{-1}, pindolol: 1–5 mg
Prevent hypotension
   dopamine: 2–15 µg·kg^{-1}·min^{-1}, dobutamine: 2–15 µg·kg^{-1}·min^{-1}
   (avoid persistent peripheral vasoconstriction)
Prevent hypertension
   Ca^{2+}-blocker (caution to intracranial hypertension)
      diltiazem: 2 mg, iv,   5–15 µg·kg^{-1}·min^{-1} (continuous infusion)
      nicardipine: 10–20 µg·kg^{-1}, iv, 0.3–3.0 µg·kg^{-1}·min^{-1} (continuous infusion)
Hemodilution
   Ht = 30%–35%, Hb = 10–12 g·dl^{-1}
Head-up tilt position
   10°–30°
Prevent excessive neck rotation, flexion, and extension

Metabolism
Plasma glucose
   80–120 mg·dl^{-1}, prevent hyperglycemia and hypoglycemia
Fluid transfusion
   Electrolytes solution: 30–50 ml·kg^{-1}·day^{-1} (infant 100 ml·kg^{-1}·day^{-1})
   pH: 7.3–7.5, Na^+: 135–145 mEq·l^{-1}
   Ca^{2+}: 1.0–1.3 mEq·l^{-1}, Mg^{2+}: 0.98–1.14 mEq·l^{-1} (Mg: 1.4–2.6 mg·dl^{-1})
   Serum osmolality: 280–320 mOsm·l^{-1}
   Colloid osmotic pressure > 15 mmHg, albumin > 4 g·dl^{-1}
Nutrition
Intravenous alimentation → nasointestinal tube feeding: 30–50 kcal·kg·day^{-1}
Body temperature: 35–37°C,
   Prefer mild hypothermia for severe cases (32°–34°C)

of muscle relaxant is prolonged, because of the slow metabolism caused by low body temperature. For example, $T_{1/2}$ of vecuronium is doubled by a 2°C reduction of core body temperature. The cardiac index must be kept higher than 3.0 l·min^{-1}·m^{-2} with hypervolemic and hyperdynamic treatments. Low cardiac output during mild hypothermia therapy is caused by bradycardia, while stroke volume and contractility of cardiac muscle are increased by mild hypothermia itself [23]. Therefore, a low dose (<5 µg·kg^{-1}·min^{-1}) of β1 catecholamine agonist, such as dobutamine and/or dopamine, is continuously infused intravenously. The cardiac index is usually kept at 3.0–6.0 l·min^{-1}·m^{-2} in this manner. Cerebral perfusion pressure, mean arterial pressure, and ICP are kept higher than 70 mmHg and 90–110 mmHg, and less than 20 mmHg, respectively, by Marion's protocol [14a]. When ICP has exceeded 20 mmHg, 200 ml of 10% glycerol is used for osmotherapy, although reduction of ICP is one of the effects of mild hypothermia [21]. If ICP increases persistently during this treatment, mannitol and/or thiopental must be used, but there is a high probability of poor outcome. Propofol may be useful as thiopental to reduce ICP. ICP was kept to less than 20 mmHg by means of mannitol and hyperventilation (SjvO$_2$ ≒ 50%, 25 mmHg < PaCO$_2$ ≦ 30 mmHg) in Clifton's group [4], and mannitol (25–50 g, every 3–4 h), ventricular drainage, and/or hyperventilation (PaCO$_2$ < 33 mmHg) and pentobarbital (60–120 mg·hr^{-1}) in Marion's group [14a].

Rewarming

The timing of patient rewarming is difficult to determine. The elements considered are the findings of brain CT, ICP, and electroencephalography. Anesthesia must be continued until the core temperature is returned to 36°–37°C. The patient should not be warmed, but the cooling is tapered off. This process takes several days: the core temperature is returned to 35°C, held there for 2–3 days, and raised to 36°–37°C. If organs and peripheral microcirculation are maintained during mild hypothermia, the rewarming period may be shortened (0.1°C, 1 h). In Clifton's group, the pace of rewarming was less than 1°C every 4 h [4].

Beneficial and Adverse Effects

We do not have any definitive conclusions of multicenter randomized crinical trials. In general, a high level of cerebral function could be protected and maintained. In clinical practice, the following beneficial effects are recognized. (1) suppression of cerebral metabolic rate for oxygen, (2) suppression of ICP [21,25], (3) maintenance of blood brain barrier function [16], (4) normalization of the elevated excitotoxic amino acids (glutamate and aspartate) in CSF [13], (5) suppression of the elevation of interleukin-1β (see the chapter by D.W. Marion, this volume), and interleukin-6 [1].

Additional beneficial effects have been demonstrated in animal experiments, and include (6) suppression of free radical reaction, (7) suppression of intracellular acidosis, (8) stabilization of the cell membrane, (9) suppression of intracellular Ca^{2+} accumulation, (10) maintenance of receptors, (11) maintenance of cytoskeltal protein, (12) suppression of translocation of protein kinase C isoforms. The adverse effects and their treatments are shown in Table 4.

Clinical Experience in Our Institute

Materials and Methods

Our mild hypothermia therapy protocol has been approved by the Yamaguchi University Hospital Ethical Committee for Human Study, and informed consent was obtained from the patients' families. The target core temperature measured in the superior jugular bulb, pulmonary artery, or bladder was 33°–34°C. We have applied the mild hypothermia therapy to five postoperative subarachnoid hemorrhage patients (SAH, Hunt and Kosnik grade 3 or 4, Fisher CT grade 3 or 4) and 37 head-injured patients (GCS ≦ 8) since 1991 [12,25]. A sedative protocol (Table 2), to maintain body functions and to prevent any adverse effects of hypothermia, should be started before cooling a patient's body. In our protocol, mild hypothermia should be maintained for 3–12 days or more after the brain insults. In addition to ordinary monitoring, special monitoring of the brain was performed.

Physiologic variables such as arterial blood pressure, heart rates, and acid–base balance were well-preserved during mild hypothermia therapy. Cardiac index was kept higher than

TABLE 4. Side effects of mild hypothermia and the treatments

Side effect	Treatment
Respiratory depression	Artificial ventilation
Arrythmia (VPC[a])	Lidocaine
Vascular constriction	Droperidol and volume load
Low cardiac output	Dobutamine and/or low-dose dopamine
Metabolic acidosis	Improve microcirculation
Electrolyte imbalance hypokalemia	Drip infusion of KCl (up to lower limit of normal range)
Bleeding tendency plt $< 5 \times 10^4 \mu l^{-1}$	Gabexate mesilate, nafamostat mesilate Platelet concentrate transfusion
Immunosuppression infection	γ-Globurin and urinastatine Antibiotics, antifungal drugs
Liver hypofunction	Maintain hepatic blood flow
Renal hypofunction	Maintain renal blood flow Low-dose dopamine
Gastrointestinal tract hypofunction	Prevent bacterial translocation, glutamine, abdominal massage
Hyperglycemia	Insulin (+KCl)
Suppress drug metabolism	Reduced dosages and monitoring plasma level

[a] VPC, ventricular premature contraction

$3.0 l \cdot min^{-1} \cdot m^{-2}$, usually $4.0–6.0 l \cdot min^{-1} \cdot m^{-2}$, with either dobutamine or low-dose dopamine support. The oxygenation index (PaO_2/FIO_2) could be maintained higher than 200 by artificial ventilation, even in the patients who had aspiration pneumonia. Hepatorenal function was maintained without major insult, probably owing to high cardiac output and good microcirculation of the organs. Plasma potassium was kept at the lower limit of the normal range by supplemental KCl drip infusion, because a low plasma level of K^+ during mild hypothermia therapy may induce cardiac arrhythmia, and the level will exceed the normal range during the rewarming period, which would cause ventricular fibrillation. Platelet counts decreased to 50000/mm³. The coagulopathy caused by the brain insult itself and by mild hypothermia was controlled with gabexate mesilate or gabexate nafamostat, and platelet concentrate. Immune suppression by mild-hypothermia-caused infection, especially pulmonary infection, was prevented or cured by antibiotics, urinastatine (inhibits leukocyte activation, leukocyte elastase, and cytokines), and immunoglobulin.

In the SAH patients, cerebrospinal fluid (CSF) excitotoxic amino acids (glutamate, glycine), and nitrite (NO_2) and nitrate (NO_3) were analyzed using a high-performance liquid chromatograph with an electrochemical detector (ECD-100, EICOM, Kyoto, Japan), and a capillary electropherograph (Waters, Milford, MA, USA), respectively [8,26].

The values were compared with those in neurologically normal groups by ANOVA and $P < 0.05$ was considered statistically significant.

Results and Discussion

Three out of five patients in SAH and 17 out of 37 patients in severe head injuries had good outcomes (good recovery or moderate disability), as evaluated by the Glasgow Outcome Scale.

In a severe head-injured patient, venous oxygen saturation measured at the superior jugular bulb ($SjvO_2$) is one of the best parameters to determine the global balance between cerebral

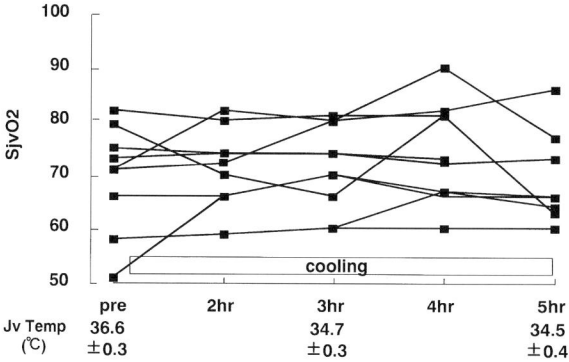

FIG. 3. Sequential changes of internal jugular venous oxygen saturation during mild hypothermia therapy in severe head-injured patients. Venous oxygen saturation ($SjvO_2$) measured in the superior jugular bulb was increased during mild hypothermia therapy, which means the balance between cerebral blood flow and cerebral metabolic rate for oxygen was preserved or improved. *JvTemp*, venous blood temperature measured at the superior jugular bulb

blood flow and cerebral metabolic rate for oxygen [17]. Recently, $SjvO_2$ can be measured continuously using an optical fiber with an oxygen saturation/cardiac output system (Oximetrix 3, SO2/CO computer, or OPT 002/RI, Abbott, USA), which can be inserted very safely [11]. If the physician is familiar with cerebral physiology and pathophysiology, the interpretations of the $SjvO_2$ changes are not difficult. The details of $SjvO_2$ are described elsewhere [17]. $SjvO_2$ was either increased or unchanged during mild hypothermia therapy, so that the balance between flow and metabolism was well maintained in the head-injured patients (Fig. 3) [25]. Intracranial pressure, measured in the subdural or intraventricular space, decreased during mild hypothermia therapy, which was demonstrated by Shiozaki [21]. Even though the reduction of core temperature was small (36.6 ± 0.3°C to 34.5 ± 0.4°C), the reduction of intracranial pressure was recorded in our cases. This phenomenon is also demonstrated noninvasively by means of near infrared spectroscopy (NIRO-500, Hamamatsu Photonics, Hamamatsu, Japan) [24], by which cerebral blood volume (oxyhemoglobin + deoxyhemoglobin) measured by NIRO-500 decreased with mild hypothermia therapy. This decrease might reflect the reduction of intracranial pressure.

Electroencephalogram traces did not disappear, because we used neurolept analgesia. Therefore, laterality could be recognized, whereas it could not be seen during barbiturate coma therapy. The latency of wave V in the auditory brain-stem-evoked response was prolonged by mild hypothermia itself, because conduction time is delayed by lowering the temperature. The prolonged latency did not recover for several days, even in the neurologically good outcome cases. The reasons for the latter need to be clarified.

Table 5 shows the concentrations of glutamate, glycine, and $NO_2 + NO_3$ in CSF in SAH patients who were treated with mild hypothermia and those in neurologically normal subjects [12,13]. High concentrations of glutamate during the prehypothermia period were normalized during the early phase of mild hypothermia therapy [12,13]. In neurologically poor outcome cases, very high concentrations of CSF glutamate were recorded. While glycine and $NO_2 + NO_3$ were significantly high during prehypothermia and hypothermia periods in SAH patients [13]. These results demonstrated that mild hypothermia therapy is effective to reduce CSF excitotoxic glutamate, but not to reduce CSF glycine and $NO_2 + NO_3$. Therefore, glycine

TABLE 5. Excitatory amino acids and NO_X concentrations in cerebrospinal fluid in subarachnoid hemorrhage patients

	Control values in patients without neurological disorder[a] ($n = 15$)	Subarachnoid hemorrhage-hypothermia ($n = 5$)	
		Prehypothermia	Hypothermia
Glutamate	2.0 ± 1.1	4.4 ± 2.2^b	3.4 ± 1.2
Glycine	4 ± 1	42 ± 20^b	33 ± 23
$NO_2 + NO_3$	6.3 ± 1.7	9.2 ± 2.7^b	9.7 ± 2.4^b

[a] Values are expressed at mean $\pm$ SD
[b] Significantly different from control, $p < 0.05$

antagonists and neuronal and inducible NO synthetase inhibitors would add protection to mild hypothermia therapy in severe brain insults during the acute phase.

Conclusions

There is no doubt that mild hypothermia has protective effects in the animal models of brain ischemia, hypoxia, and trauma. Our own recent data [12,25] and those of other investigators [4,7,14a,16,21] suggest that mild hypothermia can be applied in severe acute brain insults without major complications, and its many beneficial effects have been reconfirmed in patients. Mild hypothermia with brain-oriented intensive care is a promising new therapy for brain protection or resuscitation in stroke, severe head injury, and, probably, cardiopulmonary-resuscitated patients.

References

1. Aibiki M, Maekawa S, Ogura S, Kinoshita Y, Kawai N, Yokono S (1999) Effect of moderate hypothermia on systolic and internal jugular plasma IL-6 levels after traumatic brain injury in humans. J Neurotrauma 16:225–232
2. Busto R, Dietrich WD, Globus MY, Valdes I, Scheinberg P, Ginsberg MD (1987) Small differences in intraischemic brain temperature critically determine the extent of ischemic neuronal injury. J Cereb Blood Flow Metab 7:229–238
3. Busto R, Globus MY, Dietrich WD, Martinez E, Valdes I, Ginsberg MD (1989) Effect of mild hypothermia on ischemia-induced release of neurotransmitters and free fatty acids in rat brain. Stroke 20:904–910
4. Clifton GL (1995) Systemic hypothermia in treatment of severe brain injury: a review and update. J Neurotrauma 12:923–927
5. Coimbra C, Drake B, Boris-Moller F, Wieloch T (1996) Long-lasting neuroprotective effects of postischemic hypothermia and treatment with an anti-inflammatory/antipyretic drug. Evidence for encephalopathic processes following ischemia. Stroke 27:1578–1585
6. Colbourne F, Sutherland G, Corbett D (1997) Postischemic hypothermia. A clinical appraisal with implications for clinical treatment. Mol Neurobiol 14:171–201
7. Hayashi N (1997) Combination therapy of cerebral hypothermia, pharmacological activation of the dopamine system, and hormonal replacement in severely brain damaged patients. J Jpn Soc Intensive Care Med 4:191–197
8. Kashiwagi S, Fujisawa H, Yamashita T, Ito H, Maekawa T, Kuroda Y, Tateishi A (1994) Excitotoxic amino acid neurotransmitters are increased in human cerebrospinal fluid after subarachnoid haemorrhage. Neurol Neurosurg Psychiat 57:1442–1443

9. Kataoka K (1996) Mild hypothermia as a stroke treatment: basic examination and clinical establishment. Annual Report of Research on Cardiovascular Diseases. National Cardiovascular Center, Osaka, pp. 623–649

10. Kataoka K, Yanase H (1998) Mild hypothermia. A revived countermeasure against ischemic neuronal damages. Neurosci Res 32:103–117

11. Maekawa T, Sakabe T, Takeshita H (1984) An easy technique for catheterization of the internal jugular bulb. Stroke 15:179–180

12. Maekawa T, Tateishi A, Sadamitsu D, Kuroda Y, Soejima Y, Kashiwagi S, Yamashita T, Ito H (1994) Clinical application of mild hypothermia in neurological disorders. Minerva Anestesiol 60:537–540

13. Maekawa T, Tateishi A, Sadamitsu D, Kuroda Y, Soejima Y, Nakashima K, Kashiwagi S, Fujisawa H, Ito H (1996) Evaluation of mild hypothermia therapy with CSF excitotoxic amino acids and NOx in human neurological disorders. J Neurochem 66(Suppl 2):S-5B

14a. Marion DW, Obrist WD, Carlier PM, Penrod LE, Darby JM (1993) The use of moderate therapeutic hypothermia for patients with severe head injuries: A preliminary report. J Neurosurg 79:354–362

14b. Marion DW (1996) Critical Care Med 24:81–89

15. Minamisawa H, Smith ML, Siesjo BK (1990) The effect of mild hyperthermia and hypothermia on brain damage following 5, 10, and 15 minutes of forebrain ischemia. Ann Neurol 28:26–33

16. Naritomi H, Shimizu T, Oe H, Kinugawa H, Sawada T, Hirata T (1996) Mild hypothermia therapy in acute embolic stroke: a pilot sudy. J Stroke Cerebrovascul Dis 6 (Suppl I):193–196

17. Sadamitsu D, Maekawa T (1997) Basic and clinical meanings of oxygen saturation measured in internal jugular venous bulb. J Jpn Assoc Acute Med 8:637–649

18. Sadamitsu D, Nakashima K, Maekawa T (1996) Mild hypothermia with brain oriented intensive care for cerebral protection. Japanese experience. Bull Intensive Critical Care 3:11–14

19. Schwartz AJ, Campbell FW (1989) Cardiopulmonary resuscitation. In: Barash PG, Cullen BF, Stoelting RK (eds) Clinical anesthesia. Lippincott, Philadelphia, pp. 1477–1516

20. Shimizu T, Suzuki N (1996) Nitric oxide and central nervous system. J Jpn Soc Intensive Care Med 3:69–82

21. Shiozaki T, Sugimoto H, Taneda M, Yoshida H, Iwai A, Yoshioka T, Sugimoto T (1993) Effect of mild hypothermia on uncontrollable intracranial hypertension after severe head injury. J Neurosurg 79:363–368

22. Siesjo BK, Zhao Q, Pahlmark K, Siesjo P, Katsura K, Folbergrova J (1995) Glutamate, calcium, and free radicals as mediators of ischemic brain damage. Ann Thorac Surg 59:1316–1320

23. Suga H, Goto Y, Igarashi Y, Yasumura Y, Nozawa T, Futaki S, Tanaka N (1998) Cardiac cooling increases E_{max} without affecting relation between O_2 consumption and systolic pressure-volume area in dog left ventricle. Circ Res 63:61–71

24. Tateishi A, Maekawa T, Soejima Y, Sadamitsu D, Yamamoto M, Matsushita M, Nakashima K (1995) Qualitative comparison of carbon dioxide-induced change in cerebral near-infrared spectroscopy versus jugular venous oxygen saturation in adult with acute brain disease. Critical Care Med 23:1734–1738

25. Tateishi A, Soejima Y, Taira Y, Nakashima K, Fujisawa H, Tsuchida E, Maekawa T, Ito H (1998) Feasibility of the titration method of mild hypothermia in severely head-injured patients with intracranial hypertension. Neurosurgery 42:1065–1070

26. Ueda T, Maekawa T, Sadamitsu D, Oshita S, Ogino K, Nakamura K (1995) The determination of nitrite and nitrate in human blood plasma by capillary zone electrophoresis. Electrophoresis 16:1002–1004

Combined Therapy of Local Intraarterial Thrombolysis and Brain Hypothermia for Acute Occlusion of the Cerebral Main Trunk Arteries

Yoshio Takasato[1], Hiroyuki Masaoka[1], Hiroaki Wakimoto[1], Nobuyuki Naoe[1], Kuniyasu Saigusa[1], Miho Nagai[1], and Kemmei Kuramoto[2]

Summary. Aiming to improve the treatment results of acute cerebral main trunk artery occlusion (CMTAO), the following treatment was carried out. The factors that contribute to the treatment result were analyzed. The study was divided into two groups (A and B) with 29 patients each. In the A group (average age 67.6 years) were 21 patients with an average Glasgow Coma Scale (GCS) of 8.0 whose local neurological deficits due to CMTAO were confirmed by cerebral angiogram; cerebral hemorrhage and new infarction were ruled out by computed tomography (CT). Pro-urokinase (pro-UK) was infused intermittently while breaking up the thrombus with a microcatheter at the time of angiography immediately after the admission CT scan. In group B, after the same thrombolytic treatment, brain hypothermia treatment was added. The average age in the eight group B patients was 63.5 years with an average GCS of 9.6. Prognosis was evaluated by the Glasgow Outcome Scale (GOS) on discharge. The recanalization rate of this thrombolytic treatment was satisfactory (69.2% on average). Although a good prognosis (good recovery + moderately disabled) was seen in 10 cases (46.7%) in group A, in 7 cases (33.3%) there was death originating from hemorrhagic infarction and acute cerebral swelling. In group B no cerebral complications influenced the prognosis; five patients had a good prognosis (67%). Local intraarterial thrombolysis is effective as treatment of acute CMTAO, and a good prognosis can be expected when combining treatment with brain hypothermia.

Key words. Combined therapy, Local intraarterial thrombolysis, Brain hypothermia, Cerebral main trunk artery, Acute cerebral infarction

Introduction

Regarding treatment for an acute cerebral infarction, the use of intravenous (IV) tissue plasminogen activator (t-PA) is authorized if it is within 3 h from the onset, based on a study at the U.S. National Institutes of Health completed in 1995 [11]. Intravenous t-PA has come to be used widely [1]. However, the recanalization rate with IV t-PA infusion is low with acute cerebral main trunk artery occlusion (CMTAO) other than peripheral branch occlusion

Departments of [1] Neurosurgery and [2] Radiology, National Hospital Tokyo Disaster Medical Center, 3256 Midori-cho, Tachikawa, Tokyo 190-0014, Japan

[2,5,9,10,18]. A dispute is breaking out between the use of local intraarterial (IA) treatment and IV treatment [4,10,17]. We performed local IA thrombolysis applying pro-UK to the CMTAO, which is has had an extremely poor prognosis until now [7]. Theoretically, pro-UK is associated with little bleeding tendency with high thrombus affinity in many thrombolytic agents [7]. Furthermore, we add brain hypothermia treatment, which has a well-known brain protection effect in cerebral ischemia [3,6,13,15]. The result of each treatment was analyzed.

Materials and Methods

There was disturbed consciousness at the onset of the disease or at presentation in all 29 patients. Informed consent to the treatment was obtained for all patients. Cerebral hemorrhage and new cerebral infarction were ruled out, other than sulcal effacement and loss of gray-white matter distinction as an early ischemic change, by a CT scan and the local neurological deficit presented as motor hemiparesis. Postictal state and metabolic disease were also eliminated, as were patients who had already been recanalized and had a peripheral branch occlusion on a cerebral angiogram. Three-vessel cerebral angiography was performed as promptly as possible after CT. The pro-UK was infused intermittently (3.3 mg/20 ml saline/20 min) while breaking up the thrombus with a microcatheter after confirmation of CMTAO. The upper limit of total pro-UK dosage was 10 mg. Argatroban, a synthetic thrombin inhibitor, was used for 1 week as anticoagulant after the thrombolysis. Survey items were age, gender, consciousness on admission, CT on admission, occlusion site, collateral circulation, duration of the onset to thrombolysis, postangiographic CT, CT after 24 h, pro-UK dose, GOS estimated by CT, and GOS on discharge as an evaluation of prognosis. Duration of the onset to thrombolysis was measured at the time of the last pro-UK infusion in the patient without recanalization. The recanalization rate combined complete opening and partial opening. Characteristics of the 21 patients in whom only thrombolysis was performed were summarized in Table 1.

In eight cases, the brain hypothermia treatment was carried out after local IA thrombolysis. The cooling was carried out with whole-body water cooling by blankets (two sheets on

TABLE 1. Characteristics of 21 patients undergoing local intraarterial thrombolysis treatment only

Parameter	MCA ($n = 8$)	BA ($n = 6$)	ICA ($n = 7$)
Onset to thrombolysis (min)	244 ± 76	197 ± 46	230 ± 74
Age (years)	66.6 ± 15.9	65.2 ± 11.1	70.6 ± 5.8
Male/female	5/3	2/4	2/5
Recanalization rate (%)	62.5	83.3	57.1
pro-UK (mg)	8.1 ± 3.2	9.1 ± 1.9	8.6 ± 2.6
GCS on admission	9.6 ± 3.2	4.2 ± 1.2	9.4 ± 3.4
GOS on discharge[a]	4.0 ± 1.3	2.5 ± 1.8	1.7 ± 1.3

Data are mean values ± SD
MCA, Middle cerebral artery; BA, basilar artery; ICA, internal carotid artery; pro-UK, pro-urokinase; GCS, Glasgow Coma Scale; GOS, Glasgow Outcome Scale
[a] GOS is scored as follows: good recovery 5; moderately disabled 4; severely disabled 3; persistent vegetative state 2; dead 1

TABLE 2. Characteristics of 29 patients undergoing local intraarterial thrombolysis only or combined therapy with brain hypothermia

Parameter	Only thrombolysis ($n = 21$)	Plus hypothermia ($n = 8$)
Onset to thrombolysis (min)	226 ± 67	214 ± 44
Age (years)	67.6 ± 11.6	63.5 ± 11.7
Male/female	5/12	5/3
Recanalization rate (%)	66.7	75.0
pro-UK (mg)	8.6 ± 2.6	8.4 ± 2.3
Occlusion site	MCA 8, BA 6, ICA 7	MCA 2, BA 2, ICA 4[a]
GCS on admission	8.0 ± 2.7	9.6 ± 2.7
GOS on discharge	2.6 ± 2.7	3.0 ± 1.4

[a] The ICA occlusion was frequent in the combined treatment group

both the top and bottom of the body). The cooling was started early, preferably after thrombolysis. The temperature was controlled with a jugular bulb blood temperature. The target temperature for cooling was 35°C except for one case of 32°C. After this temperature was maintained for 3 days, the patient was rewarmed gradually to 37°C over next 4 days. The characteristics of the eight patients who had combined local IA thrombolysis and brain hypothermia are summarized in Table 2.

Results

The recanalization rate was 66.7% in group A and 75.0% in group B (69.2% on average). A good prognosis [good recovery (GR) + moderately disabled (MD)] was seen 10 patients (46.7%) in group A. There were nine deaths including seven whose trouble originated in the brain as the result of this treatment. Brain hypothermia in group B was introduced to alleviate this problem. The prognosis was good, in decreasing order, for the middle cerebral artery (MCA), basilar artery (BA), and internal carotid artery (ICA) groups (Fig. 1). All recanalized

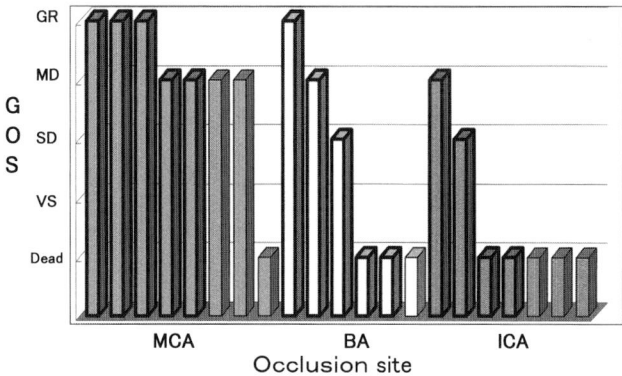

FIG. 1. Correlation between the occlusion site and prognosis on discharge in each group. Prognosis was fine, in decreasing order, for the middle cerebral artery (*MCA*), basilar artery (*BA*), and internal carotid artery (*ICA*) groups. Each bar of thick frame shows the recanalized case that had fine prognosis in all of each group in common. The average recanalization rate was 62.5% with MCA, 83.3% with BA, and 57.1% with ICA. *GOS*, Glasgow Outcome Scale; *GR*, good recovery; *MD*, moderately disabled; *SD*, severely disabled; *VS*, vegetative state

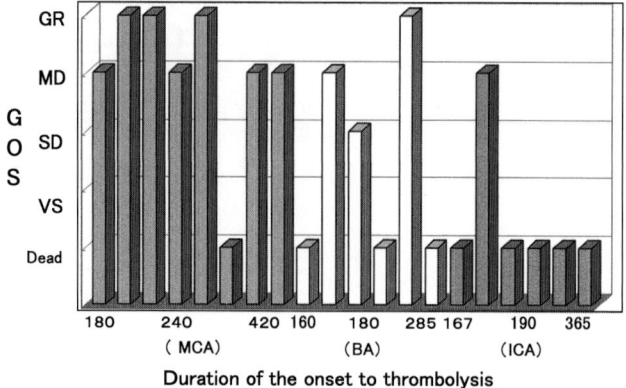

FIG. 2. Correlation between the duration of onset to thrombolysis and the prognosis in each group. The duration time is displayed in minutes. The average duration time was 244 min with MCA, 197 min with BA, and 230 min with ICA. The duration of onset to recanalization did not correlate well with the prognosis on discharge

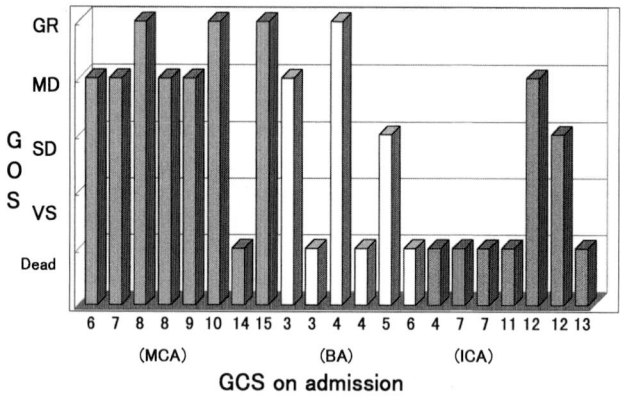

FIG. 3. Correlation between GCS on admission and prognosis in each group. Consciousness level on admission and the duration between onset to thrombolysis did not correlate well with the prognosis on discharge. The average GCS on admission was 9.6 with MCA, 4.2 with BA, and 9.4 with ICA. Low value was shown clearly with BA. GCS, Glasgow Coma Scale

patients in both groups had a good prognosis. The duration between onset to recanalization and consciousness level on arrival did not correlate well with the prognosis on discharge (Figs. 2, 3).

As the result of combining brain hypothermia with local IA thrombolysis, there was a good prognosis (GR + MD) in five of eight patients (62.5%). Whereas there were seven deaths (33%) in the group treated with local-thrombolysis only, there were deaths in group B. In other words, in group A there were seven cases of deaths in which total brain necrosis was seen on CT (Fig. 4). There were no such cases showing total brain necrosis on CT in group B (Fig. 5). Although the vertebrobasilar artery was not recanalized in case 1, brain hypothermia was

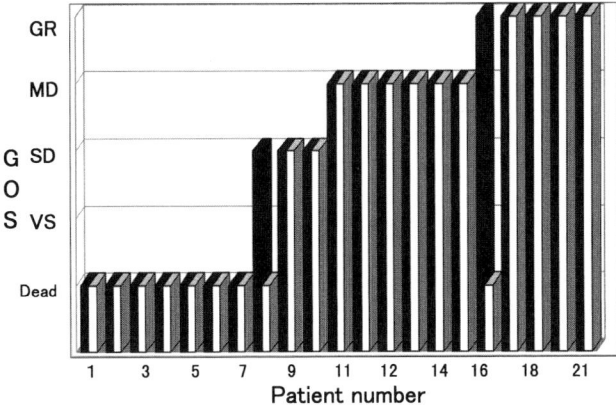

FIG. 4. GOS estimated by computed tomography (CT) and GOS on discharge in the group treated by thrombolysis alone. *Black bars*, GOS estimated by CT; *white bars* GOS on discharge. In two cases the prognosis deteriorated, in contradiction to the prediction from the CT finding. The prognosis is prescribed with the factor of brain

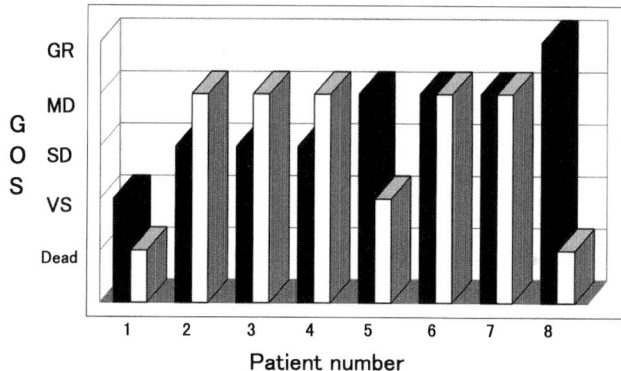

FIG. 5. GOS estimated by CT and on discharge in the group who underwent combined therapy with brain hypothermia. *Black bars*, GOS estimated by CT; *white bars*, GOS on discharge. Prognosis deteriorated in three cases due to a complication during the chronic phase

performed at 32°C. Total infarction of the brain stem was presented on the CT scan and on magnetic resmance imaging (MRI) in this case. Midriasis and respiratory arrest did not occur. He died with pneumonia 2 months from the onset of the disease. Large infarctions remained in patients 2–4, but, disturbance of the higher brain functions and motor paresis were slight. Although the early clinical course was fine for patient 5, the prognosis had deteriorated owing to a repeat infarction. Patient 8 had had chronic obstructive pulmonary disease; and although slight pneumonia occurred after the brain hypothermia treatment at 35°C the patient recovered. His imaging results and neurological findings were entirely normal, but he died with pulmonary and cardiac failure during the chronic period.

Discussion

Cumulative experience suggests a much higher recanalization rate after local IA infusion than after intravenous infusion of several plasminogen activators, especially with CMTAO [4,7,9,12]. Our 69.2% recanalization rate as a whole was a higher than has been reported in previous reports [2,7,16]. The use of pro-UK and mechanical disruption of the thrombus are credited for this high rate.

There are various opinions regarding the therapeutic time window for acute cerebral infarction [1,2,7,8,11]. The severity of the disease, occlusion site, and so on are suggested as factors that influence this judgment [3,4,17]. Our results showed that recanalization is a major influence on prognosis, even more so than time [16].

The complications of thrombolysis, intracerebral hemorrhage, and cerebral swelling are well known [7,10,17]. Although we used the pro-UK that is supported to causes the fewest complications, there were side effects in 33%. We introduced the brain hypothermia treatment to overcome these complications and to provide the brain with some protection. Since the review of efficacy of mild brain hypothermia to treat cerebral ischemia by Busto et al. in 1987, there have been many reports that brain hypothermia is effective in cerebral ischemia [3,6,15]. However, although it has been reported that temperature influences the prognosis of cerebral infarction in patients, clinical application of brain hypothermia has just begun [13]. We have been using brain hypothermia to treat severe head injury for the past 3 years in many patients. From our treatment results and the knowledge gained with this experience we can begin to understand the mechanism of the maintenance of the blood-brain barrier function and the various protective effects to the nerve cell by brain hypothermia.

The following findings were derived from our preliminary experiences in eight cases. Hemorrhagic infarction and acute brain swelling can be decreased by the brain hypothermia treatment. It reduces the size of the cerebral infarction. It also has the effect of decreasing the neurological deficit, even if the cerebral infarction remains apparent on imaging. Because there are many aged pulmonary and heart failure patients, 35°C was deemed the appropriate target temperature.

Conclusions

Combined local IA thrombolysis and brain hypothermia for treating acute CMTAO is judged effective. It is possible that this combined therapy can expand the therapeutic window of this disease. Brain protection based on maintenance of blood–brain barrier function is obtained by adding brain hypothermia to the local IA thrombolysis regimen. A good prognosis can be expected as a result.

References

1. Adams HP Jr, Brott TG, Furlan AJ, Gomez CR, Grotta J, Helgason CM, Kwiatkowski T, Lyden PD, Marler JR, Torner J, Feinberg W, Mayberg M, Thies W (1996) Guideline for thrombolytic therapy for acute stroke: a supplement to the guideline for the management of patients with acute ischemic stroke. Stroke 27:1711–1718
2. Bendszus M, Urbach H, Ries F, Solymosi L (1998) Outcome after local intra-arterial fibrinolysis compared with the natural course of patients with a dense middle cerebral artery on early CT. Neuroradiology 40:54–58
3. Busto R, Dietrich WD, Globus MYT, Valdes I, Scheinberg P, Ginsberg MD (1987) Small differ-

ence in intraischemic brain temperature critically determine the extent of ischemic neuronal injury. J Cereb Blood Flow Metabl 7:729–738

4. Caplan LR, Mohr JP, Kistler PJ, Koroshetz W (1997) Should thrombolytic therapy be the first-line treatment for acute ischemic stroke? N Engl J Med 337:1309–1310

5. Casto L, Caverni L, Camerlingo M, Censori B, Moschini L, Servalli MC, Partziguian T, Belloni G, Mamoli A (1996) Intra-arterial thrombolysis in acute ischemic stroke: experience with a superselective catheter embedded in the clot. J Neurol Neurosurg Psychiatry 60:667–670

6. Coimbra C, Wieloch T (1994) Moderate hypothermia mitigates neuronal damage in the rat brain when initiated several hours following transient cerebral ischemia. Acta Neuropathol (Berl) 87:325–331

7. Del Zoppo GJ, Higashida RT, Furlan AJ, Pessin MS, Rowley HA, Gent M, PROACT investigators (1998) PROACT: a phase II randomized trial of recombinant pro-urokinase by direct arterial delivery in acute middle cerebral artery stroke. Stroke 29:4–11

8. Gross CE, Raymond SJ, Howard DB, Bednar MM (1995) Delayed tissue-plasminogen activator therapy in a rabbit model of thromboembolic stroke. Neurosurgery 36:1172–1177

9. Hache W, Zeumer H, Ferbert A, Bruckmann H, del Zoppo GL (1988) Intra-arterial thrombolytic therapy improves outcome in patients with acute vertebrobasilar occlusive disease. Stroke 19:1216–1222

10. Jansen O, von Kummer R, Forsting M, Hache W, Sartor K (1995) Thrombolytic therapy in acute occlusion of the intracranial internal carotid artery bifurcation. Am J Neuroradiol 16:1977–1986

11. National Institute of Neurological Disorders and Stroke rt-PA Stroke Study Group (1995) Tissue plasminogen activator for acute ischemic stroke. N Engl J Med 333:1581–1587

12. Nesbit GM, Clark WM, O'Neill OR, Barnwell SL (1996) Intracranial intraarterial thrombolysis facilitated by microcatheter navigation through an occluded cervical internal carotid artery. J Neurosurg 84:387–392

13. Reith J, Jorgensen HS, Pedersen PM, Nakayama H, Raaschou HO, Jeppensen LL, Olsen TS (1996) Body temperature in acute stroke: relation to stroke severity, infarct size, mortality, and outcome. Lancet 347:422–425

14. Schwarz S, Egelhof T, Schwab S, Hacke W (1997) Basilar artery embolism. Neurology 49:1346–1352

15. Todd MM, Warner DS (1992) A comfortable hypothesis reevaluated. Anesthesiology 76:161–164

16. Von Kummer R, Holle R, Rosin L, Forsting M, Hacke W (1995) Does arterial recanalization improve outcome in carotid territiry stroke? Stroke 26:581–587

17. Wolpert SM, Bruckmann H, Greenlee R, Wechsler L, Pessin MS, del Zoppo GJ, rt-PA Acute Stroke Group (1993) Neuroradiological evaluation of patients with acute stroke treated with recombinant tissue plasminogen activator. Am J Neuroradiol 14:3–13

18. Zeumer H, Feitag HJ, Zanella F, Thie A, Arning C (1993) Local intra-arterial fibrinolysis therapy in patients with stroke: urokinase versus recombinant tissue plasminogen activator (r-TPA). Neuroradiology 35:159–162

Mild Hypothermia for Cerebral Resuscitation in Survivors of Out-of-Hospital Ventricular Fibrillation

Ken Nagao[1]*, Nariyuki Hayashi[1], Ken Arima[2], Kimio Kikushima[2], Jougi Ohtsuki[1], and Katsuo Kanmatsuse[2]

Summary. As emergency and intensive care medicine progresses, brain hypothermia is attracting attention as a therapeutic method that overcomes the limitations of cerebral protection and resuscitation. We conducted a preliminary study by preparing a protocol of mild hypothermia by coil cooling at 34°C in patients who returned to spontaneous circulation via standard advanced cardiac life support and had experienced out-of-hospital ventricular fibrillation (VF) due to suspected cardiac arrest. Primary endpoints were survival at hospital discharge and good recovery using the Glasgow Outcome Scale. This study was performed in 15 patients meeting the inclusion criteria of mild hypothermia. The average core temperature during mild hypothermia at the cooling stage was 34.4°C, and the average duration was 83.9 h. Survival rate at hospital discharge was 80%, and the good recovery rate was 67%. Multivariate analysis revealed that systemic oxygen delivery at the cooling stage was an indepedent predictor of good recovery. In conclusion, brain hypothermia (at a temperature of 34°C for 3 days and by coil cooling) in comatose survivors with out-of-hospital VF may have improved the outcome.

Key words. Hypothermia, Cerebral resuscitation, Out-of-hospital ventricular fibrillation, Sudden cardiac arrest, Good recovery

Introduction

Standard cardiopulmonary resuscitation (CPR) originated in electrical defibrillation [20] reported in 1956, rescue ventilation with mouth-to-mouth technique [17] in 1958, and closed-chest compression [13] reported in 1960. For about 40 years since then, the technique and theory of CPR have undergone changes and become the technique prevailing today, but it has not undergone much change essentially. On the other hand, the concept of CPR has developed into cardiopulmonary cerebral resuscitation (CPCR), and cerebral resuscitation after the

[1] Department of Emergency and Critical Care Medicine, Nihon University School of Medicine, 30-1 Oyaguchi Kami-machi, Itabashi-ku, Tokyo 173-8610, Japan
[2] Department of Cardiology, Nihon University School of Medicine, 1-8-13 Kanda Surugadai, Chiyoda-ku, Tokyo 101-8309, Japan
* Present address: Surugadai Nihon University Hospital, 1-8-13 Kanda Surugadai, Chiyoda-ku, Tokyo 101-8309, Japan

return of spontaneous circulation (ROSC) is being studied. However, there have been no reports of drugs found to be evidently useful for cerebral resuscitation. The therapeutic use of hypothermia in a patient with traumatic brain injury was first reported in 1943 [6], but the procedure became obsolete due to various problems involved.

In 1987 Busto et al. [1] reported that the procedure had a cerebral protective effect owing to a decrease in cerebral temperature by several degrees centigrade, and preliminary reports on three clinical trials of moderate hypothermia in patients with traumatic brain injury were published in 1993 [3,4,18]. We reported the efficacy of an alternative CPCR using emergency cardiopulmonary bypass, coronary reperfusion therapy and mild hypothermia in patients with out-of-hospital cardiac arrest [16]. The purpose of this study was to evaluate the effect of brain hypothermia in comatose survivors of out-of-hospital ventricular fibrillation (VF).

Materials and Methods

Candidates for Mild Hypothermia by Coil Cooling

The subjects were patients who fulfilled all of the following criteria:

1. Patients with a suspected cardiac cause of VF experienced out-side the hospital and aged from 18 to 74.
2. Patients whose systolic blood pressure was increased above 90 mmHg after ROSC by standard CPR [5].
3. Patients who underwent emergency coronary angiography immediately after ROSC and on whom coronary reperfusion therapy was performed in the presence of acute coronary-artery occlusion.
4. Patients whose Glasgow Coma Scale (GCS) score [19] before hypothermia was 3–5 and whose families assented informed consent to the hypothermia.

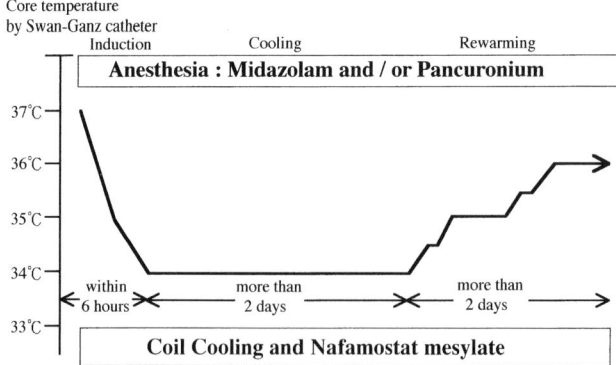

FIG. 1. Method of mild hypothermia treatment by coil cooling. For the core temperature coil cooling, which cools the blood circuit of continuous hemodialysis filtration directly, was used with pulmonary arterial blood temperature by Swan-Ganz catheter as an index. Induction and rewarming were conducted by two step-down and slow step-up methods, respectively. Midazolam and pancuronium were used for anesthesia during this period, and nafamostat mesylate was used for control of coagulant drug. Activated coagulation time was controlled at 150–200 s. (MONAN or KANEM method, see the chapter by Okamoto et al., this volume). (Modified from Hayashi 1997, with permission)

Protocol of Mild Hypothermia by Coil Cooling

Figure 1 shows the technique of mild hypothermia by coil cooling. The blood temperature in the pulmonary artery is measured continually by a Swan-Ganz catheter (model CCOTD catheter). The blood was cooled directly (see chapter by Okamoto et al., this volume). Nafamastat mesylate was used as anticoagulant, and the activated coagulation time was controlled between 150 and 200 s. The standard for controlling hypothermia conformed to the method of Hayashi [8,9]. A γ-amino butyric acid (GABA) agonist drug (midazolam) and muscle-relaxant drug (pancuronium) were used for anethesia. The two-step-down method and slow step-up method were used for induction and rewarming of hypothermia, respectively.

Cooling temperature and duration were set at 34°C and more than 2 days (usually 3 days), respectively [16]. Other standards used were as follows: systemic blood pressure >90 mmHg; hemoglobin >12 g/dl; systemic oxygen delivery >520 ml/min/m²; and oxygen extraction rate 20%–30%. Some other variables were controlled as well: complete parenteral nutrition, water and electrolytes for continuous hemodialysis filtration (CHDF), and respiration by an artificial respiratory apparatus and postural drainage.

Study of Endpoints

As the primary endpoints, the rates of survival at hospital discharge (vegetative state, severe disability, moderate disability, good recovery) and good recovery (able to return to work) were assessed using the Glasgow Outcome Scale [11]. The factors predictive of good recvovery were assessed.

Statistical Analysis

Data are expressed as the mean ± SD. Statistical comparisons were performed using Student's t-test, Fisher's exact test, and the stepwise multiple logistic regression model. P values <0.05 were considered significant.

Results

Characteristics of Patients

Sixty patients with out-of-hospital VF were transported to our emergency room from (January 1996 to December 1998). Among them, 15 patients who had an ROSC by standard advanced cardiac life support (ACLS) [5] were included in the study. Table 1 shows the backgrounds of these 15 patients. Some of the results are as follows: patients who had undergone bystander CPR, 33.3%; time elapsed from cardiac arrest to start of initiated CPR, average 9.3 min; successful defibrillation rate by paramedics, 47%; and time taken from cardiac arrest to ROSC, average 39.8 min. The cause of VF was acute coronary syndrome in 87%; of these, the successful coronary reperfusion rate for acute myocardial infarction [Thrombolysis in Myocardial Infarction Trial, phase I (TIMI) flow grade III] [2] was 89%. Some results were as follows: systolic blood pressure before induction of hypothermia, average 119 mmHg (intraaortic balloon pumping was used jointly in 87%); heart rate, average 105 bpm, Glasgow Coma Score, average 3.6; arterial blood pH, average 7.3; base excess, average −7.4 mmol/l.

Outcome after Mild Hypothermia by Coil Cooling

Table 2 shows the outcome during treatment with mild hypothermia. The core temperature at the cooling stage was on average 34.4°C, and the duration averaged 84 h. The average cardiac

TABLE 1. Baseline characteristics of the study patients

Characteristic	Study patients ($n = 15$)
Age (years)	58.6 ± 12.4
Male sex (%)	66.7
Bystander CPR (%)	33.3
Time from cardiac arrest to start of initiated CPR (min)	9.3 ± 7.9
Successful defibrillation by paramedics (%)	46.7
Time from cardiac arrest to ROSC (min)	39.8 ± 23.4
Cause of VF (%)	
Acute coronary syndrome	86.7
Hypertrophic cardiomyopathy	6.7
Idiopatic VF	6.7
Successful reperfusion (TIMI flow grade 3) by coronary intervention (%)	88.9
Systolic blood pressure before hypothermia (mmHg)	118.7 ± 21.3
Heart rate before hypothermia (bpm)	104.7 ± 16.1
Glasgow Coma Scale before hypothermia	3.6 ± 0.7
Arterial pH before hypothermia	7.30 ± 0.14
Arterial base excess before hypothermia (mmol/l)	−7.4 ± 6.1

Plus-minus values are mean ± SD
CPR, cardiopulmonary resuscitation; ROSC, return of spontaneous circulation; VF, ventricular fibrillation; TIMI, Thrombolysis in Myocardial Infarction Trial, phase I

TABLE 2. Outcome of mild hypothermia by coil cooling

Parameter	Result
Duration of induction (h)	6.6 ± 2.9
Cooling stage	
Core temperature (°C)	34.4 ± 0.5
Duration (h)	83.9 ± 40.8
Cardiax index (l/min/m²)	3.10 ± 1.41
Hemoglobin (g/dl)	14.0 ± 2.5
Platelet count (×10³/mm²)	302 ± 410
Systemic oxygen delivery (ml/min/m²)	557.5 ± 291.2
Oxygen extration ratio (%)	29.9 ± 6.7
Activated coagulation time (s)	188 ± 26
Duration of rewarming (h)	50.6 ± 6.7

Plus-minus values are mean ± SD

index at the stabilized phase of the cooling stage was 3.1 l/min/m²; the hemoglobin averaged 14 g/dl; the systemic oxygen delivery averaged 558 ml/min/m²; and the activated coagulation time averaged 188 s. The time interval for rewarming at 36°C averaged 51 h.

Neurological Outcome

Figure 2 shows the rates of survival at hospital discharge and of good recovery. The survival and good recovery rates were 80% (12/15) and 66.7% (10/15), respectively. Of the remaining patients, two (13%) died owing to pulmonary infection, which is a severe complication of hypothermia; and one (7%) died owing to low output syndrome.

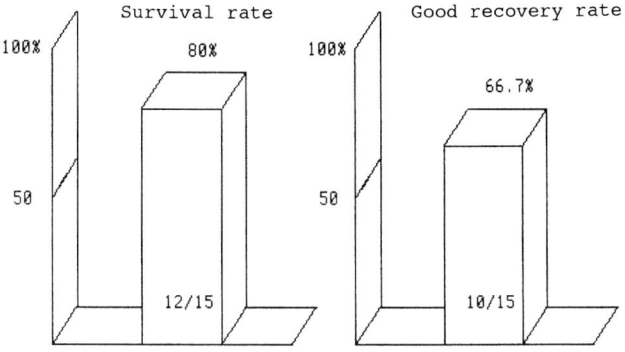

FIG. 2. Neurologic outcome of the study. Survival rate at hospital discharge (**left**) and good recovery rate (**right**). Glasgow Outcome Scale showed good recovery in 10 cases, moderate disability in 0 cases, severe disability in 0%, vegetative state in 2 cases, and death in 3 cases

TABLE 3. Comparison between patients with and without good recovery

Characteristic	With good recovery ($n = 10$)	Without good recovery ($n = 5$)	P
Age (years)	56.4 ± 12.2	63.0 ± 12.8	0.35
Bystander CPR (%)	40	20	0.43
Time from cardiac arrest to start of initiated CPR (min)	9.2 ± 9.0	9.6 ± 5.7	0.40
Successful defibrillation by paramedic (%)	50	40	0.17
Time from cardiac arrest to ROSC (min)	42.2 ± 26.5	35.0 ± 17.0	0.59
Systolic blood pressure before hypothermia (mmHg)	116.1 ± 20.6	123.8 ± 24.2	0.53
Heart rate before hypothermia (bpm)	106.5 ± 14.8	101.2 ± 19.9	0.57
Glasgow Coma Scale before hypothermia	3.6 ± 0.7	3.6 ± 0.9	1.0
Arterial pH before hypothermia	7.29 ± 0.10	7.30 ± 0.20	0.92
Arterial base excess (mmol/l) before hypothermia	-7.23 ± 6.58	-7.60 ± 5.88	0.92
Hypothermia			
Duration of induction (h)	6.7 ± 2.5	6.5 ± 3.7	0.90
Cooling stage			
Core temperature (°C)	34.4 ± 0.5	34.4 ± 0.5	1.0
Duration (h)	77.2 ± 36.2	97.4 ± 50.4	0.38
Cardiac index (l/min/m²)	3.54 ± 1.40	2.10 ± 0.85	0.05
Hemoglobin (g/dl)	14.2 ± 2.6	13.5 ± 2.6	0.64
Platelet count (10³/mm²)	364 ± 497	178 ± 61	0.43
Systemic oxygen delivery (ml/min/m²)	669 ± 293	335 ± 104	0.03
Oxygen extration ratio (%)	30.6 ± 4.6	28.6 ± 10.0	0.63
Duration of rewarming	49.0 ± 9.2	50.6 ± 7.5	0.74

Plus-minus values are mean ± SD
CPR, cardiopulmonary resuscitation; ROSC, return of spontaneous circulation

Factors Predictive of Good Recovery

Table 3 compares the improved good recovery at hospital discarge with the patients without good recovery. A significant difference was observed in systemic oxygen delivery during mild hypothermia at the cooling stage (669 ml/min/m^2 in the patients with good recovery versus 335 ml/min/m^2 in the patients without good recovery). A significant trend was observed in the cardiac index at the cooling stage. It was observed by stepwise regression analysis of the above various factors that systemic oxygen delivery at the cooling stage was an independent predictor of good recovery ($R = 0.56$).

Discussion

In 1997 Christian et al. [3] reported that the in-hospital survival rate became 38% by performing (1) immediate coronary angiography on survivors of out-of-hospital cardiac arrest and (2) percutaneous transluminal coronary angioplasty (PTCA) on patients with acute coronary-artery occlusion; successful PTCA was an independent predictor of survival. In 1998 Gueugniaud et al. [7] reported on their multicenter randomized double-blind study of epinephrine in patients with out-of-hospital cardiac arrest. If VF patients are aggregated from this groups, the survival rate at hospital discharge was 22.3% (the epinephrine dosage had no influence). Therefore, we supposed that the survival rate of the survivors with out-of-hospital VF was 22% at hospital discharge after standard CPR but would increase to 38% if immediate coronary intervention was added to standard CPR. However, there have been no reports of drugs found to evidently useful for cerebral resuscitation in comatose survivors with out-of-hospital cardiac arrest. (There was no report from Christian et al. on the cerebral resuscitation method.)

Treating patients with severe traumatic brain injury by brain hypothermia has the beneficial effect of cerebral protection [3,4,15,18]. However, there is controversy regarding to what degree and for how long the core temperature is decreased, the technique of induction of and rewarming after hypothermia, and the prevention of complications. Furthermore, the mechanism underlying the protective effects of postischemic hypothermia have not been elucidated sufficiently [12]. Regarding hypothermia techniques, it has not been clearly shown whether surface cooling (using cooling blankets) or coil cooling is better. The protocol for brain hypothermia conforms to the principles of Hayashi [8,9] regarding techniques and management. On the other hand, a coil cooling method for cooling the blood circuit of CHDF has been developed for patients with cardiac arrest (MONAN or KANEM method; see chapter by Okamoto et al., this volume). CHDF is known to be useful for controlling water and electrolytes and for removing the humoral mediators that have increased during systemic inflammatory response syndrome (SIRS) [9]. Survivors of out-of-hospital VF are considered to have SIRS that has become severe, for which CHDF can be used. Concurrently, based on the finding that vascular endothelial cells after ROSC provided hypercoagulation and antifibrinolysis (not published), it was decided to apply hypothermia by coil cooling to which CHDF using anticoagulant was added.

The results were surprising, with a survival rate at hospital discharge of 80% and a good recovery rate of 67%. This survival rate is about four times that achieved with standard CPR alone reported by Gueugniand et al. [7], about twice that for standard CPR with immediate coronary intervention added as reported by Christian et al. [3], and about 1.4 times that for CPR with vasopressin reported by Linder et al. [14]. However, this study was not randomized, and the number of cases was small; it was also expensive. It is necessary in future for developing brain hypothermia treatment of survivors of out-of-hospital VF to perform a multicenter randomized controlled study.

Conclusions

Brain hypothermia was treated by coil cooling at 34°C for 3 days with the purpose of cerebral resuscitation in survivors of out-of-hospital VF. Surprising results were obtained: The survival rate at hospital discharge was 80% (12/15), and the good recovery rate was 60% (9/15). The systemic oxygen delivery of hypothermia at the cooling stage was an independent predictor of good recovery. It is concluded that treatment of comatose survivors with out-of-hospital VF with mild brain hypothermia by coil cooling may improve the good recovery.

References

1. Busto R, Dietrich WD, Globus MYT, Valdes I, Scheinberg P, Ginsberg MD (1987) Small differences in intraischemic brain temperature critically determine the extent of ischemic neuronal injury. J Cereb Blood Flow Metab 7:729–738
2. Chesebro JH, Knatterud G, Roberts R, Borer J, Cohen LS, Dalen J, Dodge HT, Francis CK, Hillis D, Ludbrook P, Markis JE, Mueller H, Passamani ER, Powers ER, Rao AK, Robertson T, Ross A, Ryan TJ, Sobel BE, Willerson J, Williams DO, Zaret BL, Braunwald E (1987) Thrombolysis in Myocardial Infarction (TIMI) trial, phase I: comparison between intravenous tissue plasminogen activator and intravenous streptokinase; clinical findings through hospital discharge. Circulation 76:142–154
3. Christian MP, Luc-Marie J, Alain R, Mehran M, Simon NW, Jean-Francois AD, Pierre C (1997) Immediate coronary angiography in survivors of out-of-hospital cardiac arrest. N Engl J Med 336:1629–1633
4. Clifton GL, Allen S, Barrodale P, Plenger P, Berry J, Koch S, Fletcher J, Hayes RL, Choi SC (1993) A phase II study of moderate hpothermia in severe brain injury. J Neurotrauma 10:263–271
5. Emergency Cardiac Care Committee and Subcommittees (1992) American Heart Association (ECC and AHA) guidelines for cardio-pulmonary resuscitation and emergency cardiac care. JAMA 268:2171–2195
6. Fay T (1943) Observation on generalized refrigeration in cases of severe cerebral trauma. Assoc Res Nerv Ment Dis Proc 24:611–619
7. Gueugniaud PY, Mols P, Goldstein P, Pham E, Dubien PY, Deweerdt C, Vergnin M, Petit P, Carli P (1998) A comparison of repeated high doses and repeated standard doses of epinephrine for cardiac arrest outside the hospital. N Engl J Med 339:1595–1601
8. Hayashi N (1997) Combination therapy of cerebral hypothermia; pharmacological activation of the dopamine system, and hormonal replacement in severely brain damaged patients (in Japanese). J Jpn Soc Intensive Care Med 4:191–197
9. Hayashi N (1998) The adverse treatment, brain hypothermia and replacement therapy for severe brain injury. In: Abstracts of the international satellite meeting of brain hypothermia, pp 31–34
10. Hirasawa H, Matsuda K, Sugai T, Oda N (1998) Can continuous hemodiafiltration remove cytokines? Possibility of non-renal indication of continuous hemodiafiltration (in Japanese). J Jpn Soc Intensive Care Med 5:345–355
11. Jennett B, Snoek J, Bond MR, Brooks N (1981) Disability after severe head injury: observations on the use of the Glasgow Outcome Scale. J Neurol Neurosurg Psychiatry 44:285–293
12. Kataoka K, Yanase H (1997) Neuroprotective effects of hypothermia: historical considerations and contemporary basic knowledge (in Japanese). Jpn Soc Intensive Care Med 1:11–17
13. Kouwenhoven WB, Jude JR, Knickerbocker GG (1960) Closed-chest cardiac massage. JAMA 173:1064–1067

14. Lindner KH, Dirks B, Strohmenger HU, Prengel AW, Lindner IM, Lurie KG (1997) Randomised comparison of epinephrine and vasopressin in patients with out-of-hospital ventricular fibrillation. Lancet 349:535–537
15. Marion DW, Penrod LE, Kelsey SF, Obrist WD, Kochanek PM, Palmer AM, Wisniewski SR, Dekosky ST (1997) Treatment of traumatic brain injury with moderate hypothermia. N Engl J Med 226:540–546
16. Nagao K, Hayashi N, Kanmatsuse K, Arima K, Ohtsuki J, Kikushima K, Watanabe I (2000) Cardiopulmonary cerebral resuscitation using emergency cardiopulmonary bypass, coronary reperfusion therapy and mild hypothermia in patients with cardiac arrest outside the hospital. J Am Coll Cardiol (in press)
17. Safar P, Escarrage LA, Elam JO (1958) A comparison of the mouth-to-mouth and mouth-to-airway methods of artificial respiration with the chest-pressure armlift method. N Engl J Med 258:671–677
18. Shiozaki T, Sugimoto H, Taneda M, Yoshida H, Iwai A, Yoshioka T, Sugimoto T (1993) Effect of mild hypothermia on uncontrollable intracranial hypertension after severe head injury. J Neurosurg 79:363–368
19. Teasdale G, Jennett B (1974) Assessment of coma and impaired consciousness; a practical scale. Lancet 2:81–84
20. Zoll PM, Linenthal AJ, Gibson W, Paul MH, Norman LR (1956) Termination of ventricular fibrillation in man by externally applied electric countershock. N Engl J Med 254:727–732

New Hypothermia Method Using Blood Cooling System: MONAN and KANEM Method

Kazuhiko Okamoto[1], Ken Nagao[2], Takahiro Miki[1], Eiji Nitobe[1], Ken Arima[3], and Nariyuki Hayashi[2]

Summary. The main method for brain hypothermia today is surface cooling using cooling blankets. However, surface cooling has posed a problem that requires a complicated technique and manpower for controlling the core temperature of hypothermia. We have devised a blood circuit for continuous hemodiafiltration and produced and used clinically two new blood cooling systems (MONAN and KANEM methods). Compared with surface cooling, these blood cooling systems have made it easy to control the core temperature during the periods of induction, cooling, and rewarming without being influenced by the patient's body form. Moreover, postural drainage for preventing pulmonary infections, which were severe complications of hypothermia, is possible without use of a particular kinetic bed. Furthermore, it is possible improve the abnormal electrolytes seen with hypothermia, particularly hyperkalemia, at rewarming, by removing the humoral mediator that increases and courses the systemic inflammatory response syndrome. Based on our results, it is suggested that a blood cooling system using the MONAN and KANEM method is a useful technique for instituting brain hypothermia.

Key words. Hypothermia, Blood cooling system, Coil cooling, Continuous hemodiafiltration (CHDF), Surface cooling

Introduction

Half a century has elapsed since neuroprotective effects of hypothermia were recognized. Having performed hypothermia on patients with traumatic brain injury as early as 1943, Fay [4] cooled patients' entire bodies by opening windows and breaking ice on selected cold days. In 1950 Bigelow et al. [1] successfully created hypothermia by surface cooling in an experiment for cardiac surgery. Subsequently, improvements have been made of the techniques, such as the development of blankets, having made it possible to create hypothermia in a warmed

---

[1] Department of Clinical Engineering, Surugadai Nihon University Hospital, 1-8-13 Kanda Surugadai, Chiyoda-ku, Tokyo 101-8309, Japan
[2] Department of Emergency and Critical Care Medicine, Nihon University School of Medicine, 30-1 Oyaguchi Kami-machi, Itabashi-ku, Tokyo 173-8610, Japan
[3] Department of Cardiology, Surugadai Nihon University Hospital, 1-8-13 Kanda Surngadai, Chiyoda-ku, Tokyo 101-8309, Japan

room where the treatment can be easily undertaken. In 1993 there were reports on three clinical trials of moderate hypothermia (at a temperature of 32°–33°C) using cooling blankets (surface cooling) for severe brain injury. [3,8,9]. For hypothermia during cardiac surgery, Boerema et al. [2] created cooling of a femorofemoral shunt through a cooling coil in 1951, but surface cooling had been the main method until Hamilton et al. [6] developed a technique using only cardiopulmonary bypass for cooling (core cooling) in 1973.

Surface cooling using blankets is easy, but the following issues must be noted. The first is the need for those highly expert with the technique and manpower for the induction, cooling, and rewarming phoses of hypothermia. The second is the difficulty of obtaining a stabilized core temperature, which is subject to the patient's body form, as with obesity. The third is the difficulty with treating the patient because his or her whole body is covered by blankets. The fourth is deterioration of the peripheral circulation as a result of excessive cooling of the extremities. Therefore, we have devised and used clinically a blood cooling system that includes a blood circuit for continuous hemodiafiltration (CHDF).

Method

We have developed two blood cooling systems using coil cooling. Both are methods to induce hypothermia in which a contrivance was added to the blood circuit for CHDF.

Continuous Hemodiafiltration

A continuous blood purification device (TR-520; Toray Medical, Tokyo, Japan) for performing CHDF was used. Settings were as follows: blood flow 60–100 ml/min; dialysis fluid flow 300–500 ml/h; hemofiltration replacement fluid flow 300–500 ml/h; and hemofiltrate and dialysate flows more than 800 ml/h. The hemofiltration replacement fluid used for CHDF was subloood B (Fuso Pharmaceutical Industries, Osaka, Japan). Nafamostat mesylate (Futhan; Torii Pharmaceutical Co., Tokyo, Japan) was the anticoagulant used, and the activated coagulation time was controlled between 150 and 200 s. The blood circuit for CHDF that becomes a ven-ovenous shunt was devised as described below to make it the blood cooling system.

Coil Cooling by the MONAN Method

The name of the method is based on the initial letters of our five author's names (*M*iki, *O*kamoto, *N*itobe, *A*rima, *N*agao) as we development the technique jointly. Hypothermia by the MONAN method is shown in Figs. 1 and 2. The blood warming coil (BLT-500; Toray Medical, Tokyo, Japan) for quick blood transfusion was connected in series to the blood inlet side of the blood access for CHDF and the built-in CHDF circuit. The coil was sunk in the heat and cooler waterbath (MSII-51; Senko Medical Instrument, Tokyo, Japan) (Fig. 2), and the blood in this coil circuit was cooled.

Coil Cooling by KANEM Method

The KANEM method was also derived from author's names (*K*azuhiko, *A*rima, *N*agao, *E*iji, *M*iki). KANEM method is shown in Fig. 3. The twin tube (Hotline; Sims Level 1, Rockland, MA, USA) for blood cooling is shown in Fig. 4, and a cross section of the twin tube is shown in Fig. 5. The twin tube was connected in series to the blood return side of the patient for access to blood for CHDF and to the built-in CHDF circuit. The water was cooled by a temperature management products device (Meditherm; Gaymer Industries, Orchrd Park, NY,

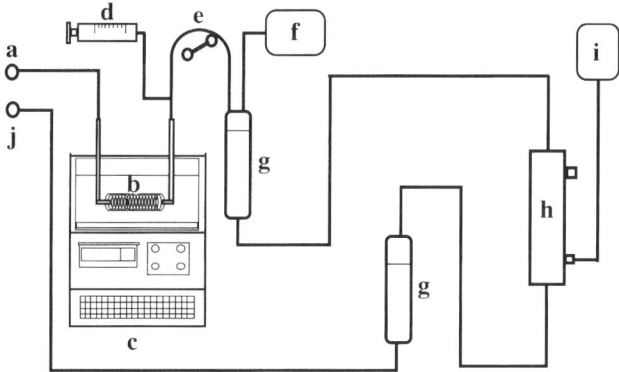

FIG. 1. Scheme of hypothemia by MONAN method. The blood warming coil (*b*) was connected in series to the blood inlet side (*a*) from the patient for blood access for continuous hemodiafiltration (CHDF). The coil (*b*) was sunk in the heat and cooler waterbath (*c*), and the blood in this coil was cooled. *a*, inlet side; *d*, injection of anticoagulant; *e*, occlusive pump; *f*, hemofiltration replacement fluid; *g*, bubble-trop air detector; *h*, hemofilter; *i*, dialysis fluid; *j*, return side

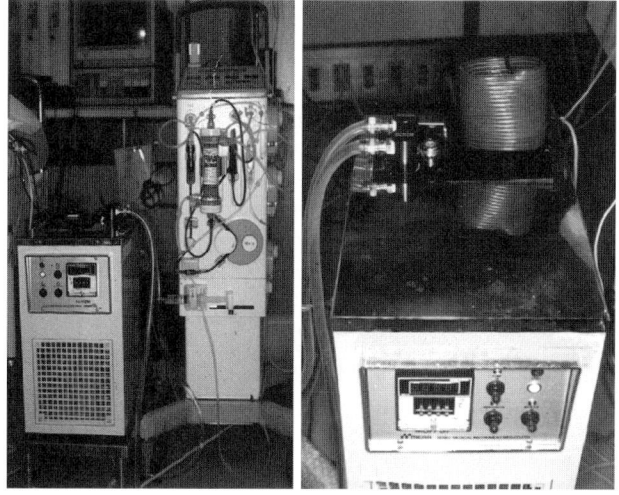

FIG. 2. Hypothermia by the MONAN method. **Left** Heat and cooler waterbath and continuous blood purification device for performing CHDF. **Right** Blood warming coil and heat and cooler waterbath

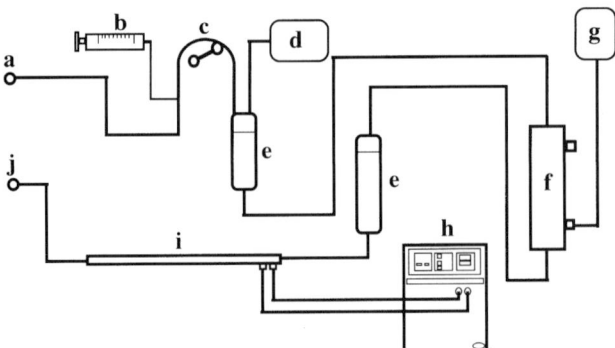

Fig. 3. Scheme of hypothermia by the KANEM method. The twin tube (*i*) was connected in series to the blood return side of the patient for access to blood for CHDF. The water cooled by the temperature management products device (*h*) was sent to the outer circumference of the twin tube, and the blood flowing in the inner cavity of the tube was cooled. *a*, inlet side; *b*, injection of anticoagulant; *c*, occlusive pump; *d*, hemofiltration replacement fluid; *e*, bubble-trop air detector; *f*, hemofilter; *g*, dialysis fluid; *j*, return side

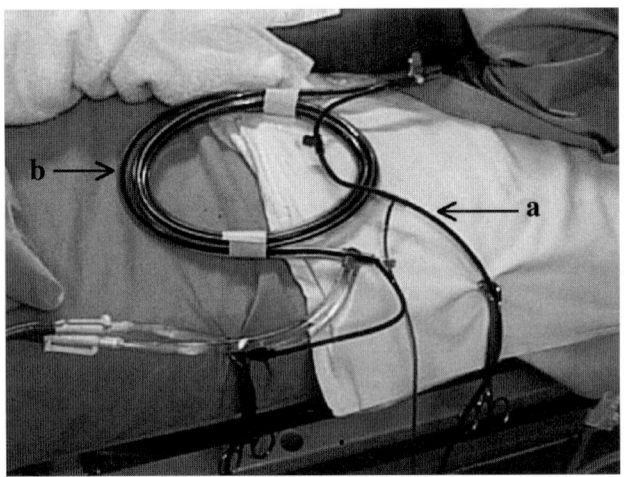

Fig. 4. Hypothermia by the KANEM method *a*, CHDF circuit; *b*, twin tube

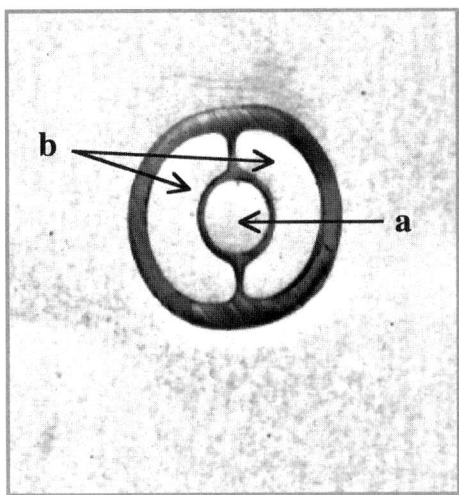

FIG. 5. Cross section of twin tube using the KANEM method. *a*, Blood flowing in the inner cavity of the tube; *b*, cooling water flowing in the outer circumference of the tube

USA); the water was sent to the outer circumference of the twin tube, and the blood flowing in the inner cavity of the tube was cooled (Figs. 4, 5).

Results

Technique for Setting the Temperature of the Cooling Device

The temperatures of the cooling device were set for five stages: induction stages I (early phase) and II (latter phase), cooling stage, and rewarming stages I (early phase) and II (latter phase). Induction of hypothermia fork about 6 h, and adjustments were made so the core temperature could be obtained by two step-downs to reach the target core temperature.

The blood temperature in the pulmonary artery was measured continually by a Swan-Ganz continuous cardiac output themodilution cathether (model 139HF-75; Baxter Healthcare Corporation, Irvine, CA, USA). During the first half of induction, the water temperature in the cooling device was set at 18°–22°C, which was changed to 20°–24°C when the target core temperature became +0.5°C. The water temperature in the cooling device was set at 22°–25°C during the cooling period. During the first rewarming period the water temperature in the cooling device was set at 25°–30°C to attain rewarming slowly by 0.5°C increments for 12 h. When the core temperature reached 35°C, the water temperature in the cooling device was set at 23°–26°C and was adjusted to maintain the core temperature at 35°C for 24 h. During the latter rewarming period the temperature was kept at 25°–33°C so the core temperature could not increase to more than 37°C. The core temperature was controlled at 36°C for some time.

Presentation of a Case

Figure 6 shows the core temperature and the temperature set in the cooling device during the period of hypothermia for a survivor of out-of-hospital ventricular fibrillation. The patient was a 55-year-old man who had had a sudden cardiac arrest during work at his office. Return

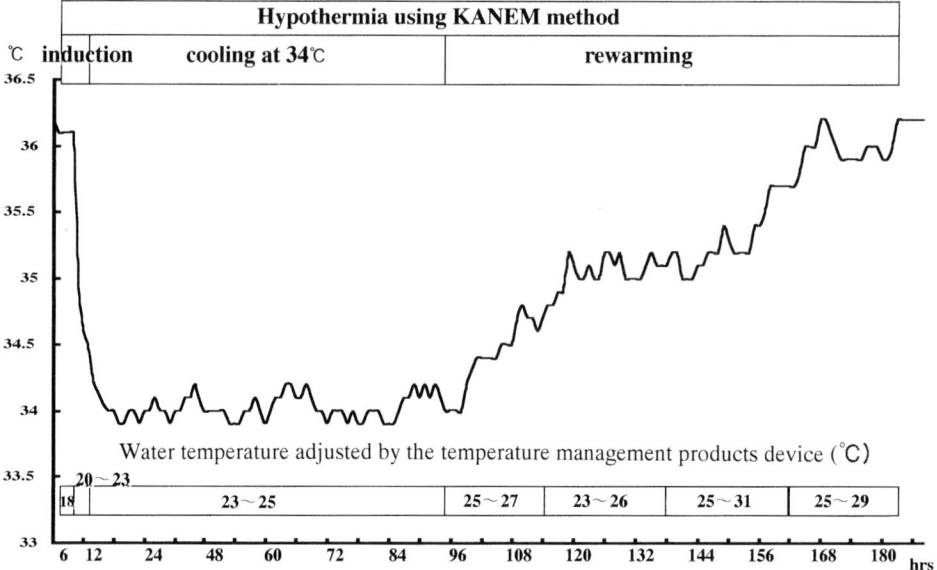

FIG. 6. Case of hypothermia using the KANEM method. As the core temperature, the pulmonary artery blood temperature was monitered by a Swan-Ganz catheter. The water temperature by the temperature management products device was adjusted to 18°–23°C during the induction period, 23°–25°C during the cooling period, and 25°–31°C during the rewarming period

of spontaneous circulation was attained by defibrillation applied by a paramedic. Coronary reperfusion therapy of the infarct-related artery was initiated immediately after hospitalization. Brain hypothermia (temperature 34°C) by the KANEM method was started within 1 h after successful coronary reperfusion. The water temperature in the cooling device was set at 18°C during the early period of hypothermia induction and at 20°C when the core temperature decreased to 34.5°C. The time interval from commencenment of the induction to the target core temperature at 34°C was 6 h. The water temperature was adjusted to 23°–25°C during the cooling period, and hypothermia at the cooling stage was maintained for 72 h at a core temperature of 34° ± 0.1°C. Subsequently, rewarming was maintained for 12 h at 0.5°C (water temperature in the cooing device 25°–27°C), with core temperature maintained at 35°C for 24 h (water temperature 23°–26°C). The water temperature during the latter half of the rewarming period was kept at 25°–31°C, and the patient's was kept at 36°C. The neurological outcome was a Glassgow Coma Scale score of 4 before induction of hypothermia and a score of 15 after the termination of hypothermia (16th morbid day).

Discussion

Today, surface cooling using cooling blankets is the popular technique for inducing brain hypothermia. However, this surface cooling poses problems, as described in the Introduction. Hence we developed a technique for cooling blood by coils useing a CHDF circuit, and we tested it in clinical cases. The MONAN and KANEM methods using CHDF, whose usefulness has been proved by clinical use from the past, were devised [5,6]. The coil (MONAN) or twin tube (KANEM), which has been used as medical material, was built into the CHDF circuit, and the blood was cooled indirectly by the cooling device. The advantages of this blood cooling system are that a good technique is available and it needs little manpower for induction, cooling, and rewarming. Moreover, it is not influenced by the patient's body fat or body form, such as height.

At the beginning, we tried the technique of cooling dialysis fluid and replacement fluid for CHDF directly. However, core temperature control by hypothermia was not sufficient because the amounts of blood flow and replacement were small. With the blood cooling system, measurement of oxygen saturation by pulse oximeter was possible, as the skin temperature of the extremities, particularly the peripheral circulation of the fingers and toes, is maintained. Furthermore, postural drainage for preventing pulmonary infections, which are severe complications of hypothermia, is possible without the use of a kinetic bed. It was also pointed out that the methods improve abnormal electrolytes during hypothermia, particularly the hyperkalemia seen at rewarming and removal of the humoral mediator that increases in SIRS [7].

Its disadvantages are that a blood cooling system that is invasive increases the possibility of infection. Moreover, some extracorporeal circulation is required that is not adequate for hemorrhagic diseases such as brain injury and cerebral hemorrhage, which require anticoagulation. Furthermore, the medical cost is higher than that for surface cooling.

Conclusions

As a technique for inducing hypothermia, the blood cooling system by coil cooling built into a CHDF circuit has been developed in the MONAN and KANEM methods. The clear advantage here is that control of core temperature has become easy.

References

1. Bigelow WG, Lindsay WK, Harrisson RC, Gordon RA, Greenwood WF (1950) Oxygen transport and utilization in dogs at low body temperatures. Am J Physiol 160:125
2. Boerema I, Wildschut A, Schmidt WJH, Broekhuysen L (1951) Experimental researches into hypothermia as an aid in the surgery of the heart. Arch Chir Neerl 3:25
3. Clifton GL, Allen S, Barrodale P, Plenger P, Berry J, Koch S, Fletcher J, Hayes RL, Choi SC (1993) A phase II study of moderate hypothermia in severe brain injury. J Neurotrauma 10:263–271
4. Fay T (1943) Observations on generalized refrigeration in caces of cerebral trauma. Assoc Res Nerv Ment Dis Proc 24:611–619
5. Forni LG, Hilton PJ (1997) Continuous hemofiltration in the treatment of acute renal failure. N Engl J Med 336:1303–1308
6. Hamilton DI, Shackleton J, Rees GJ, Abbott T (1973) Experience with deep hypothermia in infancy using core cooling. In: Barratt-Boyes BG, Neutze JM, Harris EA (eds) Heart disease in infancy. Baltimore, Williams & Wilkins, p 52
7. Hirasawa H, Matuda K, Sugai T, Oda N (1998) Can continuous hemodiafiltration remove cytokines? Possibility of non-renal indication of continuous hemodiafiltration. Jpn Soc Intensive Care Med 5:345–355
8. Marion DW, Obrist WD, Carlier PM, Penrod LE, Darby JM (1993) The use of moderate therapeutic hypothermia for patients with severe head injuries, a preliminary report. J Neurosurg 79:354–362
9. Shiozaki T, Sugimoto H, Taneda M, Yoshida H, Iwai A, Yoshioka T, Sugimoto T (1993) Effect of mild hypothermia on uncontrollable intracranial hypertension after severe head injury. J Neurosurg 79:363–368

5. Panel Discussion

Panel Discussion

NARIYUKI HAYASHI and M.R. ROSS BULLOCK

Mechanism of Action of Hypothermia

Five major candidate mechanisms have been proposed as possible routes by which hypothermia can be neuroprotective: blockage of calcium entry, prevention of glutamate release, suppression of cytokine activation and release, suppression of nitric oxide synthase activity, suppression of apoptosis, and DNA fragmentation. It was widely agreed by the discussants that hypothermia probably affects numerous different mechanisms and may do this at different times during the recovery process.

Although hyperthermia worsens axonal morphology and pathology, amyloid precursor protein immunoreactivity is unchanged with hypothermic treatment. This finding may suggest that hypothermia is less effective against axonal discontinuity mechanisms, although its effectiveness in spinal cord injury argues against this. Dr. Marion showed, using microdialysis in humans with cerebral contusion, that hypothermia therapy suppresses glutamate release in the pericontusional tissue. During rewarming, glutamate tended to rebound to precooling levels or even higher.

The panelists were agreed that more studies are needed to resolve this mechanistic question. The studies are especially important to decide about "synergistic" studies in which a neuroprotectant drug will be given simultaneously with hypothermia or immediately after hypothermia before rewarming. Such studies need to be done in the laboratory, and would include combinations of hypothermia plus glutamate antagonist, hypothermia plus calcium entry blockers, and hypothermia plus caspase inhibitors against apoptosis.

Neuronal Restoration Therapy

Dr. Hayashi proposed the concept that, before neuroprotective hypothermia initiation, it is important to restore the neuronal microenvironment to prevent ongoing brain damage. This method especially includes optimization of oxygen delivery, optimization of cerebral blood flow, and correction of metabolic imbalance in the tissue. Brain oxygen monitoring techniques such as the Paratrend 7 and Licox may offer advantages in determining when this has been achieved in the human brain during the early resuscitation process. Jugular bulb oxygen measurement may also be helpful. Measures include (1) increasing FIO_2 to 100%; (2) administering 2,3-DPG (diphosphoglycerate) to optimize hemoglobin oxygen delivery; and (3) restorating perfusion pressure with pressors. These measures are all part of acute resuscitation.

The well-recognized "catecholamine surge" that follows severe head injury or global brain ischemic events may also make the microenvironment less favorable for neurons. Changes may include promotion of brain hyperthermia caused by catecholamines, vasospasm, and alterations in energy metabolism. When catecholamine surge causes myocardial damage and subendocardial infarction, then hypothermia is <u>not safe</u>. Care needs to be taken in diagnosing possible partial-thickness myocardial infarction in this situation in the acutely traumatized patient. Although catecholamine blockers such as beta blockers are attractive on theoretical grounds, their interference with cardiac inotropic effect seems to make them contraindicated in general clinical use.

The important concept of a "prehypothermia checklist," as proposed by Dr. Hayashi, includes the following conditions. Brain hypothermia is contraindicated for patients with unstable cardiac function, arrhythmia, elongation of QT interval more than 450 mm/s on ECG, difficulty in maintaining a systolic blood pressure above 90 mmHg with fluid resuscitation, severe hypopotassemia (<3 mEq/dl), and brain death. Over lapping induction of hypothermia at the same time further accelerates unstable cardiac function because serum catecholamines are too greatly reduced. If hypothermia management is scheduled with dehydration therapy for prevention of secondary damage of brain edema, these complications especially will result in unsuccessful brain hypothermia treatment. Brain hypothermia is fundamentally important for restoration of injured neurons, control of brain tissue temperature, sufficient neuronal oxygenation, and adequate metabolic substrate with sufficient cerebral blood flow. Therefore, fluid resuscitation and accurate management of serum glucose at 120 to 140 mg/dl during brain hypothermia treatment are important in care management.

Methods for Measuring Brain Temperature

The panelists were uniformly agreed that brain temperature measurement is highly desirable for safe use of hypothermic therapy in patients because of the danger of large differences developing between core body temperature and brain temperature. Differences as large as 3°–4°C have been shown transiently by Hayashi, Sternau, and others. Many monitoring methods are available, including direct simple thermocouple sensors, thermocouples embedded in ventriculostomy catheters, and multiparameter systems such as the Paratrend 7, which also measures oxygen CO_2 and pH, and the Licox, which measures oxygen and temperature together. As yet, no "noninvasive" technique for brain temperature monitoring is available, but the new idea of brain temperature mapping using MR techniques is of interest for the future. The panelists thought that it was likely that *brain temperature gradients* may develop in different parts of the brain, depending on metabolic activity and blood flow variations in the tissue.

Techniques, of Hypothermia Establishment

Currently, all the discussants are using direct surface cooling techniques, and the kinetic concepts bed especially designed for hypothermia therapy was strongly advocated. This bed allows patients to be rotated from side to side to avoid decubiti and hypostatic pneumonia during active cooling. The patient is encased in cooling blankets front and back during this process. Dr. Maekawa presented his double-lumen gastric lavage balloon for iced saline lavage, which helps to lower core temperature more rapidly. With these techniques, most authors are able to cool patients to moderate hypothermia (32°–33°C) during a 6-h period. More rapid techniques include femorofemoral bypass with external blood cooling techniques (cardiopulmonary bypass machine), but these methods carry slightly more risk because of heparinization. Such rapid techniques may have a role to play primarily in stroke and global cerebral ischemia where the risk of intracranial bleeding may be less.

Dangers of Hypothermia

1. In the acute phase, with underlying brain hypoxia hypotension and hypoperfusion, the shift in hemoglobin oxygen dissociation to the left with hypothermia and the potential for reduced CBF around focal lesions may mean that hypothermia can worsen brain oxygen delivery. The group advocated methods such as increase of inspired oxygen fraction in the gas mix, use of allosteric hemoglobin-modifying molecules (e.g., RSR-13), and use of non-red cell hemoglobin transporters, such as perfluorocarbons, or stroma-free hemoglobin (Baxter). Hemoglobin should be kept at the optimal level of 12 mg/dl during hypothermia, if necessary with blood transfusion.
2. Hypothermia may impose major danger for the heart, especially in patients with prior cardiac ischemia events. For this reason, EKG surveillance and the ruling out of myocardial infarction are necessary. Optimal potassium management is mandatory, and requires sampling of serum electrolytes at least every 6h during the cooling and rewarming phases. Although selective brain cooling techniques have been tried in animal studies, the group believed it was very unlikely these methods will be successful in humans and that they should not be pursued further.

Reverse Jugulocarotid Perfusion

Reverse jugulocarotid perfusion has been attempted in a few patients for acute ischemic stroke, and it is in frequent use as an adjunct to high-risk thoracic aorta surgery in France. This method allows oxygenated blood to be retrogradely perfused through the jugular veins and recovered from the carotid system. Although of interest, this method was not considered appropriate for "mainstream" hypothermic therapy in the intensive care unit.

Prevention of Infection

Hypothermia, itself, suppresses the immune system, and the CD-4 count will fall. Similarly, the catecholamine surge associated with brain damage, such as neurotrauma cardiac arrest, decreases immunocompetence. To counteract this effect and to prevent systemic infection, Hayashi's group advocate early aggressive bowel toilet (enemas) during the early phases of cooling. Concomitant surveillance cultures of the blood and cerebrospinal fluid and urine are mandated daily during hypothermic therapy. Enteral feeding is highly desirable as early as possible during establishment of hypothermia, and hypothermia is not a contraindication to enteral feeding. In contrast to U.S. experience, Japanese experience suggests that low doses of morphine or other benzodiazepine sedation may be sufficient, provided the patient is kept paralyzed with neuromuscular blockers.

"Thermal Pooling Injury"

Hayashi has shown that, during the early rewarming phase, brain temperature may rise to several degrees above core temperature. The fundamental mechanism for this is unknown, but it is speculated that sudden cranial vasodilatation with warmed core blood may be responsible: this seems to be especially problematic in patients with high catecholamine levels. This phenomenon may induce a secondary brain insult by means of hyperthermic damage.

The elevation of brain tissue temperature at 40°–44°C, the brain thermopooling phenomenon, was initially recorded in herniated terminal head trauma patients. After recording hyperthermia in severe brain injury, we became interested in the mechanism of brain thermopooling and the mechanism of brain tissue temperature regulation. The answer is simple. Brain tissue temperature changes dynamically in the acute stage of severe brain injury by the influence of four major factors such as core temperature, blood pressure (or cerebral perfusion pressure, CPP), and cerebral blood flow. We recorded three causes of brain thermopooling, such as following reperfusion, elevated core temperature at higher than 38°C, systolic blood pressure lower than 90–100 mmHg or CPP reduced to less than 60–75 mmHg. These pathophysiological changes make it difficult to wash out elevated brain tissue temperature. This new pathophysiological condition starts as cerebral oxygen metabolism advances, regardless of cerebral ischemia, between 2 and 15 h after insult. Such specific pathophysiological conditions generally precede brain tissue hypoxia with luxury perfusion.

To prevent this brain thermopooling, management of unstable cardiopulmonary function, which is associated with the catecholamines surge, brain tissue temperature, and neuronal oxygenation in injured tissue, is fundamentally important. We must understand that simple hypothermia treatment is not the correct treatment.

Duration of Hypothermia Treatment

Although most U.S. studies have opted for 24 or 48 h of hypothermia, Japanese experience suggests that hypothermia may be continued much longer—up to 20 days in some cases. The average duration of hypothermia would be about 4 to 5 days. A longer duration of hypothermia means that the dangers of rewarming injury may be reduced: this makes the theoretical assumption that the damaging pathophysiology process in the brain improves spontaneously over time during the cooled period. It was common experience among the discussants that rewarming is usually associated with a rebound rise in intracranial pressure: the mechanism for this is unknown, and the group called for more research studies to identify *mediators of rewarming injury*: possible mediators may be glutamate, adenosine, or nitric oxide-mediated vasodilatation. Further studies are needed both in animal models and in humans who undergo hypothermia with rewarming. The microdialysis technique is especially suitable for this. All the authorities recommended that rewarming should be *slow*—over a period of 12 h or more. Careful repletion and correction of electrolyte imbalance is mandatory during this phase.

Pre-Conditions for Rewarming

One of the major issues in brain hypothermia treatment is complication of cytokine encephalitis at the rewarming stage, produced by blood–brain barrier dysfunction and severe systemic infections. The pathophysiological changes of cytokine encephalitis at the rewarming stage are not so simple. Difficult management of severe pulmonary infections, immune crisis with reduced growth hormone and muscle weakness, destruction of gut defense by hypoalbuminemia, severe dysfunction of the blood–brain barrier associated with systemic infection, hyperglycemia, and vasopressin release, uncontrollable increase of brain tissue glutamate, and hemoglobin dysfunction have been recorded. To prevent these complications, special considerations for ICU management are necessary at each stage of brain hypothermia treatment.

Intestinal cleaning after surgery, control of gastric juice pH below 3.5, adequate nutritional support with monitoring of serum glutamate, careful management of serum glucose between 120–140 mg/dl, oxygen delivery maintained above 800 ml/min, control of AT-III above 100%, and replacement of hypoalbuminemia are major factors for prevention of infection during brain hypothermia treatment.

However, preconditioning-care management of serum albumin above 3.5 g/dl, serum glucose below 150 mg/dl, vitamin A above 50 mg/dl, lymphocytes above 1500 mm³, Hb above 12 g/dl, AT-III above 100%, management of muscle weakness, abdominal pressure below 10 mmHg, and replacement of magnesium are especially useful to prevent worsening of rewarming-stage infections. Careful control of hypoalbuminemia is essential in preconditioning-care management because severe hypoalbuminemia (<2.5 g/dl) produces various negative factors for severe infections such as intestinal mucous edema with difficult enteral nutrition, increased free bacteria, unstable antibiotic function, easily permeable cytokines of the blood–brain barrier, no effect of mannitol for control of brain edema, and uncontrollable increase of brain-tissue glutamate by moderate brain hypothermia. For hypoalbuminemia, combination therapy with replacement of serum albumin and special-schedule nutritional support are recommended. We prefer two categories of nutritional consideration. When the blood–brain barrier dysfunction is not severely damaged with CSF/serum albumin below 0.02, we schedule early enteral administration of zinc chloride and glutamine for 3 days after trauma, followed by enteral–parenteral amino acid nutrition. In cases of severely damaged blood–brain barrier function (CSF/serum albumin ratio ≧0.02), we schedule enteral–parenteral administration of zinc chloride with replacement therapy of AT-III and albumin for 3–4 days, followed by enteral nutritional therapy through a long-intestinal abdominal decompression catheter.

If severe infection is a complication during brain hypothermia treatment, inflammatory reaction is initially suppressed by replacement of AT-III combined with low-molecular heparin, followed by replacement of albumin, activating the immune function with replacement of L-arginine, and administration of antibiotics. A combination of albekasine (IV) and digestive decontamination are useful.

The Future

Although the NIH-sponsored North American Head Injury Hypothermia study has been terminated and is undergoing data analysis at present, the group felt strongly that even if this trial were negative, future trials should continue with longer durations of hypothermia in view of the clear evidence of the beneficial effect of hypothermia on ICP, glutamate release, and outcome in numerous Phase II studies. An ongoing randomized study in Europe is examining the role of hypothermic therapy for global brain ischemic damage following cardiac arrest. The group called for a Japanese randomized controlled trial of brain hypothermia with a concept different from that of previous hypothermia treatment of severe head injury. This is because there is much expertise and enthusiasm for this form of therapy in Japan, and hypothermia is in widespread use in many neuroscience centers. Although trials of hypothermia in acute ischemic stroke may be difficult to construct, such studies are important also.

6. Summary

Summary

Nariyuki Hayashi

We have had good discussions about brain hypothermia treatment, arising from information both from experimental animal studies and from clinical trials. There is no doubt as to the effectiveness of neuroprotection from ischemic insults provided by brain hypothermia as shown in animal studies. However, in clinical studies, similar effects to animal studies have not been obtained. The benefits of hypothermia are still controversial in clinical trials of hypothermia treatment. Why are such differences recorded between animal studies and clinical results? I want to summarize the answers to this question. This answer will include the basic concept of brain hypothermia treatment in survival of patients with severe brain injuries.

Animal Studies and Their Limitations

The effect of hypothermia on neuronal protection has been discussed in terms of prevention of neurotransmitter release, free fatty acids, and membrane lipid peroxidation, reduction of free radicals, stabilization of the blood–brain barrier (BBB), reduction of brain edema, stabilization of membrane permeability, reduction of cellular Ca^{2+} uptake and neuroexcitation, downregulation of protein kinase, the protective effect on protein synthesis, gene protection, and antiischemia. Especially, neuroprotection by hypothermia is very successful in managing brain ischemic insults by means of mild to moderate brain hypothermia. However, the effects of brain hypothermia after an insult are still controversial. The restricted effect of hypothermia after brain injury means that brain edema, free radicals, neuroexcitation, and other concerns as have been previously described are not suitable targets of initial treatment. We must think about this question: "Is it true that neuroprotection from the development of secondary brain damage is the initial treatment?"

We have long accepted the concept that the primarily injured brain tissue does not survive well, and therefore prevention of secondary brain injury such as brain edema, brain ischemia, and reduced cerebral perfusion pressure (CPP) as caused by elevation of intracranial pressure (ICP) has been considered as a target of treatment. The promoting factors of these pathophysiological changes—free radicals, BBB dysfunction, excitatory amino acids, and increase of intracellular Ca^{2+} also have been considered as targets of treatment. This concept of brain injury mechanism has been supported for a long time by many experimental animal studies.

However, recent clinical studies explain three clinical issues about the previous brain injury mechanism relative to the management of severe brain injury. There is much clinical experience with the recovery of primary injured tissue as shown by CT scan and MRI studies in brain trauma. The recovery of primary brain injury without clinical deficits could be explained by such statements as "all neurons in primary injured brain tissue do not die immediately, but instead are going to die." Therefore, primary brain injury is also an initial target of treatment for neuronal recovery in the acute stage.

Before neuroprotection management, cellular shocked neurons in injured tissue need enough oxygen and suitable metabolic substrate to restore the dying neurons. It has been considered that the management of normal PaO_2, normal intracranial pressure (ICP), systolic blood pressure above 90 mmHg, and slightly increased hyperglycemia are enough to maintain cerebral oxygenation and suitable metabolic substrate. Unfortunately, as we have pointed out, this basic concept, which was derived from experimental animal studies, is not always correct for the management of severely brain-injured patients, as was shown by extremely early clinical studies. Hemoglobin dysfunction associated with harmful stress-induced hyperglycemia, brain thermopooling associated with elevation of brain tissue temperature at 40°–44°C, and circulation shift to the intestinal organs by a dopamine-dominant surge accelerates the development of brain injury more rapidly even when normal ICP, CPP, and PaO_2 are present initially. To restore shocked neurons in injured tissue, management of hemoglobin function, hyperglycemia, elevated brain tissue temperature, and catecholamine surge are necessary, starting at the initial stage. The previous neuroprotection therapy is not adequate to manage these newly defined brain injury mechanisms in the patient with severe brain injury. These brain injury mechanisms are not covered by the previous neuroprotective treatment such as management of brain edema, ICP elevation, brain ischemia, and free radical reactions. The brain injury mechanisms associated with excess neurohormone release, such as catecholamine surge, vasopressin, and growth hormone, have been found to influence the reversibility and prognosis of injured neurons. These brain injury mechanisms are difficult to determine precisely by studies in anesthetized experimental animals because anesthesia conceals the severity of neurohormonal excess release that is associated with the harmful stress.

We now understand that the mechanism of brain injury that was shown by animal studies is not similar to clinical cases, especially in severely brain-injured patients.

Clinical Studies

We Need a New Concept of Brain Hypothermia Treatment

Many clinical applications of hypothermia for the severely brain-injured patient have been tried. However, the concept of hypothermia treatment is not uniform, and is mainly divided into two types. One type is a concept of neuroprotection by hypothermia that is focused on prevention of secondary brain damage caused by brain edema and ICP elevation. Therefore, induction of hypothermia is indicated after elevation of ICP, and the duration of hypothermia is limited to 48h. The major issue associated with this concept of hypothermia treatment is that it is too late to prevent the catecholamine surge associated with brain hypoxia, brain thermopooling, vasopressin-associated BBB dysfunction, and BBB dysfunction-associated cytokine encephalitis.

In severely brain-injured patients, hypothermia for the short time of 48h is not enough to provide recovery during the cooling stage. Instead of restoration of injured neurons, the pathophysiological changes of the injured tissue are extended at the rewarming stage. At that time, brain damage becomes much worse by acceleration of primary brain damage by rewarming stress such as hypermetabolism, vascular engorgement, and neuroexcitation by glutamate, at the rewarming stage. However, it is very difficult for severely injured neurons to recover within a short time. These pitfalls in the cooling stage cannot be avoided in cases of severely brain-injured patients. Therefore, we can say that the restoration of brain injury during the cooling stage is very important and that the duration of hypothermia treatment must be changed in proportion to the severity of brain injury. To resolve these clinical issues, we need a more prolonged hypothermia treatment technique without any infections.

Why is the previous hypothermia treatment with the concept of neuroprotection not effective for critically ill patients with Glasgow Coma Scale scores of less than 5? We propose another concept of brain hypothermia treatment. Neuronal restoration therapy with the combination of brain hypothermia and sufficient cerebral oxygenation should be started initially. The major point of this concept is that restoration therapy precedes neuroprotection therapy.

What is the difference between neuronal restoration therapy and the previous neuroprotection therapy? Restoration therapy needs control of brain thermopooling, of the masking brain hypoxia that occurs even with normal PaO_2, ICP, and CPP, and management of hypothalamus–pituitary axis neurohormonal abnormality. The new concept of cerebral restoration therapy before neuroprotection therapy has not been previously proposed. Therefore, we want to summarize restoration therapy to severely brain-injured patients.

Control of brain tissue temperature at 32°–34°C is not sufficient for the restoration of injured neurons, because to allow recovery of dying neurons in injured tissue, the combination of sufficient oxygen and balanced administration of the metabolic substrate, glucose, to the dying neurons is indispensable. Metabolic suppression by hypothermia is very hazardous to the dying neurons in injured tissue, except in perifocal noninjured neurons, because dying neurons need metabolic energy, adenosine triphosphate (ATP), to maintain intracellular homeostasis and cell membrane functions. The intracellular energy crisis in injured neurons makes it difficult to maintain intracellular homeostasis. This metabolic ebb therapy is not suitable for the recovery of severely injured neurons in primary injured brain tissue.

Initial Target of Treatment

The fundamental concept of brain hypothermia treatment is control of brain tissue temperature at 32°–34°C with sufficient cerebral oxygenation and prevention of excess release of hypothalamus–pituitary axis hormones such as catecholamines, vasopressin, and growth hormones. The initial target of treatment in hypothermia treatment for severe brain injury is proposed as follows.

1. Adequate administration of oxygen and metabolic substrates. To maintain adequate microcirculation and cerebral oxygen metabolism, control of ICP below 20 mmHg, $PaO_2/FiO_2 > 300$, antithrombin-III (AT-III) > 100%, and serum glucose control between 120 and 140 mg/dl were fundamentals of management. If serum glucose is higher than 140 mg/dl, glycerol is contraindicated so as to preclude the disruption of brain tissue glucose. The core temperature is controlled at 34°C for prevention of catecholamine surge initially, and after stabilization of systolic blood pressure above 100 mmHg, brain tissue temperature is reduced to 33°–32°C with 3 to 6h intake in the criteria of moderate brain hypothermia treatment. Hemoglobin dysfunction by reduced 2,3-diphosphoglycerate (DPG) must be a concern when serum pH is higher than 7.3. Oxygen delivery is maintained at greater than 800 ml/min; CPP is controlled above 80 mmHg with sufficient fluid resuscitation. If fluid resuscitation is not successful in maintaining systolic blood pressure above 100 mmHg, temporary block of the abdominal aorta using an abdominal balloon catheter is available. Oxygen therapy is focused on management at higher than 800 ml/min/kg with a 22% to 25% oxygen extraction ration (O_2ER).

2. Control of excess release of vasopressin and growth hormone for prevention of BBB dysfunction and cytokines encephalitis. Hypothalamus–pituitary axis activation by direct injury and stimulation of the neuropeptide Y receptor with excess release of norepinephrine and hyperglycemia produces BBB dysfunction and cytokine encephalitis-associated vasopressin release. These pathophysiological changes should be prevented initially by control of brain tissue temperature at 34°C with 120 to 140 mg/dl serum glucose. To avoid the progression of catecholamine surge and hyperglycemia, 9% saline is followed by 4% saline fluid infusion. If serum glucose increases above 150 mg/dl, an insulin drop should be scheduled. Administration of AT-III alone or combined with low molecular weight heparin (LWHP) reduces vascular inflammation by activation of prostaglandin I_2 (PGI$_2$). Therefore, both BBB dysfunction and cytokine encephalitis could be treated by AT-III or AT-III combined with LWHP followed by 5% albumin drip and maintaining serum albumin above 3.5 g/dl within 2 to 3 h after injury.

3. Preclusion of selective neuronal damage of the dopamine A 10 nervous system to prevent vegetation. Brain tissue temperature control between 32° and 33°C prevent dopamine release within 3 h after trauma. The control of Hb above 11 g/dl and administration of vitamin E and C are useful for scavenging of radicals. More detailed information is presented in Chapters 1 and 4-C of this volume.

Pitfalls of Brain Hypothermia Treatment

Brain hypothermia treatment is very successful in providing recovery of injured neurons. However, the unphysiological conditions during brain hypothermia cause other negative effects. For a long time, the detailed mechanism of the negative factors in brain hypothermia were not understood. Without understanding these negative factors in hypothermia, successful treatment cannot be expected.

In our clinical experience, five major pitfalls were demonstrated in this treatment. Masking brain hypoxia, inadequate management of brain tissue temperature and hyperglycemia, undesirable duration of brain hypothermia, inadequate care management of systemic infections, and nutritional misunderstanding of the management of brain injury are nominated as major issues of brain hypothermia treatment.

1. Masking brain hypoxia: normal PaO$_2$ and ICP management are not sufficient for recovery of injured neurons in severe head trauma patients. Because of this masking brain hypoxia, produced by circulating blood shifts into the intestinal organs, release of oxygen from hemoglobin is difficult because hemoglobin enzymes are reduced, oxygen delivery is less than 800 ml/min, and there is increased demand of oxygen in the injured brain because of brain thermopooling. Masking brain hypoxia in the acute stage of severe brain injury spefically produces uncoupling of CBF and brain metabolism. To avoid this masking brain hypoxia, control of brain tissue temperature at 34°C to prevent excess release of dopamine, avoiding brain thermopooling and hemoglobin enzyme and DPG reduction, and management of oxygen delivery at more than 800 ml/min are important. Sometimes intestinal blood shift caused by excess release of dopamine is very difficult to monitor because of increasing cardiac contraction; however, intestinal vasodilatations produce normal blood pressure and normal CPP. Change of brain tissue temperature to less than bladder temperature as found by continuous monitoring of these parameters is the only way make a diagnosis of this blood shift. The most common pitfall is lower cardiac output and 90–100 mmHg of systolic blood pressure caused by reduced fluid resuscitation or cardiac dysfunction caused by catecholamine surge. This lower systolic blood pressure is not sufficient to prevent brain thermopooling without brain hypothermia. In the management of brain hypothermia,

maintaining sufficient cerebral oxygenation and adequate delivery of glucose are very important.

2. Inadequate brain temperature and hyperglycemia. In severely brain-injured patients, catecholamine surge associated with hyperglycemia is unavoidable because glycogen and ATP in liver and heart, among the major organs, metabolize to glucose by activation of epinephrine. This catecholamine surge could be prevented by brain hypothermia, and hyperglycemia is easy to control at the induction stage. However, during the cooling stage of brain hypothermia, reduction of brain tissue temperature to below 33°C sometimes increases serum glucose by systemic reduction of glucose consumption. This inadequate control of hyperglycemia increases brain tissue lactate and pyruvate with increased brain tissue glucose. The critical level to cause an increase in brain tissue lactate is above 140 mg/dl serum glucose at 33°C of brain tissue. Increased brain tissue glucose makes it possible to activate cytokines and increase BBB permeability, as described elsewhere. Therefore, in the management of moderate brain hypothermia treatment, we must control serum glucose at 120 to 140 mg/dl exactly. At the induction stage, if difficult control of hyperglycemia is experienced, brain tissue temperature should be elevated at 0.5°C increments and mild brain hypothermia treatment maintained until systemic circulation and hyperglycemia are stabilized.

3. Undesirable duration of brain hypothermia. Short-duration brain hypothermia cannot provide recovery and limits the control of pathophysiology during the cooling stage, especially in severely injured patients. Without the recovery of brain injury during the cooling stage, in these cases, rewarming promotes the progression of the pathophysiological changes stopped at the cooling stage and makes the condition much worse. Therefore, before starting rewarming, we must confirm whether the injured brain is on the way to recovery. Brain hypothermia treatment for 2 days is too short a time for recovery, especially in severely brain-injured patients. The adequate duration of brain hypothermia is theoretically variable. However, with prolonged brain hypothermia treatment, it is easy to cause an immune crisis with reduced GH and severe systemic infections. To maintain adequate duration of brain hypothermia, we need skillful care management for control of immune crisis-associated infections and diagnostic of criteria to start rewarming.

4. Cytokine encephalitis by systemic infections. The complication of severe infections during brain hypothermia decides the prognosis and success of the treatment for two reasons: one is additional brain damage by cytokine encephalitis and the other is the difficulty of the critically ill patients with brain injury in surviving prolonged brain hypothermia treatment. Severe damage of BBB function, such as a CFS/serum albumin ratio elevated to more than 0.02, is a serious condition when systemic and/or severe pulmonary infections occur because increased cytokines in the systemic circulation evoked by pulmonary infections easily penetrate the BBB and increase brain injury by cytokine encephalitis. The systemic infection itself is also a negative factor in the brain injury because it causes brain hypoxia and venous congestion with increased mediastinal pressure. Therefore, in the management of brain hypothermia treatment, severe pulmonary infections not only disturb pulmonary function but also worsen cerebral vascular inflammation, vascular permeability, brain edema, and cytokine encephalitis with BBB dysfunction. To control these pathophysiological changes, management of AT-III above 100% to prevent vascular inflammation and microembolus, which was learned from disseminated intravascular coagulability (DIC) complication studies, management of hyperglycemia to prevent increasing vascular permeability, and then control of serum albumin above 3.5 g/dl to maintain BBB function are needed. Replacement therapy of serum albumin is very successful to prevent promoting factors of infections such as intestinal mucosa edema, obstructive pancreatic dysfunction, free bacteria, and free pharmacology. Our recent

brain hypothermia treatment dramatically reduced the incidence of infections to less than 10% and improved clinical results.

5. Inadequate nutrition. In the ICU management of critically ill patients, early administration of parenteral and enteral nutrition is recommended. Recent parenteral and enteral nutrition contains much glucose, lipid, and amino acid glutamate for support of the immune functions. We wondered if such rich glucose and glutamate could permeate the BBB and produce a neuroexcitation neuronal death in cases of severe BBB dysfunction, because parenteral amino acid nutrition increased neurotoxic glutamate in the serum about twofold. In cases of CSF/serum albumin ratio higher than 0.02, which means severe BBB dysfunction, early nutrition increases neurotoxic glutamate in the injured brain tissue. The peak time of BBB dysfunction by vasopressin is 24 h; however, GH-related BBB dysfunction is 3 to 4 days after trauma. Therefore, we prefer the following criteria of nutritional management during brain hypothermia treatment. In cases in which BBB dysfunction is not severely damaged, shown as a CSF/serum albumin ratio less than 0.02, early nutrition that includes ZnCl, glutamine, and arginine for activation of the immune function is started 2 days after trauma. However, in cases of CSF/serum albumin ratio higher than 0.02, initial enteral nutrition is limited to saline with ZnCl, and 3 to 4 days later, amino acid nutrition is started with monitoring of serum glutamate. We have experienced uncontrollable increase of brain tissue glutamate, even with 32°C of moderate brain hypothermia management, with pulmonary infection. BBB dysfunction, and misunderstanding of the administration time of amino acid nutrition.

Concluding Remarks

Understanding of the mechanism of initial brain injury, adequate initial targets of treatment, neuronal restoration therapy, the mechanism of neurohormonal abnormality, intracellular neurogenic shock, and the pitfalls of hypothermia management has opened the way for successful brain hypothermia for critically ill patients with brain damage. Right now, however, the clinical results of brain hypothermia are not adequate because the concepts of brain hypothermia treatment, the duration of hypothermia, the targets of treatment, and techniques to prevent unavoidable pitfalls during hypothermia treatment are not universal and are variable.

We need a new guideline of brain hypothermia treatment that includes the new concepts of the mechanism of brain injury and of treatment. Then, we must schedule international cooperative randomized studies of brain hypothermia treatment for severe brain damage, not only that caused by brain trauma, but also cerebral apoplexy and cardiac arrest whole-brain ischemia. We have learned many things from the first international symposium of brain hypothermia treatment.

I believe that this brain hypothermia treatment will be developed into a skillful treatment to allow critically ill patients with severe brain injury to survive.

Subject Index